2014
YEAR BOOK OF
PULMONARY DISEASE®

The 2014 Year Book Series

Year Book of Endocrinology®: Drs Schott, Apovian, Clarke, Eugster, Khaodhiar, Meikle, Oetgen, Petersenn, Toth, and Willenberg

Year Book of Hand and Upper Limb Surgery®: Drs Yao, Adams, and Rizzo

Year Book of Medicine®: Drs Barker, DeVault, Garrick, Gold, Khardori, Lawton, LeRoith, and Pearson

Year Book of Neonatal and Perinatal Medicine®: Drs Fanaroff, Benitz, Donn, Neu, Papile, and Van Marter

Year Book of Ophthalmology®: Drs Rapuano, Fudemberg, Gupta, Hammersmith, Milman, Nagra, Nelson, Penne, Pyfer, Sergott, Shields, and Talekar

Year Book of Orthopedics®: Drs Morrey, Huddleston, Rose, Swiontkowski, and Trigg

Year Book of Pathology and Laboratory Medicine®: Drs Raab and Bissell

Year Book of Pediatrics®: Dr Cabana

Year Book of Plastic and Aesthetic Surgery™: Drs Miller, Gutowski, and Smith

Year Book of Pulmonary Disease®: Drs Barker, Jones, Maurer, Spradley, Tanoue, and Willsie

Year Book of Surgery®: Drs Behrns, Daly, Fahey, Hines, Howe, Huber, Klodell, Mozingo, and Pruett

Year Book of Urology®: Drs Andriole and Coplen

Year Book of Vascular Surgery®: Drs Gillespie, Bush, Passman, Starnes, and Watkins

2014

The Year Book of
PULMONARY
DISEASE®

Editor-in-Chief
James A. Barker, MD, CPE, FACP, FCCP, FAASM
*Medical Director for Quality and for Fragile Populations, S&W Health Plan,
Sr. Staff Physician, S&W Pulmonary and Sleep Disorders; Professor of Medicine,
Texas A&M SOM*

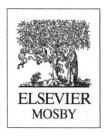

ELSEVIER
MOSBY

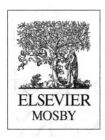

ELSEVIER
MOSBY

Vice President, Global Medical Reference: Mary E. Gatsch
Developmental Editor: Casey Jackson
Production Supervisor, Electronic Year Books: Donna M. Skelton
Electronic Article Manager: Mike Sheets
Illustrations and Permissions Coordinator: Dawn A. Vohsen

2014 EDITION
Copyright 2014, Mosby, Inc. All rights reserved.

Printed in the United States of America
Composition by TNQ Books and Journals Pvt Ltd, India
Printing/binding by Sheridan Books, Inc

Editorial Office:
Elsevier, Inc.
Suite 1800
1600 John F. Kennedy Blvd
Philadelphia, PA 19103-2899

International Standard Serial Number: 8756-3452
International Standard Book Number: 978-0-323-26487-7

Associate Editors

Shirley F. Jones, MD, FCCP, DABSM

Assistant Professor of Internal Medicine, Division of Pulmonary, Critical Care, and Sleep Medicine, Scott & White Memorial Hospital/Texas A&M Health Science Center, Temple, Texas

Janet R. Maurer, MD, MBA

Vice President, Medical Director, Health Dialog Services Corp, Scottsdale, Arizona

Christopher D. Spradley, MD, FCCP

Director, Medical Intensive Care Unit, Pulmonary Hypertension Clinic, Sleep Medicine, Scott & White Memorial Hospital, Temple, Texas

Lynn T. Tanoue, MD

Professor of Medicine, Section of Pulmonary and Critical Care Medicine, Yale School of Medicine, Yale University, New Haven, Connecticut

Sandra K. Willsie, DO, MA

Kansas City Free Clinic, Kansas City, Missouri; Medical Director, PRA International, Lenexa, Kansas

Table of Contents

JOURNALS REPRESENTED ix

1. Asthma, Allergy, and Cystic Fibrosis 1
   Introduction 1
   Asthma 5
   Cystic Fibrosis 30
2. Chronic Obstructive Pulmonary Disease 35
   Introduction 35
3. Lung Cancer 65
   Introduction 65
   Epidemiology of Lung Cancer 68
   Tobacco-related Issues 75
   Lung Cancer Screening 83
   Diagnostic Evaluation 100
   Lung Cancer Treatment 121
   Molecular Approach to Lung Cancer 127
4. Pleural, Interstitial Lung, and Pulmonary Vascular Disease ... 131
   Introduction 131
   Interstitial Lung Disease 132
   Pleural Disease 142
   Pulmonary Vascular Disease 150
5. Community-Acquired Pneumonia 163
   Introduction 163
6. Lung Transplantation 185
   Introduction 185
7. Sleep Disorders 207
   Introduction 207
   Central Sleep Apnea and Heart Failure 208
   Consequences of Sleep-Disordered Breathing 209
   CPAP Treatment and Benefits 212
   Diagnosis of Sleep-Disordered Breathing 220
   Non-CPAP Treatment of Sleep-Disordered Breathing 223

Non-Pulmonary Sleep 230
Pediatric Sleep-Disordered Breathing 232
8. Critical Care Medicine 235
Introduction 235
Acute Respiratory Disorder Syndrome................. 235
Acute Respiratory Failure 237
Airway Management 241
Cardiopulmonary Interactions 244
COPD Patients in the ICU 248
Miscellaneous...................................... 251
Pulmonary Hypertension in the ICU 262
Trauma Issues 263
Ventilator Weaning 265
Ventilator-Associated Pneumonia..................... 267

Article Index 271
Author Index 279

Journals Represented

Journals represented in this YEAR BOOK are listed below.
American Journal of Emergency Medicine
American Journal of Kidney Diseases
American Journal of Medicine
American Journal of Neuroradiology
American Journal of Public Health
American Journal of Respiratory and Critical Care Medicine
American Journal of Respiratory Cell and Molecular Biology
American Journal of Surgery
American Journal of Transplantation
Anesthesia and Analgesia
Annals of Allergy, Asthma and Immunology
Annals of Emergency Medicine
Annals of Internal Medicine
Annals of Surgery
Annals of Thoracic Surgery
Annals of the American Thoracic Society
British Medical Journal
CA: A Cancer Journal for Clinicians
Canadian Journal of Anaesthesia
Chest
Clinical Infectious Diseases
Critical Care Medicine
Drugs
European Respiratory Journal
Immunity
Journal of Allergy and Clinical Immunology
Journal of Clinical Sleep Medicine
Journal of Emergency Medicine
Journal of General Internal Medicine
Journal of Heart and Lung Transplantation
Journal of Infectious Diseases
Journal of Rheumatology
Journal of the American College of Cardiology
Journal of the American Geriatrics Society
Journal of the American Medical Association
Journal of the American Medical Association Neurology
Journal of the National Cancer Institute
Journal of Thoracic and Cardiovascular Surgery
Lancet
New England Journal of Medicine
Pediatrics
Pharmacotherapy
Radiology
Respiratory Medicine
Sleep
Thorax
Transplantation

STANDARD ABBREVIATIONS

The following terms are abbreviated in this edition: acquired immunodeficiency syndrome (AIDS), cardiopulmonary resuscitation (CPR), central nervous system (CNS), cerebrospinal fluid (CSF), computed tomography (CT), deoxyribonucleic acid (DNA), electrocardiography (ECG), health maintenance organization (HMO), human immunodeficiency virus (HIV), intensive care unit (ICU), intramuscular (IM), intravenous (IV), magnetic resonance (MR) imaging (MRI), ribonucleic acid (RNA), and ultrasound (US).

NOTE

The YEAR BOOK OF PULMONARY DISEASE is a literature survey service providing abstracts of articles published in the professional literature. Every effort is made to assure the accuracy of the information presented in these pages. Neither the editors nor the publisher of the YEAR BOOK OF PULMONARY DISEASE can be responsible for errors in the original materials. The editors' comments are their own opinions. Mention of specific products within this publication does not constitute endorsement.

To facilitate the use of the YEAR BOOK OF PULMONARY DISEASE as a reference tool, all illustrations and tables included in this publication are now identified as they appear in the original article. This change is meant to help the reader recognize that any illustration or table appearing in the YEAR BOOK OF PULMONARY DISEASE may be only one of many in the original article. For this reason, figure and table numbers will often appear to be out of sequence within the YEAR BOOK OF PULMONARY DISEASE.

1 Asthma, Allergy, and Cystic Fibrosis

Introduction

A number of pivotal articles were published in the last year that are of key importance for all health care providers caring for patients with cystic fibrosis. Among these are two manuscripts detailing outcomes following the administration of bronchial thermoplasty (BT). The medical community has been waiting for a seemingly long period to learn of the outcomes of these two studies.

Both publications report patient outcomes following BT delivered for uncontrolled severe persistent asthma. In the first study, 5-year durability of the benefits of BT were seen, impacting both asthma control and safety in 162 of the 190 treated subjects.[1] Overall, an 18% reduction was noted in ICS dose at 5 years in severe persistent asthmatics, with 12% of subjects no longer taking ICS 5 years post-BT and 7% of subjects no longer taking ICS or LABA therapy. In the second investigation, 14 subjects with severe persistent asthma were followed after BT, showing a trend but no statistical decrease in the incidence of hospitalization or ED visits.[2] These data confirm the established safety profile for BT reported at 2 years and support consideration of BT for severe persistent symptomatic asthmatics on optimal therapy with inhaled corticosteroids (ICS) and long-acting beta-agonist therapy (LABA). While few centers may possess the skills and training to safely deliver this treatment, BT represents a solid option for consideration.

Suggesting that adult-onset asthma represents a distinct phenotype,[3] an investigation suggests that adult onset asthmatics (AoA) are more likely to demonstrate peripheral neutrophilia, eosinophilia, and sputum eosinophilia than non-AoA. Additionally, the AoA subjects were more likely to be nonatopic, to have prominent nasal symptomatology and elevated exhaled nitric-oxide levels. The investigators suggest that this profile represents a distinct phenotype.

A meta-analysis of randomized, double-blind (RDB) controlled trials involving administration of heliox-(helium:oxygen) (80:20) driven nebulization vs routine nebulization (21-100% oxygen) of beta agonists was published this year, combining reports from studies inclusive of 71 children and 405 adult asthmatics.[4] The use of heliox resulted in decreased risk of hospitalizations (OR 0.49, 95% CI: 0.31-0,79, $p = 0.003$), and, in moderate-severe asthmatic exacerbations, was associated with improved pulmonary function. Citing a need for cost-effectiveness studies, the authors recommend consideration of the use of heliox to drive nebulization in moderate-severe exacerbations of acute asthma.

This report, published in the American Journal of Respiratory and Critical Care Medicine, is suggested for the busy practitioner.[5] Important issues summarized include a succinct discussion of Vitamin D's impact on the efficacy of asthma treatment. Maternal stress during pregnancy and the postnatal period is associated with a higher risk of wheeze, and there is continuing evidence that obesity is one of the most significant comorbidities experienced by asthmatics and is itself strongly associated with asthma. Also discussed are mechanisms through which various viruses enhance asthma severity and description of a new condition, "asthmatic granulomatosis," associated with difficult to control asthma (non-necrotizing granulomas); this latter condition is responsive to cytotoxic agents. In addition, the potential usefulness of FENO may help to determine patients who are adherent to ICS.

Genetics or environment—which is most important in asthma? This study of over 65 000 pregnant asthmatics-child pairs reported linkages between a wide variety of diseases occurring in childhood, some of which have not been previously reported. From the Danish National Birth Cohort (prospectively obtained data from 1996–2002),[6] various models of diseases associated with maternal asthma demonstrated that the adjusted odds ratios (OR) ranged from 0.85 for diseases of blood, immune system to 1.51 for diseases of the respiratory and nervous systems; 1.43-diseases of the skin; 1.42-infections and parasitic diseases; 1.41-diseases of the ear; and 1.35-mental disorders. There is no assessment of what it is in the asthmatic mother that leads to these disorders (medication effects; physiology, etc). Nonetheless, this is a provocative publication and a "should read."

There is evidence that omalizumab (O) improves control of severe persistent allergic asthma when used as an add-on to failed evidence-based guideline care.[7-9] An investigation that evaluated omalizumab in patients with refractory nonatopic asthma[7] reports that the secondary efficacy outcomes at week 16 of treatment with FEV1 and FEV1% predicted improved in the O group vs placebo (P) group ($p < 0.05$). No other statistically significant differences were noted for the asthma quality of life (ACQ) score or fractional excretion of nitric oxide (FE_{NO}). Changes in basophil MFI and plasmacytoid dendritic cells favored O ($p < 0.001$). This data suggests that severe nonatopic asthmatics despite guideline-directed level-4 care may stand to benefit from omalizumab. A review of the use of O is also recommended reading.[9]

The HUNT study (23 000 individuals participating in the Nord-Trondelag Health Study) followed subjects from the time they self-reported asthma.[10]

Subjects were divided into those with metabolic syndrome (MS) vs those without MS. The odds ratio (OR) for the development of asthma in subjects with increased weight circumference consistent with MS was 1.55 (CI 1.23-1.95) and for subjects with diabetes or elevated glucose was 1.64 (CI 1.07-2.52). The results of this study demonstrate that MS and two of its diagnostic criteria are risk factors for incident asthma in adults, confirming the impact of overweight and obesity on asthma.

Will my child outgrow his/her asthma? This is a common question posed to health care providers. This investigation aimed to help answer this question.[11] A questionnaire-based study of children (nearly 3500 children, ages 7-8 initially participated). Two-hundred forty eight of the participants were identified as having asthma, and they were evaluated annually with questionnaires. Between the ages of 16-17 years, pulmonary function testing (including bronchial hyperreactivity), serum IgE levels, and clinical exams were performed. The following characteristics were associated with an increased likelihood of remission of asthma: Male gender, lower asthma severity, pollen hypersensitivity, and lack of sensitization to furred animals.

As past investigations have revealed that female asthmatics require greater health care utilization and more frequent use of short-acting beta agonists, gender-related treatment approaches to asthma have been developed. There is some evidence to suggest that improved control of asthma in women is possible if specific treatment plans are used. The American Lung Association's Asthma Clinical Research Centers (ALA-ACRC) report data from four previous studies (one of well-controlled asthmatics; three with poorly controlled asthmatics).[12] These data pinpointed differences between the genders. Clinically significant differences between men and women were shown for chronic sinusitis and the use of combination therapy (LABA and ICS) (more common in women asthmatics). Women had experienced more exacerbations during the previous year and described allergies as a trigger for their asthma. They were likely to be heavier and to have gastroesophageal reflux or eczema. This investigation is worthwhile in that it underscores consideration of interventions to control gender-related differences in asthma comorbidities.

The results of a phase II, randomized, double-blind, multicenter, placebo-controlled trial of once daily Arikace, a liposome-encapsulated form of Amikacin, was published in the past year. Doses of 280 mg and 560 mg demonstrated statistically significant change in pulmonary function with maintained effect across treatment periods. Sputum density was also reduced with this investigational product. Phase III studies are required, of course, before this drug may/will reach the market, but this compound clearly shows promise for patients with cystic fibrosis and others with persistent or intractable infections with amikacin-sensitive organisms.

Other articles of interest related to cystic fibrosis, unfortunately not reviewed in this issue of the PULMONARY DISEASE YEAR BOOK, include the references below, which are recommended reading for health care providers caring for patients with cystic fibrosis. I hope that you will find the selected publications reviewed herein to be beneficial to your practice.

Sandra K. Willsie, DO, MA

References

1. Wechsler ME, Laviolette M, Rubin AS, et al. Bronchial thermoplasty: Long-term safety and effectiveness in patients with severe persistent asthma. *J Allergy Clin Immunol.* 2013;132:1295-1302.
2. Pavord ID, Thomson NC, Niven RM, et al. Safety of bronchial thermoplasty in patients with severe refractory asthma. *Ann Allergy Asthma Immunol.* 2013;111: 402-407.
3. Amelink M, de Groot JC, de Nijs SB, et al. Severe adult-onset asthma: A distinct phenotype. *J Allergy Clin Immunol.* 2013;132:336-341.
4. Rodrigo GJ, Castro-Rodriguez JA. Heliox-driven β2-agonists nebulization for children and adults with acute asthma: a systematic review with meta-analysis. *Ann Allergy Asthma Immunol.* 2014;112:29-34.
5. von Mutius E, Hartert T. Update in asthma 2012. *Am J Respir Crit Care Med.* 2013;188:150-156.
6. Tegethoff M, Olsen J, Schaffner E, Meinlschmidt G. Asthma during pregnancy and clinical outcomes in offspring: a national cohort study. *Pediatrics.* 2013; 132:483-491.
7. Garcia G, Magnan A, Chiron R, et al. A proof-of-concept, randomized, controlled trial of omalizumab in patients with severe, difficult-to-control, nonatopic asthma. *Chest.* 2013;144:411-419.
8. Hanania NA, Alpan O, Hamilos DL, et al. Omalizumab in severe allergic asthma inadequately controlled with standard therapy: a randomized trial. *Ann Intern Med.* 2011;154:573-582.
9. McKeage K. Omalizumab: a review of its use in patients with severe persistent allergic asthma. *Drugs.* 2013;73:1197-1212.
10. Brumpton BM, Camargo CA Jr, Romundstad PR, Langhammer A, Chen Y, Mai XM. Metabolic syndrome and incidence of asthma in adults: the HUNT study. *Eur Respir J.* 2013;42:1495-1502.
11. Andersson M, Hedman L, Bjerg A, Forsberg B, Lundbäck B, Rönmark E. Remission and persistence of asthma followed from 7 to 19 years of age. *Pediatrics.* 2013;132:e435-e442.
12. McCallister JW, Holbrook JT, Wei CY, et al. Sex differences in asthma symptom profiles and control in the American Lung Association Asthma Clinical Research Centers. *Respir Med.* 2013;107:1491-1500.

Asthma

Bronchial thermoplasty: Long-term safety and effectiveness in patients with severe persistent asthma

Wechsler ME, for the Asthma Intervention Research 2 Trial Study Group (Natl Jewish Health, Denver, CO; et al)
J Allergy Clin Immunol 132:1295-1302.e3, 2013

Background.—Bronchial thermoplasty (BT) has previously been shown to improve asthma control out to 2 years in patients with severe persistent asthma.

Objective.—We sought to assess the effectiveness and safety of BT in asthmatic patients 5 years after therapy.

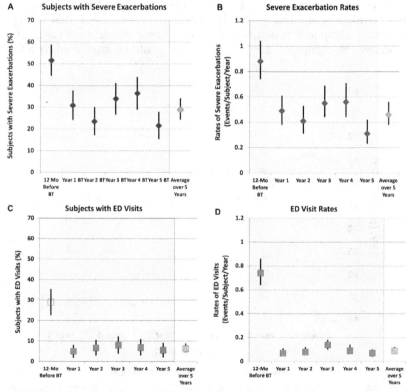

FIGURE 1.—Severe exacerbations and ED visits in the 5 years after BT. **A,** Proportion of subjects with severe exacerbations. **B,** Severe exacerbation rates. **C,** Proportion of subjects with ED visits for respiratory symptoms. **D,** ED visit rates. Values are point estimates with 95% upper and lower CIs. The 365-day period constituting year 1 began at 6 weeks after the last BT bronchoscopy. (Reprinted from The Journal of Allergy and Clinical Immunology. Wechsler ME, for the Asthma Intervention Research 2 Trial Study Group. Bronchial thermoplasty: long-term safety and effectiveness in patients with severe persistent asthma. *J Allergy Clin Immunol.* 2013;132:1295-1302.e3, Copyright, 2013, with permission from Elsevier.)

Methods.—BT-treated subjects from the Asthma Intervention Research 2 trial (ClinicalTrials.gov NCT01350414) were evaluated annually for 5 years to assess the long-term safety of BT and the durability of its treatment effect. Outcomes assessed after BT included severe exacerbations, adverse events, health care use, spirometric data, and high-resolution computed tomographic scans.

Results.—One hundred sixty-two (85.3%) of 190 BT-treated subjects from the Asthma Intervention Research 2 trial completed 5 years of follow-up. The proportion of subjects experiencing severe exacerbations and emergency department (ED) visits and the rates of events in each of years 1 to 5 remained low and were less than those observed in the 12 months before BT treatment (average 5-year reduction in proportions: 44% for exacerbations and 78% for ED visits). Respiratory adverse events and respiratory-related hospitalizations remained unchanged in years 2 through 5 compared with the first year after BT. Prebronchodilator FEV_1 values remained stable between years 1 and 5 after BT, despite a 18% reduction in average daily inhaled corticosteroid dose. High-resolution computed tomographic scans from baseline to 5 years after BT showed no structural abnormalities that could be attributed to BT.

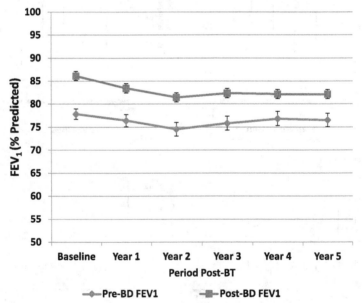

FIGURE 2.—Prebronchodilator and postbronchodilator FEV_1 over 5 years (percent predicted). Percent predicted prebronchodilator and postbronchodilator FEV_1 values (means ± SEMs) for subjects completing follow-up during each year. The percent predicted prebronchodilator FEV_1 values remained unchanged over the 5 years after BT. Postbronchodilator FEV_1 remained higher at all times; increase in percent predicted FEV_1 at baseline of 8.2% and at 5 years of 5.9%. *BD*, Bronchodilator. (Reprinted from The Journal of Allergy and Clinical Immunology. Wechsler ME, for the Asthma Intervention Research 2 Trial Study Group. Bronchial thermoplasty: long-term safety and effectiveness in patients with severe persistent asthma. *J Allergy Clin Immunol.* 2013;132:1295-1302.e3, Copyright 2013, with permission from Elsevier.)

Conclusions.—These data demonstrate the 5-year durability of the benefits of BT with regard to both asthma control (based on maintained reduction in severe exacerbations and ED visits for respiratory symptoms) and safety. BT has become an important addition to our treatment armamentarium and should be considered for patients with severe persistent asthma who remain symptomatic despite taking inhaled corticosteroids and long-acting β_2-agonists (Figs 1 and 2, Table 1).

▶ What we've been waiting for: 5-year outcomes after bronchial thermoplasty (BTP) in severe persistent asthmatics! At baseline, 72% of subjects were taking a minimum of 2 maintenance medications (long-acting β_2 agonist [LABA] and high-dose inhaled corticosteroids [ICS]), whereas 28% of subjects

TABLE 1.—Demographics and Clinical Characteristics

	All Subjects Undergoing BT at Baseline (n = 190)	Subjects Undergoing BT Completing 5-y Follow-up (n = 162)	Subjects Undergoing BT not Completing 5-y Follow-up (n = 28)
Age (y)	40.7 ± 11.9	41.5 ± 11.8	35.8 ± 11.3$
Sex	Male: 81 (42.6%)	Male: 68 (42.0%)	Male: 13 (46.4%)
	Female: 109 (57.4%)	Female: 94 (58.0%)	Female: 15 (63.6%)
Race			
White	151 (79.5%)	134 (82.7%)	17 (60.7%)
African American/black	19 (10.0%)	13 (8.0%)	6 (21.4%)
Hispanic	6 (3.2%)	4 (2.5%)	2 (7.1%)
Asian	4 (2.1%)	3 (1.9%)	1 (3.6%)
Other	10 (5.3%)	8 (4.9%)	2 (7.1%)
Weight (kg)	81.7 ± 18.4	81.4 ± 17.1	83.4 ± 24.6
ICS dose (µg)*	1960.7 ± 745.2	1958.9 ± 757.9	1900 ± 551.6
LABA dose (µg)[†]	116.8 ± 34.4	120.8 ± 47.7	108.9 ± 23.8
Symptom-free days (%)	16.4 ± 24.0	16.1 ± 24.1	18.4 ± 24.1
Asthma Control Questionnaire score	2.1 ± 0.87	2.1 ± 0.84	2.3 ± 1.02
AQLQ score	4.30 ± 1.17	4.32 ± 1.17	4.23 ± 1.16
ED visits for respiratory symptoms in prior 12 mo, [†] no. of events (no. of subjects)	141 (55)	115 (47)	26 (8)
Hospitalizations for respiratory symptoms in prior 12 mo,[†] no. of events (no. of subjects)	10 (8)	10 (8)	0 (0)
Seasonal allergies, no. (%)[‡]			
Yes	103 (54.5%)	85 (52.8%)	18 (64.3%)
No	86 (45.5%)	76 (47.2%)	10 (35.7%)
Lung function measures			
Prebronchodilator FEV_1	77.8 ± 15.65	77.8 ± 15.84	78.0 ± 14.75
Postbronchodilator FEV_1	86.1 ± 15.76	85.9 ± 15.83	87.1 ± 15.57
Morning PEF (L/min)	383.8 ± 104.3	380.9 ± 106.0	400.7 ± 93.8
Methacholine PC_{20} (mg/mL), geometric mean (range)	0.27 (0.22-0.34)	0.27 (0.21-0.35)	0.29 (0.15-0.54)

Values are means ± SDs, except when indicated otherwise.
PEF, Peak expiratory flow.
*Beclomethasone or equivalent.
[†]Salmeterol or equivalent.
[‡]Patient reported.
[$]$P = .019$ comparing subjects completing 5-year follow-up versus subjects not completing 5-year follow-up (*t* test).

required 3 maintenance medications. Although outcomes at 1 and 2 years have been published previously,[1-3] this report outlines baseline demographics (Table 1) and 5 years of annual follow-up after bronchial thermoplasty for 162 of 190 (85.3%) subjects with uncontrolled asthma (from the Asthma Intervention Research 2 trial). Fig 1 depicts results pre-BTP (pBTP) and annual follow-up for: percentage of subjects with severe exacerbations; rates of severe exacerbation (events per subject per year); percentage of subjects with emergency department (ED) visits; and ED visit rates (events per subject follow-up). Pre- and post-bronchodilator reactivity was monitored over the 5-year follow-up. For all of the above outcomes, statistically significant improvement was maintained over 5 years of annual follow-up showing essentially no change from pBTP (Fig 2). Overall, an 18% reduction was noted in ICS dose at 5 years, with 12% of subjects no longer taking ICS 5 years post-BPT, and 7% of subjects no longer taking ICS or LABA therapy. These data confirm the previously established safety profile for BTP reported at 2 years and support consideration of BTP for severe persistent symptomatic asthmatics on optimal therapy with ICS and LABA.

S. K. Willsie, DO, MA

References

1. Cox G, Thomson NC, Rubin AS, et al. Asthma control during the year after bronchial thermoplastsy. *N Engl J Med.* 2007;356:1327-1337.
2. Castro M, Rubin AS, Laviolette M, et al. Effectiveness and safety of bronchial thermoplasty in the treatment of severe asthma: a multicenter, randomized, double-blind, sham-controlled clinical trial. *Am J Respir Crit Care Med.* 2010; 181:116-124.
3. Castro M, Rubin A, Laviolette M, Hanania NA, Armstrong B, Cox G. Persistence of effectiveness of bronchial thermoplasty in patients with severe asthma. *Ann Allergy Asthma Immunol.* 2011;107:65-70.

Safety of bronchial thermoplasty in patients with severe refractory asthma
Pavord ID, for the Research in Severe Asthma Trial Study Group (Univ Hosps of Leicester NHS Trust, UK)
Ann Allergy Asthma Immunol 111:402-407, 2013

Background.—Patients with severe refractory asthma treated with bronchial thermoplasty (BT), a bronchoscopic procedure that improves asthma control by reducing excess airway smooth muscle, were followed up for 5 years to evaluate long-term safety of this procedure.

Objectives.—To assess long-term safety of BT for 5 years.

Methods.—Patients with asthma aged 18 to 65 years requiring high-dose inhaled corticosteroids (ICSs) (>750 μg/d of fluticasone propionate or equivalent) and long-acting β_2-agonists (LABAs) (at least 100 μg/d of salmeterol or equivalent), with or without oral prednisone ($\leq$30 mg/d), leukotriene modifiers, theophylline, or other asthma controller medications were enrolled in the Research in Severe Asthma (RISA) Trial. Patients had a prebronchodilator forced expiratory volume in 1 second of 50% or

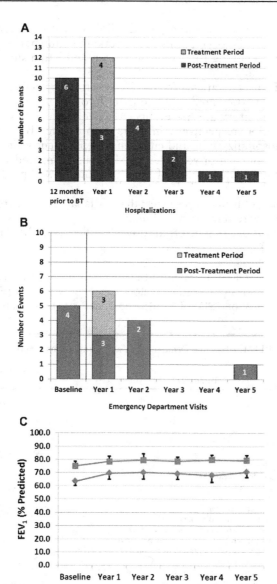

FIGURE 1.—Summary of health care utilization events. A, Hospitalizations for respiratory symptoms. B, Emergency department (ED) visits for respiratory symptoms. Bars represent number of events. Numbers within bars represent the number of patients contributing to the events. Year 1 data represent events occurring in the treatment period (day of first BT procedure until 6 weeks after the third BT procedure) and the post-treatment period (46-week period beginning 6 weeks after the last BT procedure to 12 months). $P = .16$ for the trend in the percentage of patients with hospitalizations for respiratory symptoms and $P = .22$ for the trend in the percentage of patients with ED visits for respiratory symptoms across years 1 to 5 (posttreatment period) using a repeated-measures logistic regression (generalized estimating equation), modeling the percentage of patients reporting an event. C, Prebronchodilator and postbronchodilator forced expiratory volume in 1 second (FEV_1) over time. Values represent mean (SEM) percent predicted prebronchodilator ($\diamond$) and postbronchodilator ($\square$) FEV_1 values. (Reprinted from Annals of Allergy, Asthma and Immunology. Pavord ID, for the Research in Severe Asthma Trial Study Group. Safety of bronchial thermoplasty in patients with severe refractory asthma. *Ann Allergy Asthma Immunol.* 2013;111:402-407, Copyright 2013, with permission from American College of Allergy, Asthma & Immunology.)

more of predicted, demonstrated methacholine airway hyperresponsive-ness, had uncontrolled symptoms despite taking maintenance medication, abstained from smoking for 1 year or greater, and had a smoking history of less than 10 pack-years.

Results.—Fourteen patients (of the 15 who received active treatment in the RISA Trial) participated in the long-term follow-up study for 5 years. The rate of respiratory adverse events (AEs per patient per year) was 1.4, 2.4, 1.7, and 2.4, respectively, in years 2 to 5 after BT. There was a decrease in hospitalizations and emergency department visits for respiratory symptoms in each of years 1, 2, 3, 4, and 5 compared with the year before BT treatment. Measures of lung function showed no deterioration for 5 years.

Conclusion.—Our findings suggest that BT is safe for 5 years after BT in patients with severe refractory asthma.

Trial Registration.—clinicaltrials.gov Identifier: NCT00401986 (Fig 1, Tables 1 and 2).

▶ This is a 5-year follow-up report of 14 subjects with severe persistent asthma (mean prebronchodilator forced expiratory volume in 1 second [FEV_1]: 63.5% with standard deviation [SD] of 12.5), who underwent bronchial thermoplasty

TABLE 1.—Baseline Demographics and Clinical Characteristics

Parameter	Bronchial Thermoplasty (n = 14)
Age, mean (SD), y	38.6 (13.3)
Sex, No. (%)	
Male	6 (43)
Female	8 (57)
White race, No. (%)	14 (100)
Height, mean (SD), cm	165.8 (7.9)
Weight, mean (SD), kg	90.5 (19.5)
Inhaled corticosteroid dose, mean (SD), μg^a	1,179 (421)
LABA dose, mean (SD), μg^b	127 (62)
OCS dose, mean (SD), mg (n = 7)	15 (5.8)
Symptom-free days, mean (SD), %	5.6 (14.1)
Asthma Control Questionnaire score, mean (SD)	2.8 (1.0)
Asthma Quality of Life Questionnaire score, mean (SD)	4.1 (1.3)
Rescue medication use, mean (SD), No. of puffs per 7 days	60.1 (60.1)
Emergency department visits for respiratory symptoms in prior 12 months,[c] No. of events (No. of patients)	5 (4)
Hospitalizations for respiratory symptoms in prior 12 months,[c] No. of events (No. of patients)	10 (6)
Seasonal allergies (self-reported), No. (%)	10 (71)
Lung function measures	
Morning peak expiratory flow rate, mean (SD), L/min	370.0 (82.0)
Prebronchodilator FEV_1, mean (SD), % predicted	63.5 (12.5)
Postbronchodilator FEV_1, mean (SD), % predicted	75.2 (11.9)
Methacholine PC_{20}, geometric mean (range), mg/mL	0.24 (0.1-1.1)

Abbreviations: FEV_1, forced expiratory volume in 1 second; LABA, long-acting β_2-agonist; OCS, oral corticosteroid; PC_{20}, provocative concentration causing a 20% decrease in FEV_1.
[a]Fluticasone or equivalent.
[b]Salmeterol or equivalent.
[c]Patient reported.

TABLE 2.—Adverse Events by Year

Year	Total No. of Events	Total No. (%) of Patients Reporting	No. of Events per Patient per Year
Year 1[a] (n = 14)	118	14 (100)	8.4
Year 2 (n = 14)	20	11 (78.6)	1.4
Year 3 (n = 14)	34	12 (85.7)	2.4
Year 4 (n = 12)	20	10 (83.3)	1.7
Year 5 (n = 12)	29	12 (100)	2.4

[a]Year 1 data (posttreatment period only; ie, the 46-week period beginning 6 weeks after the last bronchial thermoplasty procedure to 12 months) for 14 patients who enrolled in long-term follow-up trial. Adverse events solicited from patient during multiple office visits in year 1. In subsequent years, adverse events solicited only at annual follow-up visit.

(BT) in the Research in Severe Asthma (RISA) trial. Table 1 depicts baseline demographics and pre-BT dosing of long-acting β agonists (LABA) and inhaled corticosteroids (ICS) and Table 2 lists adverse events by year after BT. Fig 1 shows data from 12 months before BT through 5-year follow-up. As with the report of the Asthma Intervention Research 2 (AIR2) trial in which subjects with severe persistent asthma (mean prebronchodilator FEV_1 of 77.8%, SD 16.5) underwent BT,[1] pre- and postbronchodilator FEV_1 was maintained over 5 years in all subjects. The incidence of hospitalization and ED visits trended toward improvement but did not reach statistical significance. No significant change in asthma medication use was found over the monitoring period. Data from the RISA trial are additive to the AIR2 5-year outcome data concerning the safety of BT.[1]

S. K. Willsie, DO, MA

Reference

1. Wechsler ME, Laviolette M, Aalberto SR, et al. Bronchial thermoplasty: long-term safety and effectivenss in patients with severe persistent asthma. *J Allergy Clin Immunol.* 2013;132:1296-1302.

Severe adult-onset asthma: A distinct phenotype

Amelink M, de Groot JC, de Nijs SB, et al (Univ of Amsterdam, The Netherlands; Med Centre Leeuwarden, The Netherlands; et al)
J Allergy Clin Immunol 132:336-341, 2013

Background.—Some patients with adult-onset asthma have severe disease, whereas others have mild transient disease. It is currently unknown whether patients with severe adult-onset asthma represent a distinct clinical phenotype.

Objective.—We sought to investigate whether disease severity in patients with adult-onset asthma is associated with specific phenotypic characteristics.

Methods.—One hundred seventy-six patients with adult-onset asthma were recruited from 1 academic and 3 nonacademic outpatient clinics.

Severe refractory asthma was defined according to international Innovative Medicines Initiative criteria, and mild-to-moderate persistent asthma was defined according to Global Initiative for Asthma criteria. Patients were characterized with respect to clinical, functional, and inflammatory parameters. Unpaired t tests and χ^2 tests were used for group comparisons; both univariate and multivariate logistic regression were used to determine factors associated with disease severity.

Results.—Apart from the expected high symptom scores, poor quality of life, need for high-intensity treatment, low lung function, and high exacerbation rate, patients with severe adult-onset asthma were more often nonatopic (52% vs 34%, $P = .02$) and had more nasal symptoms and nasal polyposis (54% vs 27%, $P \leq .001$), higher exhaled nitric oxide levels (38 vs 27 ppb, $P = .02$) and blood neutrophil counts (5.3 vs 4.0 10^9/L, $P \leq .001$) and sputum eosinophilia (11.8% vs 0.8%, $P \leq .001$). Multiple logistic regression analysis showed that increased blood neutrophil (odds ratio, 10.9; $P = .002$) and sputum eosinophil (odds ratio, 1.5; $P = .005$) counts were independently associated with severe adult-onset disease.

Conclusion.—The majority of patients with severe adult-onset asthma are nonatopic and have persistent eosinophilic airway inflammation.

TABLE 1.—Symptoms, Medication Use, and Health Care Use

	Mild-to-Moderate Persistent Asthma (n = 98)	Severe Asthma (n = 78)	P Value
ACQ score*	1.17 (0.94)	1.91 (0.98)	<.001
AQLQ score*	5.4 (1.28)	4.8 (1.15)	.002
ICS dose (fluticasone equivalent)†	500 (250-500)	1000 (1000-1500)	<.001
OCS (%)	0	59	<.001
Anti-IgE (%)	0	11.5	.001
Exacerbations (%)			<.001
0	70	17	
1-2	18	32	
≥3	12	51	
Doctor's office visits (%)			<.001
0	14	0	
1-2	65	22	
≥3	21	78	
ED visits (%)			.04
0	90	75	
1-2	8	17	
≥3	2	8	
Hospitalizations (%)			.003
0	93	74	
1-2	5	22	
≥3	2	4	
ICU admissions (%)			.01
0	99	86	
1-2	1	10	
≥3	0	1	

Exacerbations, doctor's office visits, emergency department visits, and hospitalizations are defined as the number of events in the past 12 months. Intensive care unit admissions are the number of admissions ever to the intensive care unit.
ACQ, Asthma Control Questionnaire; AQLQ, Asthma Quality of Life Questionnaire; ED, emergency department; ICS, inhaled corticosteroids; ICU, intensive care unit; OCS, oral corticosteroids.
*Mean (SD).
†Median (first and third interquartiles).

TABLE 2.—Patients' Characteristics

	Mild-to-Moderate Persistent Asthma (N = 98)	Severe Asthma (n = 78)	P Value
Age (y)*	53.6 (11.4)	54.4 (9.8)	.6
Sex (% female)	59.2	61.5	.7
Age of onset (y)*	41.8 (13.8)	40.2 (11.9)	.4
Asthma duration (y)†	9 (3-18.5)	10 (5-21)	.07
White race (%)	82.7	87.2	.4
(Ex)smoker (%)	33.7	47.4	.08
Pack years smoked†	0 (0-4.5)	0 (0-7.6)	.3
Total IgE (kU/L)†	77.5 (26.3-277)	112 (51.7-325)	.1
Atopy (positive RAST result [%])	52	34.6	.02
IgE against Aspergillus species (%)	10	9	.7
Family history of atopy (%)	36.6	27.6	.2
Family history of asthma (%)	34.4	38.2	.6
BMI (kg/m²)†	27.3 (24.5-29.9)	28.6 (24.8-31.6)	.2
Nasal polyposis (%)	26.5	53.8	<.001
History of NSAID sensitivity (%)	11.2	16.7	.4
SNOT score*	1.15 (0.76)	1.4 (0.86)	.02
Use of nasal corticosteroids (%)	45	74.4	<.001

NSAID, Nonsteroidal anti-inflammatory drug; SNOT, 22-item Sino-Nasal Outcome Test.
*Mean (SD).
†Median (first and third interquartiles).

TABLE 4.—Inflammatory Markers

	Mild-to-Moderate Persistent Asthma (n = 98)	Severe Asthma (n = 78)	P Value
Blood eosinophils (10⁹/L)	0.18 (0.09-0.31)	0.25 (0.14-0.5)	.05
Blood neutrophils (10⁹/L)	4 (3.1-4.9)	5.3 (3.9-6.8)	<.001
FENO (ppb)	27 (16-50)	38 (19-73)	.02
Sputum eosinophils (% [n = 110])	0.8 (0.1-7.1)	11.6 (1.5-33.4)	<.001
Sputum neutrophils (% [n = 110])	73.5 (46.7-84.9)	67.2 (37.9-83.2)	.9

Values are presented as medians (first and third interquartiles).

This suggests that severe adult-onset asthma has a distinct underlying mechanism compared with milder disease (Tables 1, 2, and 4).

▶ This is an important investigation aimed at characterizing severe adult-onset asthma. A total of 176 subjects with adult-onset asthma were evaluated: 98 were characterized as mild-moderate asthmatics and 78 as severe asthmatics (forming the group upon which the study focused). More than 50% of the severe asthmatic population was receiving daily oral corticosteroids and greater than 10% were receiving anti-immunoglobulin E therapy. Tables 1 and 2 show that adult-onset severe asthmatics used higher-dose inhaled corticosteroids (ICS) (P < .001) and nasal corticosteroids (P < .001) than the mild-moderate asthmatics. Table 4 summarizes the results of inflammatory marker testing, which show that the adult-onset severe asthmatic is more likely to have peripheral neutrophilia and eosinophilia and sputum eosinophilia. They are more likely to be nonatopic and to have more nasal symptoms/nasal polyposis and higher exhaled nitric oxide levels. The investigators suggest that these data show the likelihood of a distinct phenotype, which may help to explain why adult-onset severe asthmatics often are seemingly less responsive to guideline-directed care. These data should lead to additional investigations surrounding the pathophysiology of this distinct phenotype with one result being the design of preventive steps to eliminate severe adult-onset asthma.

S. K. Willsie, DO, MA

Heliox-driven β_2-agonists nebulization for children and adults with acute asthma: a systematic review with meta-analysis
Rodrigo GJ, Castro-Rodriguez JA (Hospital Central de las Fuerzas Armadas, Montevideo, Uruguay; Pontificia Universidad Católica de Chile, Santiago)
Ann Allergy Asthma Immunol 112:29-34, 2014

Background.—The effect of heliox as a nebulizer β_2-agonist driving gas in acute asthma remains controversial.

Objective.—To perform a systematic review with a meta-analysis of randomized trials designed to evaluate the efficacy of heliox versus oxygen in driving β_2-agonist nebulization in patients with acute asthma.

Methods.—A search was conducted of all randomized controlled trials published before August 2013. Primary outcomes were change in spirometric measurements and severity composite score (pediatric studies); secondary outcomes were hospitalizations and serious adverse effects.

Results.—Eleven trials from 10 studies (697 participants) met the inclusion criteria (7 included adults and 3 included children). The mean duration of heliox therapy was 120 minutes and the most common helium-oxygen mixture used was 70:30. Patients receiving heliox presented a statistically significant difference for mean percentage of change in peak expiratory flow (17.2%; 95% confidence interval 5.2–29.2, $P = .005$). Post hoc subgroup analysis showed that patients with severe and very severe asthma showed a significant improvement in peak expiratory flow compared with those with mild to moderate acute asthma. Heliox-driven nebulization also produced significant decreases in the risk of hospitalizations (odds ratio 0.49, 95% confidence interval 0.31–0.79, $P = .003$) and severity of exacerbations (pediatric studies; standard mean difference -0.74, 95%% confidence interval -1.45 to -0.03, $P = .04$). There were no group differences for serious adverse effects.

Conclusion.—This review suggests that heliox benefits in airflow limitation and hospital admissions could be considered clinically significant. Data support the use of heliox as a nebulizing β_2-agonist driving gas in the routine care of patients with acute asthma (Fig 3).

▶ This study was a meta-analysis of randomized trials designed to determine whether a heliox oxygen mixture is efficacious in driving β_2-agonist therapy delivery in the treatment of acute asthma. The studies analyzed represent 10

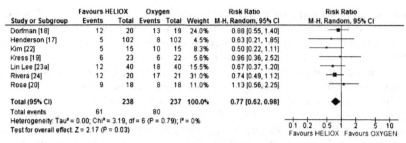

Study or Subgroup	Favours HELIOX Events	Total	Oxygen Events	Total	Weight	Risk Ratio M-H, Random, 95% CI	Risk Ratio M-H, Random, 95% CI
Dorfman [18]	12	20	13	19	24.0%	0.88 [0.55, 1.40]	
Henderson [17]	5	102	8	102	4.5%	0.63 [0.21, 1.85]	
Kim [22]	5	15	10	15	8.3%	0.50 [0.22, 1.11]	
Kress [19]	6	23	6	22	5.6%	0.96 [0.36, 2.52]	
Lin Lee [23a]	12	40	18	40	15.5%	0.67 [0.37, 1.20]	
Rivera [24]	12	20	17	21	31.0%	0.74 [0.49, 1.12]	
Rose [20]	9	18	8	18	11.0%	1.13 [0.56, 2.25]	
Total (95% CI)		**238**		**237**	**100.0%**	**0.77 [0.62, 0.98]**	
Total events	61		80				

Heterogeneity: Tau² = 0.00; Chi² = 3.19, df = 6 (P = 0.79); I² = 0%
Test for overall effect: Z = 2.17 (P = 0.03)

0.1 0.2 0.5 1 2 5 10
Favours HELIOX Favours OXYGEN

FIGURE 3.—Pooled risk ratio with 95% confidence intervals (CIs) of eligible studies comparing heliox- with oxygen-driven β_2-agonist nebulization for the outcome of hospital admissions. M-H, Mantel-Haenszel. (Reprinted from Annals of Allergy, Asthma and Immunology. Rodrigo GJ, Castro-Rodriguez JA. Heliox-driven β_2-agonists nebulization for children and adults with acute asthma: a systematic review with meta-analysis. *Ann Allergy Asthma Immunol.* 2014;112:29-34, Copyright 2014, with permission from American College of Allergy, Asthma & Immunology.)

total trials involving 71 children (3 studies) and 405 adults (7 studies). Subjects were randomly assigned to receive heliox (70:30 or 80:20) or oxygen-driven (21%−100%) β-agonist therapy for asthma exacerbations. The severity of the asthmatic exacerbations ranged from mild-moderate to very severe. Fig 3 shows the results of the meta-analysis depicting risk ratios (favoring heliox) ranging from 0.50 to 1.13. The use of heliox resulted in decreased risk of hospitalizations (odds ratio, 0.49; 95% confidence interval, 0.31−0.79; $P = .003$), and use in moderate-severe asthma showed better outcomes in spirometric measurements. The incidence of adverse events was similar between the 2 treatments. Citing a need for cost-effectiveness studies, the authors recommend consideration of the use of heliox to drive nebulization in moderate-severe exacerbations of acute asthma.

S. K. Willsie, DO, MA

Update in Asthma 2012
von Mutius E, Hartert T (Ludwig Maximilians Univ, Munich, Germany; Vanderbilt Univ School of Medicine, Nashville, TN)
Am J Respir Crit Care Med 188:150-156, 2013

Background.—Evidence from studies of asthma offers insights into the onset, risk factors, and pathogenesis of this disease, as well as how to translate the information into clinical efforts to improve health. The current state of knowledge concerning asthma was outlined.

Host and Environmental Factors.—Associations are being confirmed between asthma and factors such as obesity, stress, viruses, environmental tobacco smoke (ETS), other environmental influences, and diet. Children who develop asthma appear to be born with compromised lung function that can then be further harmed by environmental factors. In addition to ETS, links with asthma are found for the presence of atopy and allergic rhinitis in children, exposure to respiratory tract virus, and stress. Allergic

HR←

sensitization appears to predate the development of wheezing illnesses associated with the human rhinovirus (HRV), which are common in children with asthma. Respiratory syncytial virus (RSV) infection may worsen asthma, and asthma may worsen H1N1 infections. Children of mothers who smoke during pregnancy tend to have an increased risk of wheezing illness and asthma. Interestingly, maternal but not paternal atopy appears to be associated with mediator down-regulation of the upper airway mucosa in infants. Nonspecific irritants also cause respiratory symptoms, especially if there is underlying airflow obstruction. Obesity is strongly associated with asthma. Protective effects are offered by breastfeeding, even if the mother has asthma; farming; and possibly vitamin D supplementation.

Pathogenesis and Control.—Hyperventilation of hot air causes subjects with asthma to develop increased specific airway resistance and cough, although pretreatment with ipratropium can completely prevent this effect. Overexpression of nicotinamide adenine dinucleotide phosphate oxidase (NOX) 4 expression in the airway smooth muscle plays a critical role in causing hypercontractility in persons with asthma. The airways of patients with asthma and airway obstruction may not be as flexible so they cannot reverse bronchoconstriction. The increased thickness of the airway smooth muscle layer in asthmatic persons may be related to hypertrophy and hyperplasia, but duration of asthma appears noncontributory. Viruses that may contribute to asthma inception and exacerbation have also been investigated.

Conclusions.—Severe asthma is now understood to be a heterogeneous disease that exhibits various molecular, biochemical, and cellular inflammatory features as well as specific abnormalities of structure and function. Among the investigative tools and treatments studied are bronchial thermoplasty, video-assisted thoracoscopic biopsy, and the relationships between b1-integrin activation and decreased pulmonary function. About half of the patients with noneosinophilic disease respond poorly to the current anti-inflammatory treatments but not to bronchodilators. Nonadherence to inhaled corticosteroid (ICS) therapy contributes significantly to poorly controlled severe asthma, but it is difficult to identify patients who are nonadherent. ICS therapy during pregnancy may affect the health of the offspring, but more importantly it minimizes complications such as preterm labor and delivery issues; this must be weighed against the future problems that may develop.

▶ This concise review of 2012 published reports addressing issues in asthma from the *American Journal of Respiratory and Critical Care Medicine* is suggested for the busy practitioner. Particularly important issues summarized and referenced include the following: a succinct discussion of the impact of vitamin D on the efficacy of asthma treatment; maternal stress during pregnancy and the postnatal period and its association with a higher risk of wheeze; evidence that obesity is one of the most significant comorbidities experienced by asthmatics and is itself strongly associated with asthma; mechanisms through which various viruses enhance asthma severity; description of a new condition, *asthmatic granulomatosis*, associated with difficult-to-control asthma in the presence of infrequent non-necrotizing granulomas, which is responsive to cytotoxic agents; safety of bronchial thermoplasty; usefulness of fractional exhaled nitric oxide in helping to determine inhaled corticosteroid adherence; and additive effects of tiotropium to therapy in poorly controlled asthmatics.

S. K. Willsie, DO, MA

Asthma During Pregnancy and Clinical Outcomes in Offspring: A National Cohort Study

Tegethoff M, Olsen J, Schaffner E, et al (Univ of Basel, Switzerland; Univ of California at Los Angeles)

Pediatrics 132:483-491, 2013

Background and Objective.—Maternal asthma is a common pregnancy complication, with adverse short-term effects for the offspring. The objective was to determine whether asthma during pregnancy is a risk factor of offspring diseases.

Methods.—We studied pregnant women from the Danish National Birth Cohort (births: 1996—2002; prospective data) giving birth to live singletons ($n = 66\,712$ mother-child pairs), with 4145 (6.2%) women suffering from asthma during pregnancy. We estimated the associations between asthma during pregnancy and offspring diseases (*International Classification of Diseases, 10th Revision* diagnoses from national registries), controlling for potential confounders and validating findings by secondary analyses.

Results.—Offspring median age at end of follow-up was 6.2 (3.6—8.9) years. Asthma was associated with an increased offspring risk of infectious and parasitic diseases (hazard ratio [HR] 1.34; 95% confidence interval [CI] 1.23—1.46), diseases of the nervous system (HR 1.43; CI 1.18—1.73), ear (HR 1.33; CI 1.19—1.48), respiratory system (HR 1.43; CI 1.34—1.52), and skin (HR 1.39; CI 1.20—1.60), and potentially (not confirmed in secondary analyses) of endocrine and metabolic disorders (HR 1.26; CI 1.02—1.55), diseases of the digestive system (HR 1.17; CI 1.04—1.32), and malformations (odds ratio 1.13; CI 1.01—1.26), but not of neoplasms, mental disorders, or diseases of the blood and immune system, circulatory system, musculoskeletal system, and genitourinary system.

Conclusions.—To the best of our knowledge, this is the first comprehensive study of the associations between asthma during pregnancy and a wide spectrum of offspring diseases. In line with previous data on selected outcomes, asthma during pregnancy may be a risk factor for numerous offspring diseases, suggesting that careful monitoring of women with asthma during pregnancy and their offspring is important.

▶ This study of more than 65 000 pregnant asthmatic—child pairs reports linkage between several diseases occurring in childhood, some not previously reported. Follow-up ended at a median age of 6.2 years (3.6—8.9 years), and the investigators reviewed data from the Danish National Birth Cohort (prospectively obtained data from 1996—2002). Table 2 in the original article lists the results of Cox regression models of offspring diseases associated with asthma during pregnancy. Adjusted odds ratios (OR) ranged from 0.85 for diseases of blood immune system to 1.51 for diseases of the respiratory system; diseases of the nervous system (1.51), diseases of the skin (1.43), infections and parasitic diseases (1.42), diseases of the ear (1.41), and mental disorders (1.35) were estimated to be associated with maternal asthma. There was no assessment of what in the asthmatic maternal condition led to these disorders (eg, medication effects, physiology). Further research is needed about possible genetic influences vs environment to fully understand the impact and potential for intervention to prevent disease development in the offspring of asthmatic women.

S. K. Willsie, DO, MA

Omalizumab: A review of its Use in Patients with Severe Persistent Allergic Asthma
McKeage K (Adis, North Shore, Auckland, New Zealand)
Drugs 73:1197-1212, 2013

Omalizumab (Xolair®) is a subcutaneously administered monoclonal antibody that targets circulating free IgE and prevents its interaction with the high-affinity IgE receptor (FCεRI), thereby interrupting the allergic cascade. In the EU, the drug is approved as add-on therapy in adults, adolescents and children aged ≥ 6 years with severe persistent allergic asthma. In well designed clinical trials, add-on omalizumab significantly reduced the asthma exacerbation rate (primary endpoint) compared with placebo in adults, adolescents and children with severe persistent allergic asthma. Furthermore, add-on omalizumab reduced the need for inhaled corticosteroids in adults and adolescents, and improved asthma control and symptoms, and asthma-related quality of life in all age groups. The efficacy of omalizumab was also demonstrated in the real-world setting, with add-on therapy leading to reduced rates of hospitalizations, emergency room visits and unscheduled doctor's visits, as well as improvements in asthma symptom scores and the physician's overall assessment of treatment response. More data are needed to determine the optimum duration of treatment, and currently the duration is at the discretion of the treating physician. Omalizumab was generally well tolerated in clinical trials; the most common adverse event was transient injection-site reactions. In cost-utility analyses modelled over a life-time horizon, add-on omalizumab was cost effective compared with standard therapy, with incremental cost-effectiveness ratios falling within generally accepted willingness-to-pay thresholds. Thus, in difficult-to-treat patients with

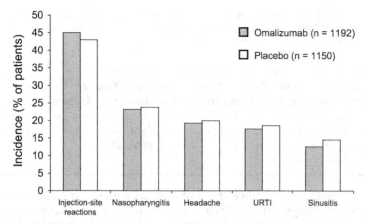

FIGURE 1.—Tolerability of add-on omalizumab in adults and adolescents with persistent allergic asthma. Results are from a review of data from several placebo-controlled trials of 16–32 weeks' duration, and include adverse events that occurred in >10 % of patients in either group [51]. Most patients had severe allergic asthma, but some studies were conducted in patients with moderate to severe disease. The omalizumab dose was based on body weight and pre-treatment total serum IgE levels. *URTI* upper respiratory tract infection. Editor's Note: Please refer to original journal article for full references. (Reprinted from McKeage K. Omalizumab: a review of its use in patients with severe persistent allergic asthma. *Drugs.* 2013;73:1197-1212, with permission from Springer International Publishing Switzerland, Copyright 2013, with permission from Adis Data Information BV.)

severe persistent allergic asthma, omalizumab provides a valuable treatment option (Fig 1).

▶ This is a comprehensive review of the use of omalizumab (subcutaneously administered recombinant DNA-derived humanized immunoglobulin E monoclonal antibody)[1] in the treatment of severe persistent allergic asthmatics. The author reviews several investigations evaluating the pharmacodynamics, pharmacokinetics, tolerability, and therapeutic uses and efficacy of omalizumab in severe persistent allergic asthma.[2] The most common adverse event attributable to omalizumab is transient injection-site reactions. Fig 1 depicts the tolerability of omalizumab vs placebo in adult and adolescent persistent allergic asthmatics. No significant differences between omalizumab vs placebo-related side effects were noted for injection site reactions, nasopharyngitis, headache, upper respiratory tract infections, and sinusitis. Omalizumab is indicated according to Global Initiative for Asthma Guidelines[3] for add-on use in patients with persistent allergic asthma that remains uncontrolled despite step 4 treatment (combinations of high-dose inhaled corticosteroids and other controller medications). Approved dosing, administration, and cost effectiveness is discussed.

S. K. Willsie, DO, MA

References

1. Soresi S, Togias A. Mechanisms of action of anti-immunoglobulin E therapy. *Allergy Asthma Proc.* 2006;27:S15-S23.
2. Corren J, Casale TB, Lanier B, Buhl R, Holgate S, Jimenez P. Safety and tolerability of omalizumab. *Clin Exp Allergy.* 2009;39:788-797.

3. Global Initiative for Asthma. *Global strategy for asthma management and prevention*. 2012. Updated, http://www.ginasthma.org/local/uploads/files/GINA_Report_2012Feb13.pdf. Accessed February 05, 2014.

A Proof-of-Concept, Randomized, Controlled Trial of Omalizumab in Patients With Severe, Difficult-to-Control, Nonatopic Asthma

Garcia G, Magnan A, Chiron R, et al (Université Paris-Sud, Faculté de Médecine, Le Kremlin Bicêtre, France; Université de Nantes, France; Hôpital Arnaud de Villeneuve, Montpellier, Cedex, France; et al)
Chest 144:411-419, 2013

Background.—While up to 50% of patients with severe asthma have no evidence of allergy, IgE has been linked to asthma, irrespective of atopic status. Omalizumab, an anti-IgE monoclonal antibody, is reported to significantly benefit a subset of patients with severe, persistent, allergic asthma. Therefore, we investigated whether omalizumab has biologic and clinical effects in patients with refractory nonatopic asthma.

Methods.—Forty-one adult patients who, despite daily treatment with or without maintenance oral corticosteroids, had severe, nonatopic, refractory asthma according to GINA (Global Initiative for Asthma) step 4, were randomized to receive omalizumab or placebo in a 1:1 ratio. The primary end point was the change in expression of high-affinity IgE receptor (FcεRI) on blood basophils and plasmacytoid dendritic cells (pDC2) after 16 weeks. The impact of omalizumab on lung function and clinical variables was also examined.

Results.—Compared with placebo, omalizumab resulted in a statistically significant reduction in FcεRI expression on basophils and pDC2 ($P < .001$). The omalizumab group also showed an overall increase in FEV_1 compared with baseline (+250 mL, $P = .032$; +9.9%, $P = .029$). A trend toward improvement in global evaluation of treatment effectiveness and asthma exacerbation rate was also observed.

Conclusions.—Omalizumab negatively regulates FcεRI expression in patients with severe nonatopic asthma, as it does in severe atopic asthma. Omalizumab may have a therapeutic role in severe nonatopic asthma. Nonetheless, our preliminary findings support further investigation to better assess the clinical efficacy of omalizumab (Tables 1 and 2).

▶ Omalizumab has been shown to improve control of severe persistent allergic asthma when used as an add-on to failed evidence-based guideline care.[1,2] This investigation evaluated omalizumab in patients with refractory nonatopic asthma. Table 1 provides the baseline demographics and treatment for the placebo (P) and omalizumab (O) groups. Table 2 provides the secondary efficacy outcomes at week 16 of treatment with forced expiratory volume in 1 second (FEV_1) and FEV_1% predicted improved in the O group vs P groups ($P < .05$). There were no other statistically significant differences between groups for asthma quality of life score or fractional excretion of nitric oxide. Fig 2 in the

TABLE 1.—Baseline Demographic and Clinical Characteristics of All Patients Who Underwent Randomization

Characteristics	Placebo (n = 21)	Omalizumab (n = 20)
Age, y	54.6 ± 12.8	55.0 ± 9.7
Female patients	13 (61.9)	13 (65.0)
Male patients	8 (38.1)	7 (35.0)
Weight, kg	70.8 ± 11.8	78.5 ± 15.1
BMI	25.7 ± 3.4	29.7 ± 5.8
IgE, IU/mL	160 ± 142	153 ± 96
IgE level < 100 IU/mL	10 (47.6)	8 (40)
FEV_1 absolute value, L	2.07 ± 0.90	1.67 ± 0.80
FEV_1 % predicted	71.3 ± 21.3%	61.2 ± 17.1%
Inhaled corticosteroids, μg/d	2,667 ± 1,111	2,710 ± 1,230
Long-acting β_2 -agonists	21 (100)	20 (100)
Oral steroids	7 (33.3)	8 (40.0)
Daily oral steroids dose, mg/d	23.0 ± 13.0	35.9 ± 53.4
Patients using leukotriene modifiers	11 (52.4)	8 (40.0)
Patients using theophylline	1 (4.8)	3 (15.0)
ACQ score	2.2 ± 1.2	2.2 ± 0.98
F_{ENO}, ppb	58.8 ± 35.4	32.5 ± 19.2
Asthma exacerbations during the previous year	5.48 ± 4.60	5.05 ± 3.10
Never smokers	15 (71.4)	15 (75.0)
Patients with aspirin- or other NSAID-related asthma	5 (23.8)	4 (20.0)

Data given as mean ± SD or No. (%). ACQ = Asthma Control Questionnaire; F_{ENO} = fraction of exhaled nitric oxide; NSAID = nonsteroidal antiinflammatory drug; ppb = parts per billion.

TABLE 2.—Clinical Secondary Efficacy Outcomes at Week 16, According to Treatment Assignment

Outcome	Placebo (n = 21)	Omalizumab (n = 20)	Difference Between Groups (95% CI)	P Value
FEV_1, mL	0 ± 200	250 ± 380	250	.032
FEV_1 % predicted	−0.2 ± 7.7	+9.7 ± 16.1	+9.5	.029
Responders[a] at visit 10, No.	5	9	4	.185
Asthma exacerbations during 16-wk treatment phase	1.43 ± 1.94	0.80 ± 1.47	...	.278
ACQ score	−0.5 ± 1.43	+0.5 ± 0.98	0	.744
F_{ENO}, ppb	0.7 ± 17.6	2.4 ± 18.2	1.7	.766

Data represent change from baseline and are given as mean ± SD unless otherwise indicated. GETE = global evaluation of treatment effectiveness.
See Table 1 legend for expansion of other abbreviations.
[a]As determined by global evaluation of treatment effectiveness scale.

original article depicts differences between O and P groups for changes in basophil mean fluorescence intensity and plasmacytoid dendritic cells. The results for both parameters were significantly changed by O ($P < .001$). Fig 4 in the original article represents cumulative numbers of asthma exacerbations per group over the 16 weeks, which trended toward but did not meet statistical significance ($P > .05$). These data suggest that severe nonatopic asthmatics, despite guideline-directed level 4 care, may stand to benefit from omalizumab. Further research is required.

S. K. Willsie, DO, MA

References

1. Humbert M, Beasley R, Ayres J, et al. Benefits of omalizumab as add-on therapy in patients with severe persistent asthma who are inadequately controlled despite best available therapy (GINA 2002 step 4 treatment): INNOVATE. *Allergy.* 2005;60: 309-316.
2. Hanania NA, Alpan O, Hamilos DL, et al. Omalizumab in severe allergic asthma inadequately controlled with standard therapy: a randomized trial. *Ann Intern Med.* 2011;154:573-582.

Metabolic syndrome and incidence of asthma in adults: the HUNT study
Brumpton BM, Camargo CA Jr, Romundstad PR, et al (Norwegian Univ of Science and Technology, Trondheim, Norway; Massachusetts General Hosp, Boston)
Eur Respir J 42:1495-1502, 2013

Obesity is a risk factor for incident asthma in adults, and obesity is a major component of metabolic syndrome. This study aimed to explore the associations of metabolic syndrome and its components with the cumulative incidence of asthma in adults.

We conducted a prospective cohort study of participants who were asthma-free at baseline (n = 23 191) in the Nord-Trøndelag Health Study from 1995 to 2008. Baseline metabolic syndrome was categorised using the definition of the Joint Interim Statement from several international organisations. Incident asthma was self-reported at follow-up, which averaged 11 years.

Metabolic syndrome was a risk factor for incident asthma (adjusted OR 1.57, 95% CI 1.31−1.87). This association was consistent in sensitivity analyses using a stricter asthma definition (adjusted OR 1.42, 95% CI 1.13−1.79). Among the components of metabolic syndrome, two remained associated with incident asthma after mutual adjustment for the other metabolic components: high waist circumference (adjusted OR 1.62, 95% CI 1.36−1.94) and elevated glucose or diabetes (adjusted OR 1.43, 95% CI 1.01−2.04).

Metabolic syndrome and two of its components (high waist circumference and elevated glucose or diabetes) were associated with an increased risk of incident asthma in adults (Tables 1 and 3).

▶ Over the last decade, several studies have evaluated a link between obesity and asthma.[1-3] This prospective study evaluated more than 23 000 individuals participating in the Nord-Trondelag Health Study; individuals were excluded from the study if they had asthma or a history of asthma. Individuals were followed up at 11 years, at which time they self-reported asthma (have or ever had

TABLE 1.—Characteristics of the Analysis Cohort Participants, Nord-Trøndelag Health Study, Norway

Baseline Characteristics	With Metabolic Syndrome[#]	Without Metabolic Syndrome[#]
Subjects	2971	20 220
Age years		
19–29	280 (9.4)	3374 (16.7)
30–39	715 (24.1)	6227 (30.8)
40–49	1328 (44.7)	7849 (38.8)
50–55	648 (21.8)	2770 (13.7)
Sex		
Female	1434 (48.3)	11 326 (56.0)
Male	1537 (51.7)	8894 (44.0)
Family history of asthma	446 (16.4)	2931 (15.6)
Smoking	931 (33.0)	5752 (30.0)
Physical activity[¶] h per week		
<1	857 (31.6)	4395 (24.3)
1–2	1124 (41.4)	7235 (40.0)
≥3	735 (27.0)	6459 (35.7)
Education years		
≤10	856 (29.2)	3803 (19.0)
11–12	1537 (52.4)	10 750 (53.6)
≥13	542 (18.4)	5505 (27.5)
Social benefit recipient	626 (26.3)	3337 (20.4)
Economic difficulties	909 (36.4)	5465 (31.6)
Allergic rhinitis	572 (24.1)	3795 (23.9)
Gastro-oesophageal reflux disease	1206 (52.6)	6324 (40.5)
Waist circumference ≥88 cm in females, ≥102 cm in males	1779 (59.9)	1384 (6.8)
Triglycerides ≥1.7 mmol·L^{-1}	324 (91.9)	4843 (24.0)
HDL cholesterol <1.3 mmol·L^{-1} in females, <1.0 mmol·L^{-1} in males	2213 (74.5)	2715 (13.4)
Elevated blood pressure[+] or use of anti-hypertensive medication	2644 (89.0)	8765 (43.3)
Elevated glucose[§] or diabetes	271 (9.1)	328 (1.6)

Total n=23 191. Data are presented as n or n (%). HDL: high-density lipoprotein.
[#]Metabolic syndrome was defined according to the Joint Interim Statement clinical criteria including alternate indicators anti-hypertensive medication and diabetes; glucose was nonfasting and ≥4 h since last meal.
[¶]Number of observations does not include total cohort due to missing data.
[+]Systolic blood pressure ≥130 mm Hg or diastolic blood pressure ≥ 85 mm Hg.
[§]≥5.6 mmol·L^{-1} and ≥ 4 h since last meal.

asthma). Table 1 depicts baseline characteristics of metabolic syndrome (MS) subjects and the non-MS subjects: age, education, gender, family history of asthma, comorbidities, and defining characteristics of MS. The odds ratio (OR) for the development of asthma in subjects with increased weight circumference consistent with MS was 1.55 (confidence interval [CI], 1.23–1.95) and the OR for diabetes or elevated glucose was 1.64 (CI, 1.07–2.52). Even after the investigators performed mutual adjustment for other metabolic components of MS (Table 3), the associations between MS, high waist circumference, elevated glucose or diabetes, and incident asthma remained. The results of this study show that MS and 2 of its diagnostic criteria are risk factors for incident asthma in adults, confirming results of a previous study,[4] which found a moderate association between MS and asthma. The reasons for these associations remain to be fully elucidated.

S. K. Willsie, DO, MA

TABLE 3.—Sensitivity Analysis: Association (Odds Ratios) of Metabolic Syndrome and its Components with Incident Asthma on Medication

Metabolic Components	Total n	Incident Asthma on Medication[#]	Model 1[¶] OR (95% CI)	Model 2[+] OR (95% CI)	Model 3[§] OR (95% CI)
Waist circumference ≥88 cm in females, ≥102 cm in males	2 563	119	1.80 (1.46–2.23)	1.66 (1.34–2.06)	1.55 (1.23–1.95)
Triglycerides ≥1.7 mmol·L⁻¹	6401	195	1.30 (1.08–1.57)	1.21 (1.01–1.46)	1.05 (0.86–1.29)
HDL cholesterol <1.3 mmol·L⁻¹ in females, <1.0 mmol·L⁻¹ in males	4106	150	1.39 (1.15–1.69)	1.30 (1.07–1.58)	1.18 (0.96–1.46)
Elevated blood pressure[f] or use of anti-hypertensive medication	9859	269	1.10 (0.92–1.31)	1.07 (0.89–1.28)	0.99 (0.82–1.19)
Elevated glucose[##] or diabetes	501	24	1.87 (1.23–2.85)	1.76 (1.15–2.68)	1.64 (1.07–2.52)
Metabolic syndrome[¶¶] ≥3 components	2413	95	1.55 (1.23–1.94)	1.42 (1.13–1.79)	NA

Total n = 20 155. HDL: high-density lipoprotein; NA: not applicable.
[#]Incident asthma definition requires use of an asthma medication at follow-up and excludes those with wheezing from at-risk group at baseline and follow-up.
[¶]Adjusted for age, sex and family history of asthma.
[+]Adjusted for age, sex, family history of asthma, smoking, physical activity, education, social benefit and economic difficulties at baseline.
[§]Adjusted for all covariates and other metabolic risk factors.
[f]Systolic blood pressure ≥130 mm Hg or diastolic blood pressure ≥85 mm Hg.
[##]Elevated glucose was ≥5.6 mmol·L⁻¹ and ≥4 h since last meal.
[¶¶]Metabolic syndrome was defined according to the Joint Interim Statement clinical criteria including alternate indicators anti-hypertensive medication and diabetes; glucose was nonfasting and ≥4 h since last meal.

References

1. Ford ES. The epidemiology of obesity and asthma. *J Allergy Clin Immunol.* 2005; 115:897-909.
2. Lessard A, Turcotte H, Cormier Y, Boulet LP. Obesity and asthma: a specific phenotype? *Chest.* 2008;134:317-323.
3. Lugogo NL, Kraft M, Dixon AE. Does obesity produce a distinct asthma phenotype? *J Appl Physiol.* 2010;108:729-734.
4. Lee EJ, In KH, Ha ES, et al. Asthma-like symptoms are increased in the metabolic syndrome. *J Asthma.* 2009;46:339-342.

Remission and Persistence of Asthma Followed From 7 to 19 Years of Age

Andersson M, Hedman L, Bjerg A, et al (The OLIN Studies, Luleå, Sweden; et al)
Pediatrics 132:e435-e442, 2013

Background and Objective.—To date, a limited number of population-based studies have prospectively evaluated the remission of childhood asthma. This work was intended to study the remission and persistence of childhood asthma and related factors.

Methods.—In 1996, a questionnaire was distributed to the parents of all children aged 7 to 8 years in 3 municipalities in northern Sweden, and 3430 (97%) participated. After a validation study, 248 children were identified as having asthma; these children were reassessed annually until age 19 years when 205 (83%) remained. During the follow-up period lung function, bronchial challenge testing, and skin prick tests were performed. Remission was defined as no use of asthma medication and no wheeze during the past 12 months as reported at endpoint and in the 2 annual surveys preceding endpoint (ie, for ≥3 years).

Results.—At age 19 years, 21% were in remission, 38% had periodic asthma, and 41% persistent asthma. Remission was more common among boys. Sensitization to furred animals and a more severe asthma (asthma score ≥2) at age 7 to 8 years were both inversely associated with remission, odds ratio 0.14 (95% confidence interval 0.04—0.55) and 0.19 (0.07—0.54), respectively. Among children with these 2 characteristics, 82% had persistent asthma during adolescence. Asthma heredity, damp housing, rural living, and smoking were not associated with remission.

Conclusions.—The probability of remission of childhood asthma from age 7- to 8-years to age 19 years was largely determined by sensitization status, particularly sensitization to animals, asthma severity, and female gender, factors all inversely related to remission (Table 4).

▶ You'll outgrow your asthma! This is a common quote in the lay press, which is much less commonly espoused by health care providers. This questionnaire-based study of Swedish children had a 97% participation rate with nearly 3500 children, ages 7 to 8 years initially participating. All children underwent skin prick testing for common allergens. A total of 248 children were identified as having asthma; these children were evaluated annually with questionnaire testing until the age of 19 with 83% participating until the end of the monitoring period. Between the ages of 16 and 17 years, all subjects underwent pulmonary function testing (including bronchial hyperreactivity), serum immunoglobulin

TABLE 4.—Factors Related to Remission and Periodic Asthma, Respectively, Analyzed by Multinomial Logistic Regression With Persistent Asthma as Reference

Independent Baseline Variables	Remission OR (95%CI)	Remission OR (95%CI)[a]	Periodic Asthma OR (95%CI)	Periodic Asthma OR (95%CI)[a]
Male gender	2.66 (1.00-7.03)	2.53 (1.04—6.15)	1.01 (0.46—2.25)	
Positive SPT to any animal	0.14 (0.04—0.55)	0.17 (0.06—0.48)	0.21 (0.07—0.66)	0.22 (0.09—0.58)
Positive SPT to any pollen	1.84 (0.41—8.37)		1.29 (0.35—4.80)	
Positive SPT to any mold	1.44 (0.16—12.9)		0.64 (0.06—7.40)	
Physician-diagnosed rhinitis	0.41 (0.14—1.20)		0.71 (0.29—1.72)	
Physician-diagnosed eczema	0.51 (0.19—1.42)		0.30 (0.12—0.73)	0.28 (0.12—0.64)
Asthma score ≥2/5	0.19 (0.07—0.54)	0.22 (0.08—0.57)	0.24 (0.10—0.57)	0.23 (0.10—0.52)
Living in an apartment	1.05 (0.32—3.50)		3.12 (1.15—8.44)	3.86 (1.51—9.86)
Mother smokes	0.75 (0.22—2.54)		1.84 (0.68—4.97)	
Mother smoked during pregnancy	1.87 (0.52—6.80)		1.08 (0.36—3.26)	

[a]Results from the stepwise backward multinomial regression model.

E, levels and clinical examinations. Persistent asthmatics were differentiated from asthmatics who underwent remission or had periodic asthma. Table 4 delineates odds ratios (OR) for asthmatics undergoing remission. Remission occurred in 43 subjects. The following were associated with an increased likelihood of remission: male gender, lower asthma severity, pollen hypersensitivity, and lack of sensitization to furred animals. Female children with sensitization to furred animals and more severe asthma should receive greater attention and closer follow-up, as they are at the greatest risk of development of persistent asthma.

S. K. Willsie, DO, MA

Sex differences in asthma symptom profiles and control in the American Lung Association Asthma Clinical Research Centers

McCallister JW, for the American Lung Association Asthma Clinical Research Centers (Wexner Med Ctr at The Ohio State Univ, Columbus; et al)
Respir Med 107:1491-1500, 2013

Objective.—Important differences between men and women with asthma have been demonstrated, with women describing more symptoms and worse asthma-related quality of life (QOL) despite having similar or better pulmonary function. While current guidelines focus heavily on assessing asthma control, they lack information about whether sex-specific approaches to asthma assessment should be considered. We sought to determine if sex differences in asthma control or symptom profiles exist in the well-characterized population of participants in the American Lung Association Asthma Clinical Research Centers (ALA-ACRC) trials.

TABLE 2.—Juniper Asthma Control Questionnaire (ACQ) Responses for Poorly-Controlled Subjects. Individual Item Responses were Analyzed by Sex of Respondent, and Describe the Preceding Seven Days. ACQ7 = Seven-Question Asthma Control Questionnaire; SD = Standard Deviation; CI = 95% Confidence Interval; FEV_1 = Forced Expiratory Volume in One Second; p = p-Value Adjusted for Trial, Age, Race and Body Mass Index; p* = p-Value Adjusted for Trial, Age, Race, Body Mass Index, Gastroesophageal Reflux Disease, Eczema, Sinusitis, and Rhinitis

	Women N = 952 (72%)			Men N = 372 (28%)				
	Mean	SD	95% CI	Mean	SD	95% CI	p	p*
ACQ7	1.9	0.8	1.9, 2.0	1.8	0.8	1.8, 1.9	0.54	0.36
Woken by asthma past week?	1.5	1.3	1.4, 1.6	1.3	1.2	1.1, 1.4	<0.01	0.02
How bad were symptoms?	1.9	1.1	1.9, 2.0	1.8	1.1	1.7, 1.9	0.08	0.11
How limited in activities?	1.8	1.2	1.7, 1.9	1.5	1.2	1.4, 1.6	0.001	0.02
How much shortness of breath did you experience?	2.5	1.1	2.4, 2.5	2.3	1.1	2.1, 2.4	0.03	0.07
How much time did you wheeze?	2.0	1.3	1.9, 2.1	1.9	1.2	1.8, 2.0	0.89	0.68
How many puffs of short-acting bronchodilator each day?	1.5	1.0	1.5, 1.6	1.5	1.1	1.4, 1.6	0.91	0.75

Methods.—We reviewed baseline data from four trials published by the ALA-ACRC to evaluate individual item responses to three standardized asthma questionnaires: the Juniper Asthma Control Questionnaire (ACQ), the multi-attribute Asthma Symptom Utility Index (ASUI), and Juniper Mini Asthma Quality of Life Questionnaire (mini-AQLQ). *Results.*—In the poorly-controlled population, women reported similar overall asthma control (mean ACQ 1.9 vs. 1.8; $p = 0.54$), but were more likely to report specific symptoms such as nocturnal awakenings, activity limitations, and shortness of breath on individual item responses. Women reported worse asthma-related QOL on the mini-AQLQ (mean 4.5 vs. 4.9;

TABLE 3.—Mini Asthma Quality of Life Questionnaire (AQLQ) in Poorly-Controlled Subjects. Individual Item Responses were Analyzed by Sex of Respondent, and Describe the Preceding Two Weeks. $p = p$-Value Adjusted for Age, Race, and Body Mass Index; $p^* = p$-Value Adjusted for Trial, Age, Race, Body Mass Index, Gastroesophageal Reflux Disease, Eczema, Sinusitis, and Rhinitis; SD = Standard Deviation

AQLQ Score		Women Mean (SD) 4.5 (1.2) Women	Median 4.5 %	Men Mean (SD) 4.9 (1.1) Men	Median 5.0 %	p <0.0001	p^* 0.001
Feel short of breath as a	No time	148	16	76	20	0.08	0.20
result of your asthma?	Any time	804	84	296	80		
Feel bothered by or have to	No time	139	15	100	27	<0.0001	<0.0001
avoid dust in the environment?	Any time	813	85	272	73		
Feel frustrated as a result of	No time	340	36	147	40	0.44	0.94
your asthma?	Any time	612	64	225	60		
Feel bothered by coughing?	No time	264	28	149	40	<0.001	0.01
	Any time	688	72	223	60		
Feel afraid of not having	No time	431	45	151	41	0.09	0.04
your asthma medication?	Any time	521	55	221	59		
Experience a feeling of	No time	245	26	113	30	0.11	0.86
chest tightness or chest heaviness?	Any time	707	74	259	70		
Feel bothered by or have to	No time	180	19	118	32	<0.0001	<0.001
avoid cigarette smoke in the environment?	Any time	772	81	254	68		
Have difficulty getting a	No time	406	43	193	52	0.01	0.10
good night's sleep as a result of your asthma?	Any time	546	57	179	48		
Feel concerned about	No time	343	36	140	38	0.98	0.58
having asthma?	Any time	609	64	232	62		
Experience a wheeze in	No time	276	29	119	32	0.62	0.68
your chest?	Any time	676	71	253	68		
Feel bothered by or have to	No time	327	34	198	53	<0.0001	<0.001
avoid going outside because of weather or air pollution?	Any time	625	66	174	47		
Limitations with strenuous	No time	235	25	139	37	<0.001	<0.01
activities?	Any time	717	75	233	63		
Limitations with moderate	No time	400	42	228	61	<0.0001	<0.001
activities?	Any time	552	58	144	39		
Limitations with social	No time	644	68	282	76	0.04	0.06
activities?	Any time	308	32	90	24		
Limitations with work-related activities?	No time	631	66	270	73	0.17	0.46
	Any time	321	34	102	27		

$p < 0.001$) and more asthma-related symptoms with a lower mean score on the ASUI (0.73 vs. 0.77; $p \leq 0.0001$) and were more likely to report feeling bothered by particular symptoms such as coughing, or environmental triggers.

Conclusions.—In participants with poorly-controlled asthma, women had outwardly similar asthma control, but had unique symptom profiles on detailed item analyses which were evident on evaluation of three standardized asthma questionnaires (Tables 2 and 3).

▶ Several studies have documented that women asthmatics require greater health care utilization and more frequent use of short-acting β agonists.[1-3] In addition, gender-related treatment approaches to asthma have been developed, and some evidence exists to suggest improved control of asthma in women using specific treatment plans.[4,5] The American Lung Association's Asthma Clinical Research Centers' data from 4 previous studies (one of well-controlled asthmatics, 3 of poorly controlled asthmatics) were reviewed with regard to response differences between genders. Clinically significant differences between men and women were shown in the incidence of chronic sinusitis, which is more common in women ($P = .001$), and the use of combination therapy with long-acting β agonists and inhaled corticosteroids: more common in women vs men ($P = .05$). Women additionally had more exacerbations during the previous year ($P < .0001$) and listed allergies as a trigger for their asthma ($P = 0.01$), were more likely to be heavier ($P < .0001$), and were more likely to have gastroesophageal reflux disease ($P = .03$) or eczema ($P = .03$). Table 2 lists the results of the Asthma Control Questionnaire, which showed similar overall scores between men and women; however, women were more likely to have been awakened by asthma the last week ($P < .01$) and to report limited activity ($P = .001$). Results of the Mini Asthma Quality of Life Questionnaire provided in Table 3, showed again, similar overall numerical scores and key differences between the genders. These data, in total, support data of previous reports of gender-related differences in asthma and support the need for health care providers to design evaluation and treatment plans to address these gender-related differences. Doing so may limit undertreatment of female asthmatics who have uncontrolled disease.

S. K. Willsie, DO, MA

References

1. Akinbami LJ, Moorman JE, Liu X. Asthma prevalence, health care use, and mortality: United States, 2005–2009. *Natl Health Stat Report.* 2011;32:1-14.
2. Lee JH, Haselkorn T, Chipps BE, Miller DP, Wenzel SE. Gender differences in IgE-mediated allergic asthma in the epidemiology and natural history of asthma: outcomes and Treatment Regimens (TENOR) study. *J Asthma.* 2006;43:179-184.
3. Osborne ML, Vollmer WM, Linton KL, Buist AS. Characteristics of patients with asthma within a large HMO: a comparison by age and gender. *Am J Respir Crit Care Med.* 1998;157:123-128.
4. Clark NM, Gong ZM, Wang SJ, Lin X, Bria WF, Johnson TR. A randomized trial of a self-regulation intervention for women with asthma. *Chest.* 2007;132:88-97.
5. Clark NM, Gong ZM, Wang SJ, Valerio MA, Bria WF, Johnson TR. From the female perspective: long-term effects on quality of life of a program for women with asthma. *Gend Med.* 2010;7:125-136.

Prescription fill patterns in underserved children with asthma receiving subspecialty care

Bollinger ME, Mudd KE, Boldt A, et al (Univ of Maryland, Baltimore)

Ann Allergy Asthma Immunol 111:185-189, 2013

Background.—Children with asthma receiving specialty care have been found to have improved asthma outcomes. However, these outcomes can be adversely affected by poor adherence with controller medications.

Objective.—To analyze pharmacy fill patterns as a measure of primary adherence in a group of underserved minority children receiving allergy subspecialty care.

Methods.—As part of a larger 18-month nebulizer use study in underserved children (ages 2-8 years) with persistent asthma, 53 children were recruited from an urban allergy practice. Pharmacy records were compared with prescribing records for all asthma medications.

Results.—Allergist controller prescriptions were written in 30-day quantities with refills and short-acting β-agonists (SABAs) with no refills. Only 49.1% of inhaled corticosteroid (ICS), 49.5% of combination ICS and long-acting β-agonist, and 64.5% of leukotriene modifier (LTM) initial and refill prescriptions were ever filled during the 18-month period. A mean of 5.1 refills (range, 0-14) for SABAs were obtained during 18 months, although only 1.28 SABA prescriptions were prescribed by the allergist. Mean times between first asthma prescription and actual filling were 30 days (range, 0-177 days) for ICSs, 26.6 days (range, 0-156 days) for LTMs, and 16.8 days (range, 0-139 days) for SABAs.

Conclusion.—Underserved children with asthma receiving allergy subspecialty care suboptimally filled controller prescriptions, yet filled abundant rescue medications from other prescribers. Limiting albuterol prescriptions to one canister without additional refills may provide an opportunity to monitor fill rates of both rescue and controller medications and provide education to patients about appropriate use of medications to improve adherence (Fig 1).

▶ We prescribe guideline-directed care for our asthmatics and wonder why our patients' asthma is not improving! Underserved pediatric asthmatics receiving allergist subspecialty care were monitored over 18 months for prescription filling practices. Initial allergist-prescribed medications included a 30-day supply of controller medication (with refills) and 1 canister of short-acting β agonist (SABA) (no refill). Over the 18-month period of monitoring, patients refilled primarily the SABAs (mean 5.1 refills over 18 months, while allergists prescribed a mean of only 1.28 SABA refills). These data (Fig 1) indicate that the asthmatics are filling and refilling additional SABA prescriptions from nonsubspecialists. The increased filling/refilling of SABAs occurred in the face of less than 50% of controller prescriptions ever being filled or refilled and approximately 65% of leukotriene modifier prescriptions being filled or refilled. This clearly represents a need for better education of the parties caring for the asthmatics in the home as well as the referring providers

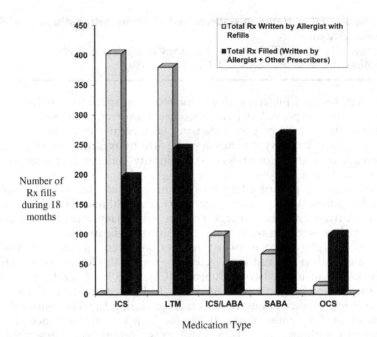

FIGURE 1.—Number of prescriptions written by an allergist (initial and refills) vs prescriptions filled in underserved children with asthma. (Reprinted from Annals of Allergy, Asthma and Immunology. Bollinger ME, Mudd KE, Boldt A, et al. Prescription fill patterns in underserved children with asthma receiving subspecialty care. *Ann Allergy Asthma Immunol*. 2013;111:185-189, Copyright 2014, with permission from American College of Allergy, Asthma & Immunology.)

(should coordinate care with specialists). Successful education and changed prescription-filling practices have great potential to improve control of asthma in children.

S. K. Willsie, DO, MA

Cystic Fibrosis

Phase II studies of nebulised Arikace in CF patients with *Pseudomonas aeruginosa* infection

Clancy JP, for the Arikace Study Group (Cincinnati Children's Hosp Med Ctr, OH)

Thorax 68:818-825, 2013

Rationale.—Arikace is a liposomal amikacin preparation for aerosol delivery with potent *Pseudomonas aeruginosa* killing and prolonged lung deposition.

Objectives.—To examine the safety and efficacy of 28 days of once-daily Arikace in cystic fibrosis (CF) patients chronically infected with *P aeruginosa*.

Methods.—105 subjects were evaluated in double-blind, placebo-controlled studies. Subjects were randomised to once-daily Arikace (70, 140, 280 and 560 mg; n=7, 5, 21 and 36 subjects) or placebo (n=36) for 28 days. Primary outcomes included safety and tolerability. Secondary outcomes included lung function (forced expiratory volume at one second (FEV_1)), *P aeruginosa* density in sputum, and the Cystic Fibrosis Quality of Life Questionnaire-Revised (CFQ-R).

Results.—The adverse event profile was similar among Arikace and placebo subjects. The relative change in FEV_1 was higher in the 560 mg dose group at day 28 ($p = 0.033$) and at day 56 (28 days post-treatment, $0.093L \pm 0.203$ vs $-0.032L \pm 0.119$; $p = 0.003$) versus placebo. Sputum *P aeruginosa* density decreased >1 log in the 560 mg group versus placebo (days 14, 28 and 35; $p = 0.021$). The Respiratory Domain of the CFQ-R increased by the Minimal Clinically Important Difference (MCID) in 67% of Arikace subjects (560 mg) versus 36% of placebo ($p = 0.006$), and correlated with FEV_1 improvements at days 14, 28 and 42 ($p < 0.05$). An open-label extension (560 mg Arikace) for 28 days followed

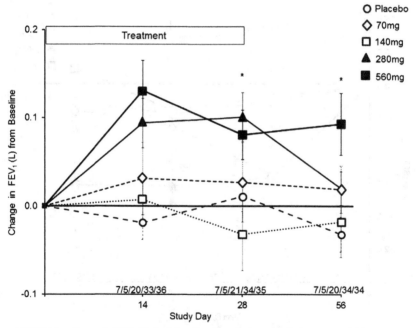

FIGURE 2.—Change in FEV_1 (L) from baseline through day 56. Filled squares, solid line=Arikace 560 mg, *$p = 0.033$ at day 28, *$p = 0.003$ at day 56 (compared with placebo). Filled triangles, solid line=Arikace 280 mg, *$p = 0.009$ at day 28 (compared with placebo). Open squares, dashed line=Arikace 140 mg. Open diamonds, dashed line=Arikace 70 mg. Open circles, dashed line=placebo. The values above the abscissa are the number of subjects in each dose cohort providing data at each time point (70 mg/140 mg/280 mg/560 mg/ placebo). (Reprinted from Clancy JP, for the Arikace Study Group. Phase II studies of nebulised Arikace in CF patients with Pseudomonas aeruginosa infection. *Thorax.* 2013;68:818-825, with permission from the BMJ Publishing Group Ltd.)

by 56 days off over six cycles confirmed durable improvements in lung function and sputum *P aeruginosa* density (n=49).

Conclusions.—Once-daily Arikace demonstrated acute tolerability, safety, biologic activity and efficacy in patients with CF with *P aeruginosa* infection (Figs 2-4).

▶ This is a phase II, randomized, double-blind, multicenter, placebo-controlled trial of once-daily Arikace, a liposome-encapsulated form of Amikacin, showing safety and tolerability. Fig 2 depicts the change in forced expiratory volume at one second (FEV_1) from baseline; the 280- and 560-mg dose showed statistically significant change with maintained effect across treatment periods. Fig 3 evaluated sputum density showing reduction with the 280- and 560-mg dose. Fig 4 shows continuous statistically significant % FEV_1 improvement after 6 treatments, administered every 28 days with a 56-day washout period between treatments (open-label extension phase of study). Phase III studies are planned to evaluate the 560-mg dose delivered via rapid-delivery nebulizer, but not the 70-, 140-, or 280-mg dose of Arikace. This new compound, with demonstrated

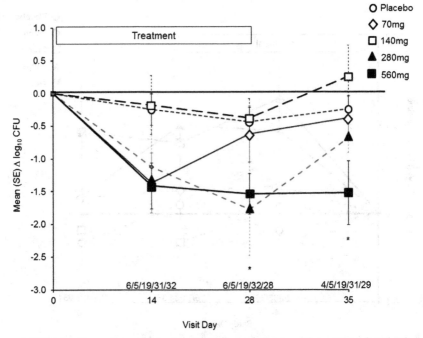

FIGURE 3.—Change in sputum density of *Pseudomonas aeruginosa* ($\log_{10}$ CFU/g) from baseline through day 35. Filled squares, solid line=Arikace 560 mg, *$p = 0.007$ at day 28, *$p = 0.021$ at day 35. Filled triangles, solid line=Arikace 280 mg. Open squares, dashed line=Arikace 140 mg. Open diamonds, dashed line=Arikace 70 mg. Open circles, dashed line=placebo. The values above the abscissa are the number of subjects in each dose cohort providing data at each time point (70 mg/140 mg/280 mg/560 mg/placebo). (Reprinted from Clancy JP, for the Arikace Study Group. Phase II studies of nebulised Arikace in CF patients with Pseudomonas aeruginosa infection. *Thorax*. 2013;68:818-825, with permission from the BMJ Publishing Group Ltd.)

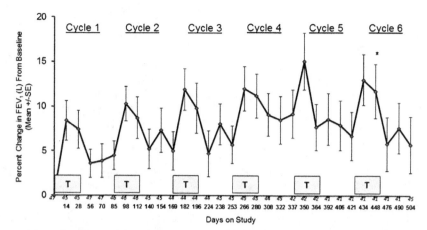

FIGURE 4.—Change in FEV_1 (% predicted) from baseline through cycle 6 of Arikace. Each cycle consisted of 28 days of once daily Arikace (560 mg) followed by 56 days off study drug. Each shaded box is a treatment cycle. Study days (every 2 weeks) are as shown on the abscissa, with the number of subjects at each time point as noted immediately above the study days. $*p < 0.0001$ for FEV_1 at end of treatment following six cycles compared with baseline; $**p = 0.0001$ for FEV_1 at 56 days post-treatment following six cycles compared with baseline. (Reprinted from Clancy JP, for the Arikace Study Group. Phase II studies of nebulised Arikace in CF patients with Pseudomonas aeruginosa infection. *Thorax.* 2013;68:818-825, with permission from the BMJ Publishing Group Ltd.)

high sputum and low systemic concentration, shows promise for cystic fibrosis patients and others who have persistent infection with *Pseudomonas aeruginosa* or other Amikacin-sensitive organisms. Stay tuned!

S. K. Willsie, DO, MA

2 Chronic Obstructive Pulmonary Disease

Introduction

Data concerning the comorbidities in many patients with COPD and the impact of comorbidities on morbidity and mortality are increasingly appreciated. In 2013, a number of studies addressing COPD and cardiac disease were published. These studies include assessment of various management strategies and risks associated with COPD and coronary artery or generalized vascular disease and heart failure. The study included in this section by Patel et al is an attempt to better quantify cardiac events that occur in the setting of COPD exacerbations, an often underdiagnosed and underappreciated relationship. Another comorbidity receiving increased attention are mental changes related to COPD, both during exacerbations and hospitalizations and during periods of stable disease. The study by Dodd et al addresses cognitive declines identified in up to 50 percent of patients discharged after a COPD exacerbation and the persistence of those declines over an extended period. Atlantis et al present a systematic review and meta-analysis of anxiety and depression in COPD. The review emphasizes the prevalence and bidirectional impact of these mood disorders on management, complications, and personal impact of COPD. A corollary to anxiety and depression and yet rarely noted or appreciated in patients with chronic respiratory disease is chronic pain. Roberts et al reported chronic pain as well as narcotic medication in the COPD population at a significantly higher rate than in the general population, thereby identifying a concern that should be assessed in all COPD patients.

In 2013, the Centers for Disease Control and Prevention updated its original 2002 surveillance report on COPD in the United States with data from 2000 through 2011. This report authored by Ford et al documented a slight decrease in the death rate for men and a decrease in hospitalizations for both men and women.

A wide-ranging group of studies about the role of various medications in obstructive were reported. A meta-analysis of the currently available studies of use of macrolide antibiotics to prevent COPD exacerbations by Donath et al again confirmed a reduction in exacerbations, but at the expense of some significant and sometimes intolerable side effects. Tse et al reported a randomized, placebo-controlled trial using n-acetyl cysteine in a relatively high dose. The trial did not demonstrate a difference in hospitalizations or functional parameters. Statins have for the last decade been suggested and studied as potential drugs to decrease exacerbation rates purportedly through their immunomodulatory mechanism. Most studies are small and not methodologically robust. Wang et al abstracted an insurance database of 14,000 COPD patients and found an impact on exacerbation rate as well. The last mediation article is about the concerns of cardiac events and potential mortality with tiotropium products. Wise et al assess Respimat, the soft mist inhaler formulation of tiotropium, with respect to cardiac events and found similar event rates and death rates compared with the Handihaler formulation.

In the 2011 update of the Global Obstructive Lung Disease guidelines, the authors made fundamental changes in the classification of disease in response to concerns that the guidelines needed to more accurately reflect the functional status of the patient—symptoms and exacerbations—rather than pulmonary function numbers. This revision has resulted in a flurry of studies such as that by Agusti et al to evaluate the usefulness of the new classification system. Other authors addressing slightly different questions with respect to COPD, eg, the severity and indicators of progression, have also started to move away from just using pulmonary function or existing indexes to using multicomponent parameters that reflect patient function and risk (Mannino et al). Generally, clinicians are recognizing the need to have and use better prediction models for various clinical COPD scenarios. For example, multiple outcome prediction models exist for patients presenting with community-acquired pneumonia; however, until recently no such models exist for COPD patients presenting with acute exacerbations. Singanayagam et al have initiated this process by doing a meta-analysis of known risk factors in the COPD patient in exacerbation.

Part of the improved classification of COPD patients is to better characterize phenotypes that may be better served by tailored management approaches. The recent recognition of an acquired defect in the cystic fibrosis transmembrane receptor (CFTR) function in chronic bronchitic patients with bronchiectasis (Dransfield et al) might respond to a CFTR function-directed therapy. Similarly, COPD patients with allergic symptoms may represent a phenotype that responds primarily to management of the allergic symptoms (Jamieson et al). Another very different phenotype, but one that may also require very individualized management strategies is the COPD patient with significant pulmonary hypertension. Clinically, these patients resemble primary pulmonary hypertension patients, are functionally very disabled (Hurdman et al), and may be functionally limited mostly by the pulmonary hypertension, which requires a different management strategy from COPD.

The final article in this section is a systematic review of supervised exercise programs after rehabilitation for COPD. Patients tend to improve functionally significantly while doing rehabilitation programs; however, as with anyone doing training programs, if the level of activity is not maintained, the gains are soon lost. Beauchamp et al found that even when supervised exercise programs are prescribed following a formal rehabilitation program, the initial gains wane over a year-long period.

Janet R. Mauer, MD, MBA

Cardiovascular Risk, Myocardial Injury, and Exacerbations of Chronic Obstructive Pulmonary Disease
Patel ARC, Kowlessar BS, Donaldson GC, et al (Univ College London, UK)
Am J Respir Crit Care Med 188:1091-1099, 2013

Rationale.—Patients with chronic obstructive pulmonary disease (COPD) have elevated cardiovascular risk, and myocardial injury is common during severe exacerbations. Little is known about the prevalence, magnitude, and underlying mechanisms of cardiovascular risk in community-treated exacerbations.

Objectives.—To investigate how COPD exacerbations and exacerbation frequency impact cardiovascular risk and myocardial injury, and whether this is related to airway infection and inflammation.

Methods.—We prospectively measured arterial stiffness (aortic pulse wave velocity [aPWV]) and cardiac biomarkers in 98 patients with stable COPD. Fifty-five patients had paired stable and exacerbation assessments, repeated at Days 3, 7, 14, and 35 during recovery. Airway infection was identified using polymerase chain reaction.

Measurements and Main Results.—COPD exacerbation frequency was related to stable-state arterial stiffness (rho = 0.209; $P = 0.040$). Frequent exacerbators had greater aPWV than infrequent exacerbators (mean ± SD aPWV, 11.4 ± 2.1 vs. 10.3 ± 2.0 ms^{-1}; $P = 0.025$). Arterial stiffness rose by an average of 1.2 ms^{-1} (11.1%) from stable state to exacerbation (n = 55) and fell slowly during recovery. In those with airway infection at exacerbation (n = 24) this rise was greater (1.4 ± 1.6 vs. 0.7 ± 1.3 ms^{-1}; $P = 0.048$); prolonged; and related to sputum IL-6 (rho = 0.753; $P < 0.001$). Increases in cardiac biomarkers at exacerbation were higher in those with ischemic heart disease (n = 12) than those without (n = 43) (mean ± SD increase in troponin T, 0.011 ± 0.009 vs. 0.003 ± 0.006 μg/L, $P = 0.003$; N-terminal pro-brain natriuretic peptide, 38.1 ± 37.7 vs. 5.9 ± 12.3 pg/ml, $P < 0.001$).

Conclusions.—Frequent COPD exacerbators have greater arterial stiffness than infrequent exacerbators. Arterial stiffness rises acutely during COPD exacerbations, particularly with airway infection. Increases in arterial stiffness are related to inflammation, and are slow to recover. Myocardial injury is common and clinically significant during COPD exacerbations, particularly in those with underlying ischemic heart disease.

▶ Chronic obstructive pulmonary disease (COPD) is now well recognized as a systemic inflammatory process that is often accompanied by other medical conditions. It remains the third leading cause of death worldwide, ranking behind ischemic cardiovascular and cerebrovascular disease. Smoking is frequently a common risk factor in all these processes; therefore, vasculopathy and other cardiac disease and obstructive lung disease often go hand in hand. In addition, several studies have documented that patients with COPD are at increased risk for cardiac events or increased mortality in various medical situations, particularly in the setting of COPD exacerbations. This study attempts to better quantify the risk of myocardial events in the peri-exacerbation period and begins to study the mechanisms that lie behind this risk, a first step to designing prevention measures. Several other studies were published in 2013 that further defined cardiac risks associated with comorbid COPD. Almassi et al[1] reported a large, randomized trial in which cardiac bypass graft surgery was performed either on-pump or off-pump in patients with comorbid COPD. The reason for the study was the known high risk of cardiac events in COPD patients undergoing cardiac surgery. In this study, patients who had surgery off pump had more complications at the time of surgery; however, long-term outcomes were not different between the 2 approaches. Gunter et al[2] reported a study of aortic valve replacement with or without bypass grafting in COPD patients. Of the 2379 patients reported, more than one-fifth had varying severities of COPD. COPD did not seem to impact the early perioperative mortality, but long-term survival (> 3 years) was worse across all levels of COPD, with severe disease carrying the worst odds ratio of 2.28. Stone et al[3] addressed the outcomes of patients undergoing abdominal aortic aneurysm (AAA) repair, both endovascular and open, who also had COPD. Smoking is a well-described risk factor for AAA, so it is not surprising that more than a third of patients coming for repair have a COPD diagnosis. Both types of repair were associated with higher in-hospital morbidity and mortality in oxygen-requiring COPD patients. Five-year survival was diminished in all levels of COPD; however, oxygen-dependency was an independent predictor of death.

Brenner et al[4] tried to assess the impact of COPD on survival in patients with systolic heart failure. They found, however, that it was very difficult to tell which patients had COPD because obstruction was variable in this population except when serial pulmonary functions were done in stable patients. Congestion was hard to separate from fixed obstruction except in patients shown to have hyperinflation. Only proven COPD was associated with increased mortality. Finally, Jensen et al[5] used the Copenhagen City Heart Study, a population-based study covering more than 35 years of follow-up, to define a relationship between resting heart rate and mortality in COPD patients. Higher resting heart rate was associated with reduced survival across all levels of COPD. The authors found that when resting heart rate was added to the Global Obstructive Lung Disease Guidelines, risk prediction was significantly enhanced. Resting heart rate levels can, in some cases, change survival predictions by years according to this study. Each of these studies provides some additional information about the impact of COPD as a comorbidity on management or survival. The better we understand these interactions, the easier it will be to treat our COPD patients.

J. R. Maurer, MD

References

1. Almassi GH, Shroyer AL, Collins JF, et al. Chronic obstructive pulmonary disease impact upon outcomes: the veterans affairs randomized on/off bypass trial. *Ann Thorac Surg.* 2013;96:1302-1309.
2. Gunter RL, Kilgo P, Guyton RA, et al. Impact of preoperative chronic lung disease on survival after surgical aortic valve replacement. *Ann Thorac Surg.* 2013;96: 1322-1328.
3. Stone DH, Goodney PP, Kalish J, et al; Vascular Study Group of New England. Severity of chronic obstructive pulmonary disease is associated with adverse outcomes in patients undergoing elective abdominal aortic aneurysm repair. *J Vasc Surg.* 2013;57:1531-1536.
4. Brenner S, Guder G, Berliner D, et al. Airway obstruction in systolic heart failure—COPD or congestion? *Int J Cardiol.* 2013;168:1910-1916.
5. Jensen MT, Marott JL, Lange P, et al. Resting heart rate is a predictor of mortality in COPD. *Eur Respir J.* 2013;42:341-349.

Cognitive Dysfunction in Patients Hospitalized With Acute Exacerbation of COPD

Dodd JW, Charlton RA, van den Broek MD, et al (St. George's Univ of London, England, UK; Univ of Illinois, Chicago)
Chest 144:119-127, 2013

Background.—Cognitive impairment is one of the least well-studied COPD comorbidities. It is known to occur in hypoxemic patients, but its presence during acute exacerbation is not established.

Objectives.—The purpose of this study was to assess neuropsychological performance in patients with COPD who were awaiting discharge from hospital following acute exacerbation and recovery and to compare them with stable outpatients with COPD and with healthy control subjects.

Methods.—We recruited 110 participants to the study: 30 inpatients with COPD who were awaiting discharge following an exacerbation, 50 outpatients with stable COPD, and 30 control subjects. Neuropsychological tests measured episodic memory, executive function, visuospatial function, working memory, processing speed, and an estimate of premorbid abilities. Follow-up cognitive assessments for patients who were stable and those with COPD exacerbation were completed at 3 months.

Results.—Patients with COPD exacerbation were significantly worse ($P < .05$) than stable patients over a range of measures of cognitive function, independent of hypoxemia, disease severity, cerebrovascular risk, or pack-years smoked. Of the patients with COPD exacerbation, up to 57% were in the impaired range and 20% were considered to have suffered a pathologic loss in processing speed. Impaired cognition was associated with worse St. George's Respiratory Questionnaire score ($r = -0.40$-0.62, $P \leq .02$) and longer length of stay ($r = 0.42$, $P = .02$). There was no improvement in any aspect of cognition at recovery 3 months later.

Conclusions.—In patients hospitalized with an acute COPD exacerbation, impaired cognitive function is associated with worse health status and longer hospital length of stay. A significant proportion of patients are discharged home with unrecognized mild to severe cognitive impairment, which may not improve with recovery.

▶ To achieve the better value (outcomes) in patient care mandated by the Patient Protection and Affordable Care Act, 2010, it is necessary to take a more holistic approach to the management plan of patients with chronic illness. A patient with a chronic obstructive pulmonary disease (COPD) exacerbation, for example, needs an evaluation and management of all his or her other comorbidities as well as his or her psychosocial situation to determine necessary interventions are in place that will result in a good outcome after an acute exacerbation or other acute event. One of the comorbidities that has received little attention but is possibly one of the highest contributors to treatment failure across chronic illness is the presence of cognitive impairment. It is and will continue to be an increasingly common issue as the population ages. The problem has been little studied in COPD patients, and the results of this study suggest a need for considerable attention to this issue. Although this is a relatively small study, fairly sophisticated neuropsychological testing was performed. The results are sobering. At least half of the patients discharged home had at least significant cognitive deficits, and many had considerably more severe deficits. Furthermore, these did not resolve after 3 months. Early studies have suggested an increase in white matter in the brains of COPD patients, a marker of small vessel disease.[1] Lahousse et al[2] reported a sobering study in which they assessed the role of cerebral microbleeding as a cause of cognitive decline in older COPD patients. In 165 patients with COPD, this group found an increase in microbleeds (45%) compared with normal controls (31%), and these bleeds tended to be in deep or infratentorial regions suggesting arteriolosclerotic or hypertensive pathology. Smoking is a known risk factor for this process. Cerebral small vessel disease is probably only one of several causes. One of the first steps in addressing this issue will be to try to determine if there are causes of the cognitive deficits that are remediable, for example, overuse of corticosteroids, and address them. It may be much harder to address issues such as microbleeding.

J. R. Maurer, MD

References

1. Dodd JW, Chung AW, van den Broek MD, Barrick TR, Charlton RA, Jones PW. Brain structure and function in chronic obstructive pulmonary disease: a multimodal cranial magnetic resonance imaging study. *Am J Respir Crit Care Med.* 2012; 186:240-245.
2. Lahousse L, Vernooij MW, Darweesh SKL, et al. Chronic obstructive pulmonary disease and cerebral microbleeds: the Rotterdam study. *Am J Respir Crit Care Med.* 2013;188:783-788.

Bidirectional Associations Between Clinically Relevant Depression or Anxiety and COPD: A Systematic Review and Meta-analysis
Atlantis E, Fahey P, Cochrane B, et al (Univ of Western Sydney, Penrith, New South Wales, Australia)
Chest 144:766-777, 2013

Background.—The longitudinal associations between depression or anxiety and COPD, and their comorbid effect on prognosis, have not been adequately addressed by previous reviews. We aimed to systematically assess these associations to inform guidelines and practice.

Methods.—We searched electronic databases for articles published before May 2012. Longitudinal studies in adult populations that reported an association between clinically relevant depression or anxiety and COPD, or that reported their comorbid effect on exacerbation and/or mortality, were eligible. Risk ratios (RRs) were pooled across studies using random-effects models and were verified using fixed-effects models. Heterogeneity was explored with subgroup and metaregression analyses.

Results.—Twenty-two citations yielded 16 studies on depression or anxiety as predictors of COPD outcomes (incident COPD/chronic lung disease or exacerbation) and/or mortality, in 28,759 participants followed for 1 to 8 years, and six studies on COPD as a predictor of depression in 7,439,159 participants followed for 1 to 35 years. Depression or anxiety consistently increased the risk of COPD outcomes (RR, 1.43; 95% CI, 1.22-1.68), particularly in higher-quality studies and in people aged ≤66 years. Comorbid depression increased the risk of mortality (RR, 1.83; 95% CI, 1.00-3.36), particularly in men. Anxiety (or psychologic distress) increased the risk of COPD outcomes/mortality in most studies (RR, 1.27; 95% CI, 1.02-1.58). Finally, COPD consistently increased the risk of depression (RR, 1.69; 95% CI, 1.45-1.96).

Conclusions.—Depression and anxiety adversely affect prognosis in COPD, conferring an increased risk of exacerbation and possibly death. Conversely, COPD increases the risk of developing depression. These bidirectional associations suggest potential usefulness of screening for these disease combinations to direct timely therapeutic intervention.

▶ Just a few years ago, there was almost no literature on anxiety and depression and their impact on patients with chronic obstructive pulmonary disease (COPD).[1] So it is great to see that enough research now exists to do a systematic review! The estimated prevalence of clinically relevant mood disorder in the COPD population is estimated to be around 40% (compared with around 10% in the normal population). In various chronic illnesses, the presence of significant anxiety or depression impairs adherence with medication regimens and perceived quality of life. In COPD patients, reports also have identified lost productivity, increased use of health care resources, increased risk of exacerbation, and pneumonia.[2-4] This study confirms many of these findings across studies and also emphasizes that mood disorders exacerbate the personal impact of the disease; however, COPD limitations and symptoms also precipitate the development of anxiety and depression. One of the difficulties in studying anxiety, in particular, in COPD has been the lack of an appropriate tool to screen for and measure anxiety. The reason for this is that actual COPD symptoms, such as shortness of breath, can overlap with anxiety symptoms or medication side effects, such as overmedication with β2 agonists. Thus, a very welcome addition to the pulmonary literature in 2013 was the publication of an Anxiety Inventory for Respiratory Disease.[5] This tool now needs to be validated by other centers and in other geographic locations to ensure it is useful across COPD and other pulmonary disease populations. Such a tool is necessary to have a consistent measure for use in clinical trials of assessment and intervention. For example, another 2013 observational study about anxiety in COPD concluded that patients with higher activity levels have higher levels of anxiety.[6] This needs to be further studied prospectively (using a tool such as that described above) because the current literature suggests that significant anxiety increases morbidity, whereas higher levels of physical activity are associated with improved outcomes.[7]

J. R. Maurer, MD

References

1. Maurer J, Rebbpragada V, Borson S, et al; ACCP Workshop Panel on Anxiety and Depression in COPD. Anxiety and depression in COPD: current understanding, unanswered questions, and research needs. *Chest.* 2008;134:43S-56S.
2. Dalal AA, Shah M, Lunacsek O, Hanania NA. Clinical and economic burden of depression/anxiety in chronic obstructive pulmonary disease patients within a managed care population. *COPD.* 2011;8:293-299.
3. Fan VS, Ramsey SD, Giardino ND, et al; National Emphysema Treatment Trial (NETT) Research Group. Sex, depression, and risk of hospitalization and mortality in chronic obstructive pulmonary disease. *Arch Intern Med.* 2007;167: 2345-2353.
4. Laurin C, Moullec G, Bacon SL, Lavoie KL. Impact of anxiety and depression on chronic obstructive pulmonary disease exacerbation risk. *Am J Respir Crit Care Med.* 2012;185:918-923.
5. Willgoss TG, Goldbart J, Fatoye F, Yohannes AM. The development and validation of the anxiety inventory for respiratory disease. *Chest.* 2013;144:1587-1596.
6. Nguyen HQ, Fan VS, Herting J, et al. Patients with COPD with higher levels of anxiety are more physically active. *Chest.* 2013;144:145-151.
7. Waschki B, Kirsten A, Holz O, et al. Physical activity is the strongest predictor of all-cause mortality in patients with COPD: a prospective cohort study. *Chest.* 2011;140:331-342.

Chronic Pain and Pain Medication Use in Chronic Obstructive Pulmonary Disease: A Cross-Sectional Study

Roberts MH, Mapel DW, Hartry A, et al (Health Services Res Division, Albuquerque, NM; Health Economics & Outcomes Res, Malvern, PA)
Ann Am Thorac Soc 10:290-298, 2013

Rationale.—Pain is a common problem for patients with chronic obstructive pulmonary disease (COPD). However, pain is minimally discussed in COPD management guidelines.

Objectives.—The objective of this study was to describe chronic pain prevalence among patients with COPD compared with similar patients with other chronic diseases in a managed care population in the southwestern United States (age ≥ 40 yr).

Methods.—Using data for the period January 1, 2006 through December 31, 2010, patients with COPD were matched to two control subjects without COPD but with another chronic illness based on age, sex, insurance, and healthcare encounter type. Odds ratios (OR) for evidence of chronic pain were estimated using conditional logistic regression. Pulmonary function data for 200 randomly selected patients with COPD were abstracted.

Measurements and Main Results.—Retrospectively analyzed recurrent pain-related utilization (diagnoses and treatment) was considered evidence of chronic pain. The study sample comprised 7,952 patients with COPD (mean age, 69 yr; 42% male) and 15,904 patients with other chronic diseases (non-COPD). Patients with COPD compared with non-COPD patients had a higher percentage of chronic pain (59.8 vs. 51.7%; $P < 0.001$), chronic use of pain-related medications (41.2 vs. 31.5%; $P < 0.001$), and chronic use of short-acting (24.2 vs. 15.1%; $P < 0.001$) and long-acting opioids (4.4 vs. 1.9%; $P < 0.001$) compared with non-COPD patients. In conditional logistic regression models, adjusting for age, sex, Hispanic ethnicity, and comorbidities, patients with COPD had higher odds of chronic pain (OR, 1.56; 95% confidence interval [CI], 1.43−1.71), chronic use of pain-related medications (OR, 1.60; 95% CI, 1.46−1.74), and chronic use of short-acting or long-acting opioids (OR, 1.74; 95% CI, 1.57−1.92).

Conclusions.—Chronic pain and opioid use are prevalent among adults with COPD. This finding was not explained by the burden of comorbidity.

▶ Anxiety and depression have been shown to be prevalent in nearly half of all patients with chronic obstructive pulmonary disease (COPD) and significantly impact quality of life in that population. The increasing attention to these mood disorders has prompted numerous studies in the last few years so that patients are now routinely screened, and many get appropriate interventions. Pain, especially chronic pain, is much less often associated with COPD; most patients are not systematically assessed for pain. However, a few studies suggest that pain may be quite common in these patients and that, on average, they are more apt to be using more narcotics than age-matched controls.[1] Interestingly, there is virtually no discussion of pain assessment or approaches to treatment in COPD guidelines.[2] Pain can be a major factor in the development of anxiety and depression and in impaired quality of life. The risk for pain in these patients may be more related to the multiple comorbidities that are related to smoking, for example, cardiac disease and osteoporosis. The current cross-sectional study sought to better define the prevalence of pain, risk factors for pain, and the use of pain medications. In almost 8000 COPD patients, this study confirmed the high rates of pain when compared with almost 16 000 people with other chronic illnesses (Fig 1 in the original article). More COPD patients complained of pain and had higher use of narcotic pain medications as had been noted previously; the COPD patients range across the spectrum of airflow obstruction. The types of pain were primarily inflammatory and mechanical/compressive back pain. Adding pain into the mix with mood disorders undoubtedly reduces further the quality of life for COPD patients and may even impact survival. Very little is known about the best approaches to management of pain in this population, the risk factors, or preventive strategies.

This poorly studied and rarely discussed area deserves attention in clinical trials aimed at an overall better understanding and improved outcomes.

J. R. Maurer, MD

References

1. Blinderman CD, Homel P, Billings JA, Tennstedt S, Portenoy RK. Symptom distress and quality of life in patients with advanced chronic obstructive pulmonary disease. *J Pain Symptom Manage.* 2009;38:115-123.
2. Gold. Global strategy for the diagnosis, management, and prevention of copd, global initiative for chronic obstructive lung disease (GOLD). www.goldcopd.org. Accessed January 8, 2014.

COPD Surveillance—United States, 1999-2011
Ford ES, Croft JB, Mannino DM, et al (Ctrs for Disease Control and Prevention, Atlanta, GA; Univ of Kentucky College of Public Health, Lexington)
Chest 144:284-305, 2013

This report updates surveillance results for COPD in the United States. For 1999 to 2011, data from national data systems for adults aged ≥25 years were analyzed. In 2011, 6.5% of adults (approximately 13.7 million) reported having been diagnosed with COPD. From 1999 to 2011, the overall age-adjusted prevalence of having been diagnosed with COPD declined ($P = .019$). In 2010, there were 10.3 million (494.8 per 10,000) physician office visits, 1.5 million (72.0 per 10,000) ED visits, and 699,000 (32.2 per 10,000) hospital discharges for COPD. From 1999 to 2010, no significant overall trends were noted for physician office visits and ED visits; however, the age-adjusted hospital discharge rate for COPD declined significantly ($P = .001$). In 2010 there were 312,654 (11.2 per 1,000) Medicare hospital discharge claims submitted for COPD. Medicare claims (1999-2010) declined overall ($P = .045$), among men ($P = .022$) and among enrollees aged 65 to 74 years ($P = .033$). There were 133,575 deaths (63.1 per 100,000) from COPD in 2010. The overall age-adjusted death rate for COPD did not change during 1999 to 2010 ($P = .163$). Death rates (1999-2010) increased among adults aged 45 to 54 years ($P < .001$) and among American Indian/Alaska Natives ($P = .008$) but declined among those aged 55 to 64 years ($P = .002$) and 65 to 74 years ($P < .001$), Hispanics ($P = .038$), Asian/Pacific Islanders ($P < .001$), and men ($P = .001$). Geographic clustering of prevalence, Medicare hospitalizations, and deaths were observed. Declines in the age-adjusted prevalence, death rate in men, and hospitalizations for COPD since 1999 suggest progress in the prevention of COPD in the United States.

▶ In 2002 the Centers for Disease Control released its first chronic obstructive pulmonary disease (COPD) surveillance report. It was recognition of the increasing burden of this disease in the United States population and the cost of managing the disease. That report included disease prevalence, data about hospitalizations, outpatient visits, emergency room visits, and mortality. By 2008, chronic lower respiratory diseases, of which the principal component is COPD, became the third most common cause of death in the United States. This happened primarily because deaths from cerebrovascular disease, previously number 3, have continued a steady decline over a number of years.[1] In 2008, it was estimated that the direct economic cost of COPD and asthma was almost $54 billion per year including prescription medications (largest component at $20.4 billion); outpatient, emergency, and hospital stays; and home health care. The information presented in this report is expanded considerably. For the report, a large group of data sources were accessed. These included Behavioral Risk Factor Surveillance System (BRFSS), National Health Interview Survey, National Ambulatory Medical Care Survey, National Hospital Ambulatory Medical Care Survey, National Hospital Discharge Survey, death certificates from the National Vital Statistics System, and Medicare Part A hospital claims administrative data. The primary message of the report is a slight decrease in death rate for men and a decrease in hospitalization rates in both men and women since 1999. Another 2013 study using Medicare data reported a decrease in respiratory hospitalizations from 58 to 44 per 100 person-years, while the prevalence of COPD in Medicare patients did not change; in addition, the rate of hospitalization for multiple COPD exacerbations also decreased.[2] These changes may be related to the ongoing decline in smoking in this country. Between 1965 and 2010, in both men and women, the number of smokers decreased by half—to 21.5% in men and 17.3% in women. Or it may be a combination of the decline in smoking, increased awareness of COPD, and better management. No matter what the cause, this is a glimmer of hope in the war against COPD.

J. R. Maurer, MD

References

1. Minino AM, Xu J, Kochanek KD. Division of Vital Statistics. Deaths: preliminary data for 2008. *Natl Vital Stat Rep*. 2010;59:1-52.
2. Baillargeon J, Wang Y, Kuo YF, Holmes HM, Sharma G. Temporal trends in hospitalization rates for older adults with chronic obstructive pulmonary disease. *Am J Med*. 2013;126:607-613.

A meta-analysis on the prophylactic use of macrolide antibiotics for the prevention of disease exacerbations in patients with Chronic Obstructive Pulmonary Disease

Donath E, Chaudhry A, Hernandez-Aya LF, et al (Univ of Miami Miller School of Medicine — Regional Campus, Atlantis, FL; Univ of Michigan School of Medicine, Ann Arbor; et al)
Respir Med 107:1385-1392, 2013

Introduction.—Macrolides are of unique interest in preventing COPD exacerbations because they possess a variety of antibacterial, antiviral and anti-inflammatory properties. Recent research has generated renewed interest in prophylactic macrolides to reduce the risk of COPD exacerbations. Little is known about how well these recent findings fit within the context of previous research on this subject. The purpose of this article is to evaluate, via exploratory meta-analysis, whether the overall consensus favors prophylactic macrolides for prevention of COPD exacerbations.

Methods.—EMBASE, Cochrane and Medline databases were searched for all relevant randomized controlled trials (RCTs). Six RCTs were identified. The primary endpoint was incidence of COPD exacerbations. Secondary endpoints including mortality, hospitalization rates, adverse events and likelihood of having at least one COPD exacerbation were also examined.

Results.—There was a 37% relative risk reduction (RR = 0.63, 95% CI: 0.45–0.87, p value = 0.005) in COPD exacerbations among patients taking macrolides compared to placebo. Furthermore, there was a 21% reduced risk of hospitalization (RR = 0.79, 95% CI: 0.69–0.90, p-value = 0.01) and 68% reduced risk of having at least one COPD exacerbation (RR = 0.34, 95% CI 0.21–0.54, p-value = 0.001) among patients taking macrolides versus placebo. There was also a trend toward decreased mortality and increased adverse events among patients taking macrolides but these were not statistically significant.

Conclusions.—Prophylactic macrolides are an effective approach for reducing incident COPD exacerbations. There were several limitations to this study including a lack of consistent adverse event reporting and some degree of clinical and statistical heterogeneity between studies.

▶ Macrolide antibiotics are unique among antibiotics because of their multiple types of activity. They are also antiviral and, particularly, immunomodulatory. These multiple actions have resulted in their use in a wide variety of circumstances, including the successful treatment of panbronchiolitis and prevention of cystic fibrosis exacerbations as well as reduction in development of bronchiolitis obliterans syndrome in lung transplant patients. It has also been used to prevent chronic obstructive pulmonary disease (COPD) exacerbations. Clinical trials have been conducted in each of these diseases, usually with success in reducing symptoms, preventing acute events, or generally improving patient quality of life. Probably the most cited trial in COPD was a multicenter study published in 2011. Albert et al[1] reported in a placebo-controlled trial that patients taking daily azithromycin had a longer period to first exacerbation; however, some hearing loss side effects were reported in this study. What remained unclear was the impact of potential development of microbial resistance patterns using a continuous prophylaxis regimen such as this. The meta-analysis presented here reviews the Albert et al[1] trial, but also 6 other randomized, controlled trials to assess consistency in findings. The authors found that all but one of the studies reported a reduction in COPD exacerbations when using prophylactic macrolides. However, this benefit is offset by adverse events. The one measure of adverse events that was relatively constant—and relatively common—across trials was discontinuation of the trial because of the adverse event. The authors found it difficult to capture the emergence of antibiotic resistance, although they note this is a worldwide concern. The evidence for reduction of acute exacerbations is compelling; however, the literal cost and the cost in adverse events and resistance are considerable. This argues for studies to assess different approaches in a robust, controlled way, such as intermittent administration or administration of lower doses of drug.

J. R. Maurer, MD

Reference

1) *ɒʄʃ/i mu las t*
2) *MC*   3) *N p C*

1. Albert R, Connett J, Bailey W, et al. Azithromycin for prevention of exacerbations of COPD. N Engl J Med. 2011;365:689-698.

High-Dose N-Acetylcysteine in Stable COPD: The 1-Year, Double-Blind, Randomized, Placebo-Controlled HIACE Study

Tse HN, Raiteri L, Wong KY, et al (Kwong Wah Hosp, Hong Kong, China; Wong Tai Sin Hosp, Hong Kong, China; Zambon Company SpA, Bresso, Italy)

Chest 144:106-118, 2013

Background.—The mucolytic and antioxidant effects of N-acetylcysteine (NAC) may have great value in COPD treatment. However, beneficial effects have not been confirmed in clinical studies, possibly due to insufficient NAC doses and/or inadequate outcome parameters used. The objective of this study was to investigate high-dose NAC plus usual therapy in Chinese patients with stable COPD.

Methods.—The 1-year HIACE (The Effect of High Dose N-acetylcysteine on Air Trapping and Airway Resistance of Chronic Obstructive Pulmonary Disease—a Double-blinded, Randomized, Placebo-controlled Trial) double-blind trial conducted in Kwong Wah Hospital, Hong Kong, randomized eligible patients aged 50 to 80 years with stable COPD to NAC 600 mg bid or placebo after 4-week run-in. Lung function parameters, symptoms, modified Medical Research Council (mMRC) dyspnea and St. George's Respiratory Questionnaire (SGRQ) scores, 6-min walking distance (6MWD), and exacerbation and admission rates were measured at baseline and every 16 weeks for 1 year.

Results.—Of 133 patients screened, 120 were eligible (93.2% men; mean age, 70.8 ± 0.74 years; %FEV$_1$ 53.9 ± 2.0%). Baseline characteristics were similar in the two groups. At 1 year, there was a significant improvement in forced expiratory flow 25% to 75% ($P =.037$) and forced oscillation technique, a significant reduction in exacerbation frequency (0.96 times/y vs 1.71 times/y, $P =.019$), and a tendency toward reduction in admission rate (0.5 times/y vs 0.8 times/y, $P =.196$) with NAC vs placebo. There were no significant between-group differences in mMRC dypsnea score, SGRQ score, and 6MWD. No major adverse effects were reported.

Conclusion.—In this study, 1-year treatment with high-dose NAC resulted in significantly improved small airways function and decreased exacerbation frequency in patients with stable COPD.

Trial Registry.—ClinicalTrials.gov; No.: NCT01136239; URL: www.clinicaltrials.gov.

▶ N-acetyl cysteine (NAC) has for decades been considered a potential treatment in obstructive lung disease and other lung diseases. Not only is it a mucolytic, it also has antioxidant and anti-inflammatory properties. It scavenges reactive oxygen species and is a precursor of reduced glutathione. However, previous clinical trials assessing NAC treatment of chronic obstructive pulmonary disease (COPD) has been inconsistent. A Cochrane systematic review of 30 studies and a meta-analysis suggested a small, but inconsistent, benefit of NAC in reducing exacerbations[1,2]; however, the 3-year Bronchitis Randomized On NAC Cost-Utility Study (BRONCUS), which was a double-blinded randomized, controlled study, did not show either a reduction of exacerbations or an improvement in flow rates.[3] The Chinese investigators conducting the current study reasoned that the BRONCUS study may have been negative because (1) the dose of NAC used was too small or (2) no tool was used to measure small airway function and, therefore, measurements were not sensitive enough to actually detect the impact of the treatment. So they used more than twice the dose of NAC than BRONCUS investigators did, and they implemented 2 small airway measurements: forced expiratory flow 25 to 75 and forced external oscillation, which can detect airflow in the small airways. This was a relatively small study with a total of 120 patients and 58 in the NAC arm. Although the authors were able to show a significant difference in the rate of exacerbations and small airway function (barely), they were unable to show a difference in hospitalizations or other functional parameters. This leaves in question the clinical significance of the findings. Although intriguing, the use of NAC at this high dosage requires a larger, longer study to justify its place in COPD management.

J. R. Maurer, MD

References

1. Poole P, Black PN. Mucolytic agents for chronic bronchitis or chronic obstructive pulmonary disease. *Cochrane Database syst Rev.* 2010;(2):CD001287.
2. Grandjean EM, Berthet P, Ruffmann R, Leuenberger P. Efficacy of oral long-term N-acetylcysteine in chronic bronchopulmonary disease: a meta-analysis of published double-blind, placebo-controlled clinical trials. *Clin Ther.* 2000;22:209-221.
3. Decramer M, Rutten-van Molken M, Dekhuijzen PN, et al. Effects of N-acetylcysteine on outcomes in chronic obstructive pulmonary disease (Bronchitis Randomized on NAC Cost-Utility Study, BRONCUS): a randomised placebo-controlled trial. *Lancet.* 2005;365:1552-1560.

Statin Use and Risk of COPD Exacerbation Requiring Hospitalization

Wang M-T, Lo Y-W, Tsai C-L, et al (School of Pharmacy, Taipei, Taiwan, Republic of China; Natl Defense Med Ctr, Taipei, Taiwan, Republic of China; et al)

Am J Med 126:598-606.e2, 2013

Background.—Despite recent studies that suggested statins' beneficial effects on chronic obstructive pulmonary disease (COPD) outcomes, the impact, if any, of statins on COPD exacerbations remains unclear. This study aimed to examine the association between statin use and risk of hospitalized COPD exacerbation, and to assess whether the association varied by statin initiation, dose, or duration of use.

Methods.—A retrospective nested case-control study among patients with COPD was conducted analyzing a nationwide health insurance claims database in Taiwan. Cases were subjects hospitalized for COPD exacerbations; each case was matched to 4 randomly selected controls on age, sex, cohort entry, and number of COPD-related outpatient visits by an incident-density sampling approach. Conditional logistic regressions were employed to quantify the COPD exacerbation risk associated with statin use.

Results.—The study cohort comprised 14,316 COPD patients, from which 1584 cases with COPD exacerbations and 5950 matched controls were identified. Any use of statins was associated with a 30% decreased risk of COPD exacerbation (95% confidence interval [CI], 0.56-0.88), and current use of statins was related to a greater reduced risk (adjusted odds ratio [OR] 0.60; 95% CI, 0.44-0.81). A dose-dependent reduced risk of COPD exacerbation by statins was observed (medium average daily dose: adjusted OR 0.60; 95% CI, 0.41-0.89; high daily dose: adjusted OR 0.33; 95% CI, 0.14-0.73). The reduced risk remained significant for either short or long duration of statin use.

Conclusions.—Statin use was associated with a reduced risk of COPD exacerbation, with a further risk reduction for statins prescribed more recently or at high doses.

▶ Several publications in the last 10 years purportedly showed a significant benefit of statins in reducing the rates of chronic obstructive pulmonary disease (COPD) exacerbations by as much as 40% and even have shown a substantial decreased mortality risk.[1,2] The proposed reasons for this impact are anti-inflammatory and immunomodulary effects, which have been identified both in human and in animal models.[3,4] In some cases, this seems to be a greater benefit than the commonly used inhaled medications that are recommended in major COPD management guidelines.[5] In the 2013 edition of the Global Initiative for Chronic Obstructive Lung Disease guidelines, one paragraph is devoted to immunomodulary drugs (not statins) and does not make any recommendations for their use.[5] Certainly, the lack of attention to statins cannot be because of adverse side effects or cost: Statins are one of the most widely used drugs for control of cholesterol in the world, and generic versions are much lower in cost than many of the pulmonary inhaled medications. The reasons that statins have not been incorporated into the armamentarium of COPD management are probably best stated by 1 of 2 systematic reviews that both came to the same general conclusion: "...the majority of published studies have inherent methodological limitations of retrospective studies and population-based analyses. There is a need for prospective interventional trials designed specifically to assess the impact of statins on clinically relevant outcomes in COPD."[6,7] The study abstracted here is not that definitive prospective study; it is a study based on information from a nationwide health insurance database of pharmacy and medical encounters. The authors were able to study more than 14 000 COPD patients during the period from January 2000 through December 2008. Again, there was a strong association between statin use and reduced exacerbations. But is this relationship causal? We continue to await that definitive prospective trial.

J. R. Maurer, MD

References

1. Blamoun AI, Batty GN, DeBari VA, Rashid AO, Sheikh M, Khan MA. Statins may reduce episodes of exacerbation and the requirement for intubation in patients with COPD: evidence from a retrospective cohort study. *Int J Clin Pract.* 2008; 62:1373-1378.
2. Mancini GB, Etminan M, Zhang B, Levesque LE, FitzGerald JM, Brophy JM. Reduction of morbidity and mortality by statins, angiotensin-converting enzyme inhibitors, and angiotensin receptor blockers in patients with chronic obstructive pulmonary disease. *J Am Coll Cardiol.* 2006;47:2554-2560.
3. Takahashi S, Nakamura H, Seki M, et al. Reversal of elastase-induced pulmonary emphysema and promotion of alveolar epithelial cell proliferation by simvastatin in mice. *Am J Physiol Lung Cell Mol Physiol.* 2008;294:L882-L890.
4. Arnaud C, Veillard NR, Mach F. Cholesterol-independent effects of statins in inflammation, immunomodulation and atherosclerosis. *Curr Drug Targets Cardiovasc Haematol Disord.* 2005;5:127-134.
5. Gold. Global strategy for the diagnosis, management, and prevention of COPD, global initiative for chronic obstructive lung disease (GOLD). www.goldcopd. org. Accessed January 8, 2014.
6. Dobler CC, Wong KK, Marks GB. Associations between statins and COPD: a systematic review. *BMC Pulm Med.* 2009;9:32.
7. Janda S, Park K, FitzGerald JM, Etminan M, Swiston J. Statins in COPD: a systematic review. *Chest.* 2009;136:734-743.

Tiotropium Respimat Inhaler and the Risk of Death in COPD

Wise RA, for the TIOSPIR Investigators (Johns Hopkins Univ School of Medicine, Baltimore, MD; et al)

N Engl J Med 369:1491-1501, 2013

Background.—Tiotropium delivered at a dose of 5 µg with the Respimat inhaler showed efficacy similar to that of 18 µg of tiotropium delivered with the HandiHaler inhalation device in placebo-controlled trials involving patients with chronic obstructive pulmonary disease (COPD). Although tiotropium HandiHaler was associated with reduced mortality, as compared with placebo, more deaths were reported with tiotropium Respimat than with placebo.

Methods.—In this randomized, double-blind, parallel-group trial involving 17,135 patients with COPD, we evaluated the safety and efficacy of tiotropium Respimat at a once-daily dose of 2.5 μg or 5 μg, as compared with tiotropium HandiHaler at a once-daily dose of 18 μg. Primary end points were the risk of death (noninferiority study, Respimat at a dose of 5 μg or 2.5 μg vs. HandiHaler) and the risk of the first COPD exacerbation (superiority study, Respimat at a dose of 5 μg vs. HandiHaler). We also assessed cardiovascular safety, including safety in patients with stable cardiac disease.

Results.—During a mean follow-up of 2.3 years, Respimat was noninferior to HandiHaler with respect to the risk of death (Respimat at a dose of 5 μg vs. HandiHaler: hazard ratio, 0.96; 95% confidence interval [CI], 0.84 to 1.09; Respimat at a dose of 2.5 μg vs. HandiHaler: hazard ratio, 1.00; 95% CI, 0.87 to 1.14) and not superior to HandiHaler with respect to the risk of the first exacerbation (Respimat at a dose of 5 μg vs. Handi-Haler: hazard ratio, 0.98; 95% CI, 0.93 to 1.03). Causes of death and incidences of major cardiovascular adverse events were similar in the three groups.

Conclusions.—Tiotropium Respimat at a dose of 5 μg or 2.5 μg had a safety profile and exacerbation efficacy similar to those of tiotropium HandiHaler at a dose of 18 μg in patients with COPD.

▶ Numerous trials evaluating the long-acting anticholinergic drug tiotropium have consistently shown its benefit in patients with chronic obstructive pulmonary disease both in terms of pulmonary function and reduction in exacerbations using different formulations.[1-4] The drug is delivered by the HandiHaler, a single-dose dry powder inhaler, or by a novel delivery system, Respimat Soft Mist Inhaler, which delivers an aqueous dose without a propellant. In 2008, reports began to appear suggesting that tiotropium, delivered initially by HandiHaler and later by Respimat, appeared to increase the risk of cardiovascular and cerebrovascular events and even possibly death. These data were reported to the Federal Drug Administration by the drug manufacturer after review of adverse event information from a large pool of clinical trials of the drug, a meta-analysis, and a cohort study.[5] Of note, the trials from which these data were drawn tended to be of short duration, typically a year or less. These reports initiated a large and ongoing controversy about the safety of tiotropium (both formulations) and whether it should be used, especially in patients who had known vascular disease. Shortly after, the Understanding Potential Long-Term Impacts on Function with Tiotropium study was published, which was a 4-year study of the drug, which showed an actual decrease in death risk compared with placebo with the HandiHaler version of tiotropium.[6] Because there has been less reported trial experience with Respimat compared with HandiHaler, it has been more difficult to establish for certain if there is a difference in vascular event risk between these 2. This study, Tiotropium Safety and Performance in Respimat was designed to compare in a randomized, controlled prospective way the safety and efficacy of HandiHaler and Respimat at 2 different doses. Adverse vascular events were not different between groups. Death rates were similar in the 3 groups. And the respiratory impact in terms of exacerbations was similar. So why do studies show such a variable pattern, especially with respect to adverse vascular events? The authors say this may suggest a role for caution in interpretation of some trial results. In a number of the tiotropium trials, more patients dropped out of the placebo arms, potentially biasing the data. Meta-analysis reports and observational studies often were based on data that did not include the initial methodology assessment of vascular events as an end point so may have had multiple biases and confounders, for example, increased participants with some pre-existing cardiac disease, influencing the data. Also, the short timeframe of many studies could have captured impending vascular events that had no relationship to the respiratory drugs. So, in sum, the controversy about adverse vascular impacts of tiotropium seems to be winding down but is not quite yet settled.[7]

J. R. Maurer, MD

References

1. Vogelmeier C, Hederer B, Glaab T, et al. Tiotropium versus salmeterol for the prevention of exacerbations of COPD. *N Engl J Med.* 2011;364:1093-1103.
2. Bateman ED, Tashkin D, Siafakas N, et al. A one-year trial of tiotropium Respimat plus usual therapy in COPD patients. *Respir Med.* 2010;104:1460-1472.
3. Cooper CB, Celli BR, Jardim JR, et al. Treadmill endurance during 2-year treatment with tiotropium in patients with COPD: a randomized trial. *Chest.* 2013; 144:490-497.
4. Briggs DD Jr, Covelli H, Lapidus R, Bhattycharya S, Kesten S, Cassino C. Improved daytime spirometric efficacy of tiotropium compared with salmeterol in patients with COPD. *Pulm Pharmacol Ther.* 2005;18:397-404.
5. Michele TM, Pinheiro S, Iyasu S. The safety of tiotropium—the FDA's conclusions. *N Engl J Med.* 2010;363:1097-1099.
6. Tashkin DP, Celli B, Senn S, et al. A 4-year trial of tiotropium in chronic obstructive pulmonary disease. *N Engl J Med.* 2008;359:1543-1554.
7. Verhamme KMC, Afonso A, Romio S, Stricker BC, Brusselle GGO, Sturkenboom MCJM. Use of tiotropium Respimat Soft Mist Inhaler versus Handi-Haler and mortality in patients with COPD. *Eur Respir J.* 2013;42:606-615.

Characteristics, stability and outcomes of the 2011 GOLD COPD groups in the ECLIPSE cohort

Agusti A, on behalf of the ECLIPSE investigators (Universitat de Barcelona and CIBER Enfermedades Respiratorias, Mallorca, Spain; et al)
Eur Respir J 42:636-646, 2013

The 2011 Global Initiative for Chronic Obstructive Lung Disease (GOLD) classifies patients with chronic obstructive pulmonary disease (COPD) into four groups (A to D).

We explored the characteristics, stability and relationship to outcomes of these groups within the ECLIPSE study (Evaluation of COPD Longitudinally to Identify Predictive Surrogate End-points) (n = 2101).

Main results showed that: 1) these groups differed in several clinical, functional, imaging and biological characteristics in addition to those used for their own definition; 2) A and D groups were relatively stable over time, whereas groups B and C showed more temporal variability; 3) the risk of exacerbation over 3 years increased progressively from A to D, whereas that of hospitalisation and mortality were lowest in A, highest in D and intermediate and similar in B and C, despite the former having milder airflow limitation. The prevalence of comorbidities and persistent systemic inflammation were highest in group B.

The different longitudinal behaviour of group A *versus* B and C *versus* D (each pair with similar forced expiratory volume in1 s (FEV_1) values supports the 2011 GOLD proposal of assessing COPD patients by more than FEV_1 only. However the assumption that symptoms do not equate to risk appears to be naïve, as groups B and C carry equally poor clinical outcomes, though for different reasons.

▶ The Global Obstructive Lung Disease (GOLD) Guidelines of 2011 took a fundamentally different approach to the assessment of patients with chronic obstructive pulmonary disease (COPD).[1] Prior versions of the guideline generally assessed patients with obstructive disease primarily by forced expiratory volume in 1 second (FEV_1) values. In the 2011 document, the new COPD assessment system suggested segmenting COPD patients according to 2 areas: symptoms and risk within the already defined objective stages of airflow limitation (Fig 1 in the original article). For symptom assessment, they suggested using the patient perception of symptoms (recommending the modified Medical Research Council scale of breathlessness or the COPD Assessment Test). For risk assessment (meaning risk of future exacerbation), they suggested using previous history of exacerbations combined with severity of airflow obstruction. This method was an attempt to incorporate patient-level factors into the assessment of the impact of the disease on an individual to better tailor management to that person. This approach was similar to the intent of incorporation of risk and level of control in the 2007 asthma guidelines, EPR-3.[1] As was expected and encouraged (as this assessment system was based on the best guesses of its authors), many investigators quickly relooked at existing cohorts of patients from recent clinical trials to determine how applicable and accurate the classifications are. Whether they add to the management of COPD patients in terms of achieving better outcomes for the patients remains a question for future studies. The study abstracted here is one of the studies that quickly followed in the wake of the GOLD 2011 changes. A recent review of this and 3 other studies by the authors of the GOLD 2011 symptom/risk classification made the following observation: "The most salient findings [of the studies] were that: 1) the prevalence of these four [see Fig in the original article] groups depends on the specific population studied, C being least prevalent; 2) comorbidities are particularly prevalent in the two 'high symptom' groups (B and D); 3) patients classified as A or D tend to remain in the same group over time, whereas those classified as B or C change substantially during follow-up; 4) mortality at 3 years was lowest in A and worst in D but surprisingly similar (and intermediate) in B and C; and 5) the incidence of exacerbations during follow-up increases progressively from A to D but that of hospitalizations behave similarly to mortality."[2] This seems to me to be a great deal of new and helpful information gained from this classification system with some very important new insights into the disease. As the GOLD authors digest the information and revise the classification, potentially creating versions for specific populations, I believe it will become a very useful tool in management, improving outcomes, and determining prognosis.

J. R. Maurer, MD

References

1. Guidelines for the Diagnosis and Management of Asthma (EPR-). http://www. nhlbi.nih.gov/guidelines/asthma/. Accessed January 4, 2014.
2. Agusti A, Hurd S, Jones P, et al. FAQs about the GOLD 2011 assessment proposal of COPD: a comparative analysis of four different cohorts. *Eur Respir J*. 2013;42: 1391-1401.

A New Approach to Classification of Disease Severity and Progression of COPD
Mannino DM, Diaz-Guzman E, Pospisil J (College of Medicine, Univ of Kentucky, Lexington)
Chest 144:1179-1185, 2013

Background.—Most current classification schemes for COPD use lung function as the primary way of classifying disease severity and monitoring disease progression. This approach misses important components of the disease process.

Methods.—We evaluated existing data to develop a classification scheme for COPD using measures beyond lung function, including respiratory symptoms, exacerbation history, quality-of-life assessment, comorbidity, and BMI. We then applied this scheme to data from the Lung Health Study, calculating a score for study subjects in year 1 and year 5 of the study, along with the difference between year 1 and year 5.

Results.—We developed a four-point scale ranging from 1.00 (mild) to 4.00 (very severe). In year 1 of the study, the mean COPD score was 1.76; in year 5 it was 1.82. The mean difference from year 1 to year 5 was an increase (worsening) of 0.06 and a range from −1.0 to 1.6. The COPD score at year 1, year 5, and the difference between these scores were all predictive of mortality at follow-up. For example, the 14.0% of subjects whose score improved by at least 0.25 between year 1 and 5 had decreased mortality compared with those with stable scores (between −0.25 and 0.25; hazard ratio, 0.6; 95% CI, 0.4, 0.8).

Conclusions.—A COPD severity score that includes components in addition to lung function and allows for both improvement and worsening of disease may provide additional guidance to COPD classification, management, and prognosis.

▶ As far back as the 1960s, pulmonary physicians have tried to model the progression of chronic obstructive pulmonary disease (COPD) to understand the prognosis and to help patients in planning for the future.[1] In the 1980s, when lung transplant became an option for patients with advanced disease, the need for a clearer understanding of COPD progression became even more critical as a guideline for choosing candidates for transplantation at the appropriate time in the course of their disease. At that time, lung function and, to some extent, exercise capacity were the primary components used to assess disease severity and progression. But that approach was imprecise. In 2004, the BODE Index, based on body mass index, pulmonary function, dyspnea, and exercise capacity, was published and widely recognized as a major step forward in categorizing severity of disease and, in addition, was reasonably predictive of death in most cohorts.[2] However, since then, the BODE Index has been modified to apply to different populations, and somewhat simplified indexes have been created.[3] However, all these models depend on having measurements of lung function as a central component. Models for asthma severity, as contrasted to COPD, have recently moved toward a multicomponent approach incorporating symptoms, level of impairment, and exacerbation risk to determine severity. The authors endeavored to create a model that emulates that approach, including comorbidities, and to identify the worst component as the focus of determining therapy. In this model, worsening disease is not based solely on declining lung function but on a worsening score, which is a composite measure. Other authors have also sought to simplify the BODE index, as it is often hard to apply to population data where one or more of the critical measures are missing. Roberts et al[4] created a quasi-BODE Index that uses body mass index, shortness of breath/no shortness of breath, and simple questions about the ability to walk a block and lift 10 pounds in addition to a peak expiratory flow to assess severity. These elements are easier to obtain than BODE elements, especially in the elderly, and are used to create a score. The higher the score, the worse the prognosis. These ongoing refinements in prognostic models for COPD are a welcome refinement that reflects a greater understanding of the disease and its heterogeneity. In particular, incorporating symptomatology as the Mannino study should help to guide more appropriate individual therapy.

J. R. Maurer, MD

References

1. Burrows B, Strauss RH, Niden AH. Chronic obstructive lung disease. Interrelationships of pulmonary function data. *Am Rev Respir Dis.* 1965;91:861-868.
2. Celli BR, Cote CG, Marin JM, et al. The body-mass index, airflow obstruction, dyspnea, and exercise capacity index in chronic obstructive pulmonary disease. *N Engl J Med.* 2004;350:1005-1012.
3. Puhan MA, Hansel NN, Sobradillo P, et al. Large-scale international validation of the ADO index in subjects with COPD: an individual subject data analysis of 10 cohorts. *BMJ Open.* 2012;2. pii:e002152.

4. Roberts MH, Mapel DW, Bruse S, Petersen H, Nyunoya T. Development of a Modified BODE Index as a mortality risk measure among older adults with and without chronic obstructive pulmonary disease. *Am J Epidemiol.* 2013;178: 1150-1160.

Predictors of Mortality in Hospitalized Adults with Acute Exacerbation of Chronic Obstructive Pulmonary Disease: A Systematic Review and Meta-analysis

Singanayagam A, Schembri S, Chalmers JD (St. Mary's Hosp, London, UK; Ninewells Hosp, Dundee, Scotland, UK)
Ann Am Thorac Soc 10:81-89, 2013

Rationale.—There is a need to identify clinically meaningful predictors of mortality following hospitalized COPD exacerbation.

Objectives.—The aim of this study was to systematically review the literature to identify clinically important factors that predict mortality after hospitalization for acute exacerbation of chronic obstructive pulmonary disease (COPD).

Methods.—Eligible studies considered adults admitted to hospital with COPD exacerbation. Two authors independently abstracted data. Odds ratios were then calculated by comparing the prevalence of each predictor in survivors versus nonsurvivors. For continuous variables, mean differences were pooled by the inverse of their variance, using a random effects model.

Measurements and Main Results.—There were 37 studies included (189,772 study subjects) with risk of death ranging from 3.6% for studies considering short-term mortality, 31.0% for long-term mortality (up to 2 yr after hospitalization), and 29.0% for studies that considered solely intensive care unit (ICU)—admitted study subjects. Twelve prognostic factors (age, male sex, low body mass index, cardiac failure, chronic renal failure, confusion, long-term oxygen therapy, lower limb edema, Global Initiative for Chronic Lung Disease criteria stage 4, cor pulmonale, acidemia, and elevated plasma troponin level) were significantly associated with increased short-term mortality. Nine prognostic factors (age, low body mass index, cardiac failure, diabetes mellitus, ischemic heart disease, malignancy, FEV_1, long-term oxygen therapy, and Pao_2 on admission) were significantly associated with long-term mortality. Three factors (age, low Glasgow Coma Scale score, and pH) were significantly associated with increased risk of mortality in ICU-admitted study subjects.

Conclusion.—Different factors correlate with mortality from COPD exacerbation in the short term, long term, and after ICU admission. These parameters may be useful to develop tools for prediction of outcome in clinical practice.

▶ Exacerbations are serious events in the life of a patient with chronic obstructive pulmonary disease (COPD). Not only might they presage an ongoing decline in lung function and worsening quality of life, but they also bring an increased risk of short-term and long-term mortality. Community-acquired pneumonia (CAP) is also a serious event, particularly in the life of an elderly patient also potentially with negative impacts on survival and postpneumonia morbidity. Unlike COPD exacerbations, however, tools have been developed that are used to predict, at the time of presentation of patients with CAP, what the prognosis of that particular patient is. Those tools not only provide information for the patient and the physician; they also help to determine the most appropriate approach to care. Pulmonary physicians have recently recognized the need to develop tools such as those that exist for CAP; however, before the tools can be designed, it is necessary to sort through existing evidence to determine if there is adequate information about risk factors in specific populations of COPD patients (for example, differing phenotypes) to develop useable tools. That was the purpose of this meta-analysis. The authors were successful in identifying from 37 studies, 12 short-term risk factors and 9 long-term risk factors. This is a great first step toward developing predictive tools. The next steps are harder, that is, to simplify the factors (eliminate those that add little, for example) to the extent they can be easily used by primary care and emergency department physicians and to properly weight the chosen factors to provide valuable prognostic and management guidance.

J. R. Maurer, MD

Acquired Cystic Fibrosis Transmembrane Conductance Regulator Dysfunction in the Lower Airways in COPD
Dransfield MT, Wilhelm AM, Flanagan B, et al (Univ of Alabama at Birmingham)
Chest 144:498-506, 2013

Background.—Cigarette smoke and smoking-induced inflammation decrease cystic fibrosis transmembrane conductance regulator (CFTR) activity and mucociliary transport in the nasal airway and cultured bronchial epithelial cells. This raises the possibility that lower airway CFTR dysfunction may contribute to the pathophysiology of COPD. We compared lower airway CFTR activity in current and former smokers with COPD, current smokers without COPD, and lifelong nonsmokers to examine the relationships between clinical characteristics and CFTR expression and function.

Methods.—Demographic, spirometry, and symptom questionnaire data were collected. CFTR activity was determined by nasal potential difference (NPD) and lower airway potential difference (LAPD) assays. The primary measure of CFTR function was the total change in chloride transport (Δchloride-free isoproterenol). CFTR protein expression in endobronchial biopsy specimens was measured by Western blot.

Results.—Compared with healthy nonsmokers (n = 11), current smokers (n = 17) showed a significant reduction in LAPD CFTR activity (Δchloride-free isoproterenol, −8.70 mV vs −15.9 mV; P =.003). Similar reductions were observed in smokers with and without COPD. Former smokers with COPD (n = 7) showed a nonsignificant reduction in chloride conductance (−12.7 mV). A similar pattern was observed for CFTR protein expression. Univariate analysis demonstrated correlations between LAPD CFTR activity and current smoking, the presence of chronic bronchitis, and dyspnea scores.

Conclusions.—Smokers with and without COPD have reduced lower airway CFTR activity compared with healthy nonsmokers, and this finding correlates with disease phenotype. Acquired CFTR dysfunction may contribute to COPD pathogenesis.

▶ Airway mucus stasis with hyperviscous mucus is part of the pathology described in chronic obstructive pulmonary disease (COPD).[1] The finding of mucus stasis is important, as it has been associated with increased loss of lung function and, in many cases, bronchiectasis.[2] As in cystic fibrosis, the mucus stasis in COPD allows for bacterial colonization and inflammation resulting in bronchitis symptomatology and recurrent exacerbations. The most common phenotype of this segment of COPD patients is combined chronic bronchitis and bronchiectasis.[3] It has been speculated that the mucus stasis seen in these patients may be an issue with epithelial chloride transfer similar to the defect in cystic fibrosis. In fact, it has been shown that in smokers, the cystic fibrosis transmembrane conductance regulator (CFTR) function is suppressed.[4] It is now thought that acquired abnormalities in the CFTR may be important in several diseases. This report shows that CFTR activity is reduced in patients with COPD with a consistent phenotype. This finding is important, as there are several available and investigational drugs that modulate CFTR function and provide the potential for therapeutic intervention.

J. R. Maurer, MD

References

1. Hogg JC, Chu F, Utokaparch S, et al. The nature of small-airway obstruction in chronic obstructive pulmonary disease. *N Engl J Med.* 2004;350:2645-2653.
2. Sethi S, Maloney J, Grove L, Wrona C, Berenson CS. Airway inflammation and bronchial bacterial colonization in chronic obstructive pulmonary disease. *Am J Respir Crit Care Med.* 2006;173:991-998.
3. Martinez-Garcia MA, Soler-Cataluna JJ, Donat Sanz Y, et al. Factors associated with bronchiectasis in patients with COPD. *Chest.* 2011;140:1130-1137.
4. Cantin AM, Hanrahan JW, Bilodeau G, et al. Cystic fibrosis transmembrane conductance regulator function is suppressed in cigarette smokers. *Am J Respir Crit Care Med.* 2006;173:1139-1144.

Effects of Allergic Phenotype on Respiratory Symptoms and Exacerbations in Patients with Chronic Obstructive Pulmonary Disease

Jamieson DB, Matsui EC, Belli A, et al (Johns Hopkins Univ, Baltimore, MD)

Am J Respir Crit Care Med 188:187-192, 2013

Rationale.—Chronic obstructive pulmonary disease (COPD) guidelines make no recommendations for allergy diagnosis or treatment.

Objectives.—To determine whether an allergic phenotype contributes to respiratory symptoms and exacerbations in patients with COPD.

Methods.—Two separate cohorts were analyzed: National Health and Nutrition Survey III (NHANES III) and the COPD and domestic endotoxin (CODE) cohort. Subjects from NHANES III with COPD (n = 1,381) defined as age >40 years, history of smoking, FEV_1/FVC <0.70, and no diagnosis of asthma were identified. The presence of an allergic phenotype (n = 296) was defined as self-reported doctor diagnosed hay fever or allergic upper respiratory symptoms. In CODE, former smokers with COPD (n = 77) were evaluated for allergic sensitization defined as a detectable specific IgE to perennial allergens. Bivariate and multivariate models were used to determine whether an allergic phenotype was associated with respiratory symptoms and exacerbations.

Measurements and Main Results.—In NHANES III, multivariate analysis revealed that individuals with allergic phenotype were more likely to wheeze (odds ratio [OR], 2.1; $P < 0.01$), to have chronic cough (OR, 1.9; $P = 0.01$) and chronic phlegm (OR, 1.5; $P < 0.05$), and to have increased risk of COPD exacerbation requiring an acute doctor visit (OR, 1.7; $P = 0.04$). In the CODE cohort, multivariate analysis revealed that sensitized subjects reported more wheeze (OR, 5.91; $P < 0.01$), more nighttime awakening due to cough (OR, 4.20; $P = 0.03$), increased risk of COPD exacerbations requiring treatment with antibiotics (OR, 3.79; $P = 0.02$), and acute health visits (OR, 11.05; $P < 0.01$). An increasing number of sensitizations was associated with a higher risk for adverse health outcomes.

Conclusions.—Among individuals with COPD, evidence of an allergic phenotype is associated with increased respiratory symptoms and risk of COPD exacerbations.

▶ The authors state that the purpose of this study is to assess whether the presence of allergies in patients with chronic obstructive pulmonary disease (COPD) worsens their respiratory health. They correctly identify that upper airway allergic disease as a comorbidity is rarely addressed in patients with fixed obstructive lung disease but is commonly assessed in asthmatics. And it is widely accepted that upper airway disease related to allergies contributes to issues with asthma control and asthma exacerbations. In fact, the Global Obstructive Lung Disease Guidelines (GOLD), a widely used international guideline, does not have any recommendations about the assessment and management of allergic disease. The study used 2 database cohorts to examine the overlap of COPD and allergic symptoms. In one, clinical symptoms indicative of hay fever—type allergies were captured, and, in the second, specific immuno-globulin E testing was performed. As in asthma patients, COPD patients who had milder disease and those with more significant disease had increased respiratory symptoms, including more exacerbations in the more severe patients. Some issues with the study should be acknowledged. Using databases, especially the National Health and Nutrition Survey database used in this study, for example, could result in capturing some asthmatic patients who were misclassified as COPD patients. Nevertheless, the important question posed here is: If we treated these allergic symptoms, could we reduce morbidity related to lung disease? This is the question that needs to be studied prospectively.

J. R. Maurer, MD

Pulmonary hypertension in COPD: results from the ASPIRE registry
Hurdman J, Condliffe R, Elliot CA, et al (Royal Hallamshire Hosp, Sheffield, UK; et al)
Eur Respir J 41:1292-1301, 2013

The phenotype and outcome of severe pulmonary hypertension in chronic obstructive pulmonary disease (COPD) is described in small numbers, and predictors of survival are unknown. Data was retrieved for 101 consecutive, treatment-naïve cases of pulmonary hypertension in COPD.

Mean ± SD follow-up was 2.3 ± 1.9 years. 59 patients with COPD and severe pulmonary hypertension, defined by catheter mean pulmonary artery pressure ≥40 mmHg, had significantly lower carbon monoxide diffusion, less severe airflow obstruction but not significantly different emphysema scores on computed tomography compared to 42 patients with mild-moderate pulmonary hypertension. 1- and 3-year survival for severe pulmonary hypertension, at 70% and 33%, respectively, was inferior to 83% and 55%, respectively, for mild-moderate pulmonary hypertension. Mixed venous oxygen saturation, carbon monoxide diffusion, World Health Organization functional class and age, but not severity of airflow obstruction, were independent predictors of outcome. Compassionate treatment with targeted therapies in 43 patients with severe pulmonary hypertension was not associated with a survival benefit, although improvement in functional class and/or fall in pulmonary vascular resistance >20% following treatment identified patients with improved survival.

Standard prognostic markers in COPD have limited value in patients with pulmonary hypertension. This study identifies variables that predict outcome in this phenotype. Despite poor prognosis, our data suggest that further evaluation of targeted therapies is warranted (Fig 2).

▶ Pulmonary hypertension is common in advanced lung disease. However, severely elevated pulmonary pressures tend to be much more common in patients with fibrotic interstitial disease like pulmonary fibrosis than in patients

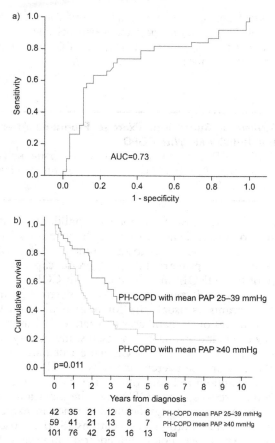

FIGURE 2.—a) Receiver operating characteristics curve analysis of survival at 2 years for mean pulmonary arterial pressure (PAP) in pulmonary hypertension associated with chronic obstructive pulmonary disease (COPD); b) cumulative survival from date of diagnosis in pulmonary hypertension associated with COPD by mean PAP. AUC: area under the curve. (Reprinted from Hurdman J, Condliffe R, Elliot CA, et al. Pulmonary hypertension in COPD: results from the ASPIRE registry. *Eur Respir J*. 2013;41:1292-1301, Copyright 2013, with permission from European Respiratory Society.)

with obstructive disease like cystic fibrosis or emphysema. In chronic obstructive pulmonary disease (COPD), pulmonary hypertension tends to develop slowly as the patients become more hypoxemic, and they usually have preserved cardiac output. For the 1% or so of COPD patients who seem to have severe pulmonary hypertension, this is not the case. They can develop the same types of cardiac dysfunction and functional debility that any patient with severely elevated pulmonary pressures experiences. The aim of this study was to better characterize this group of COPD patients, as the center is a large referral center with a large registry of patients with coexistent parenchymal and vascular disease. Not surprisingly, the phenotype of this group is relatively worse diffusion capacity compared with the level of obstruction. And the prognosis is much worse than that of COPD patients who do not have severe pulmonary hypertension. Targeted pulmonary hypertension strategies were not particularly helpful. These data suggest these patients have a disease course more like pulmonary fibrosis patients than typical COPD patients who have similar FEV_1s but better diffusing capacities (Fig 2).

J. R. Maurer, MD

Systematic Review of Supervised Exercise Programs After Pulmonary Rehabilitation in Individuals With COPD
Beauchamp MK, Evans R, Janaudis-Ferreira T, et al (Spaulding Rehabilitation Hosp, Boston, MA; West Park Healthcare Centre, Toronto, Ontario, Canada)
Chest 144:1124-1133, 2013

Background.—The success of pulmonary rehabilitation (PR) is established, but how to sustain benefits over the long term is less clear. The aim of this systematic review was to determine the effect of supervised exercise programs after primary PR on exercise capacity and health-related quality of life (HRQL) in individuals with COPD.

Methods.—Randomized controlled trials of postrehabilitation supervised exercise programs vs usual care for individuals with COPD were identified after searches of six databases and reference lists of appropriate studies. Two reviewers independently assessed study quality. Standardized mean differences (SMDs) with 95% CIs were calculated using a fixed-effect model for measures of exercise capacity and HRQL.

Results.—Seven randomized controlled trials, with a total of 619 individuals with moderate to severe COPD, met the inclusion criteria. At 6-month follow-up there was a significant difference in exercise capacity in favor of the postrehabilitation interventions (SMD, −0.20; 95% CI, −0.39 to −0.01), which was not sustained at 12 months (SMD, −0.09; 95% CI, −0.29 to 0.11). There was no difference between postrehabilitation interventions and usual care with respect to HRQL at any time point.

Conclusions.—Supervised exercise programs after primary PR appear to be more effective than usual care for preserving exercise capacity in the medium term but not in the long term. In this review, there was no effect on HRQL. The small number of studies precludes a definitive conclusion as to the impact of postrehabilitation exercise maintenance on longer-term benefits in individuals with COPD.

▶ In 2013, the American Thoracic Society and the European Respiratory Society published a statement updating the 2006 document.[1] This updated report noted the following advances: (1) evidence now supports a variety of types of exercise in rehabilitation programs; (2) pulmonary rehabilitation has been shown to improve symptoms, exercise tolerance, and quality of life in a variety of chronic pulmonary diseases; (3) symptomatic chronic obstructive pulmonary disease (COPD) patients with less-severe pulmonary functions may benefit similarly to those with worse pulmonary function; (4) pulmonary rehabilitation started shortly after a hospitalization is effective; (5) exercise rehabilitation started during acute or critical illness reduces functional decline and hastens recovery; (6) home-based exercise training is effective in reducing dyspnea and increasing exercise performance; (7) new technologies are being tested to support pulmonary rehabilitation activities; (8) the scope of outcomes assessment has broadened to include knowledge and self-efficacy, muscle function, balance, and physical activity; (9) anxiety and depression are prevalent, may affect outcomes, and can be helped by intervention. Among those elements identified as necessary to address in the future is "to effect behavior change and to optimize and maintain outcomes." This is one of the big gaps still in pulmonary rehabilitation. The early significant gains in function, quality of life, and even possibly reduced risk of exacerbation begins to wane at 6 to 12 months. This is painfully obvious in the systematic review presented here of 6 studies of ongoing exercise programs after a formal pulmonary rehabilitation program. The authors conclude that benefits wane in the long term (defined as 12 months), even with these programs. However, this literature is not very robust: different frequencies of exercise were used, different types of maintenance exercise were used, and drop out from the programs was common. This is an important area that deserves robust, controlled trials. Even though important benefits are achieved in initial pulmonary rehabilitation programs, the cost is harder to justify if the benefits cannot be sustained over a longer period.

J. R. Maurer, MD

Reference

1. Spruit MA, Singh SJ, Garvey C, et al; ATS/ERS Task Force on Pulmonary Rehabilitation. An official American Thoracic Society/European Respiratory Society statement: key concepts and advances in pulmonary rehabilitation. *Am J Respir Crit Care Med.* 2013;188:e13-e64.

3 Lung Cancer

Introduction

Lung cancer is the leading cause of cancer death around the world. In 2013, lung cancer claimed an estimated 159 480 lives, more than breast, colon, and prostate cancers combined.[1] In contrast to substantial improvement in outcomes for these other common solid tumors over the past quarter century, the overall 5-year survival rate for lung cancer has changed very little, remaining abysmally low at approximately 16%. The good news is that the lung cancer death rate in women finally seems to be declining somewhat, though it still far exceeds the death rate from breast cancer. The mortality gains made in both men and women largely reflect efforts aimed at curtailing cigarette smoking. The enormous benefits reaped by smoking cessation, including gain of life years, are indisputable.[2,3] However, approximately 20% of adult Americans are habitual smokers, despite public health awareness and regulatory interventions. This makes the scientific efforts aimed at understanding lung cancer biology all the more important, as lung cancer will continue to be an enormous challenge for the foreseeable future if the major risk factor, cigarette smoking, remains so widely prevalent.

2013 saw the publication of the 3rd edition of the American College of Chest Physicians Evidence-Based Clinical Practice Guidelines for the Diagnosis and Management of Lung Cancer.[4] The 24 articles in the guidelines provide concise and practical recommendations for all aspects of lung cancer. Most importantly, detailed discussions are provided of the evidence base supporting those recommendations. While only a few articles could be highlighted in this compendium, all are worth reading.[5-7] The guidelines serve as a comprehensive reference, probably the best available for practicing clinicians.

2013 was a banner year for lung cancer screening. At the very end of the year, the United States Preventive Services Task Force (USPSTF) finalized its revised lung cancer screening statement.[8] The USPSTF now recommends "annual screening for lung cancer with low-dose computed tomography in adults aged 55 to 80 years who have a 30 pack-year smoking history and currently smoke or have quit within the past 15 years." This is a huge change from the prior statement, which did not recommend "for or against" lung cancer screening with any modality. Comprehensive modeling studies were performed by the Cancer Intervention and Surveillance Modeling Network (CISNET) to inform the USPSTF recommendation.[9] The CISNET centers evaluated the impact of screening in populations of varying ages and smoking exposure, using data from the National Lung Screening Trial (NLST) as well as other large screening studies to develop their models. In the NLST, participants were all between the ages of 55 to 74 years and had a 30 pack-year smoking history, either currently smoking or having quit within the prior 15 years.[10] The CISNET analysis included groups that varied with respect to the age at which screening should begin, the duration of cigarette cessation in patients who had quit smoking, and the intensity of smoking (measured as pack-years). Their modeling demonstrated that the NLST population is not the only group that can benefit from screening, but emphasized that a balance of harms and benefits ensues depending on the age and smoking characteristics of a given group. Along these same lines, Kovalchik and colleagues used a lung cancer prediction model to demonstrate that, even within the NLST population, groups at higher as well as lower risk for developing lung cancer can be identified, and it is the higher risk groups who truly benefit from low-dose CT screening.[11] Targeting screening to the higher risk individuals could increase the cost effectiveness of screening. Moreover, targeting screening away from lower risk individuals will decrease the multitude of false positive findings that inevitably are found on the screening CTs in this cigarette-exposed population. As lung cancer screening propagates to the general community, we will have to tackle the difficult questions as to which individuals outside the NLST criteria merit screening based on risk, as well as which individuals who meet the NLST criteria are actually at such low lung cancer risk that they might be better served by not undergoing CT scanning and incurring harm related to false positive findings.[12,13] Risk predictive tools such as those developed by Tammemagi and colleagues will need to be incorporated in clinical practice to help objectively inform those difficult decisions.[11,14]

Lung cancer screening brings to the forefront the perennial challenge of evaluation of pulmonary nodules. With the high rate of discovery of nodules on low-dose screening CTs, and the knowledge that the vast majority of these are false positives, a structured approach to nodule evaluation becomes all the more important.[6,15,16] Clinicians historically have been quite good at predicting the likelihood that nodules discovered incidentally on CT scans are malignant. However, whether we will be as accurate evaluating the plethora of nodules that will inevitably be found with screening CTs is not known. Fortunately, tools for predicting both lung cancer risk per se and lung cancer risk for a nodule identified on CT have been developed, are easily accessible, and will likely continue to be refined in the future.[11,14,17]

Most lung cancers found by screening will be early stage. We may eventually see a shift in stage distribution as a result, but for the present the majority of lung cancers diagnosed are Stage III or IV. Treatment options for patients with advanced stage disease are still limited. For these patients, systemic treatment is necessary, and the burgeoning scientific interest in translating genomic information to targeted therapies is rapidly transforming the therapeutic paradigm. It has been only a decade since the discovery that mutations in the *EGFR* gene in a small but significant percentage of adenocarcinomas identified a group of patients whose tumors responded to targeted inhibition of the EGFR receptor tyrosine kinase. Since then, intense research has demonstrated that more than half of all adenocarcinomas and squamous cell carcinomas harbor mutations, all of which theoretically are targetable for treatment. Staying informed about lung cancer requires an understanding of this change in approach to treatment, and an appreciation that those of us involved in obtaining diagnostic tissue have a responsibility to include mutational testing in the algorithm.[18,19] All of this new information has led us to an exciting time in lung cancer care, with the hope that the combination of primary prevention efforts curtailing tobacco exposure, better early detection with screening, and scientific discovery informing new lines of treatment will lead to better outcomes for our patients.

Lynn T. Tanoue, MD

References

1. Siegel R, Naishadham D, Jemal A. Cancer statistics, 2013. *CA Cancer J Clin.* 2013;63:11-30.
2. Thun MJ, Lopez AD, Hartge P. Smoking-related mortality in the United States. *N Engl J Med.* 2013;368:1753.
3. Jha P, Ramasundarahettige C, Landsman V, et al. 21st-century hazards of smoking and benefits of cessation in the United States. *N Engl J Med.* 2013;368: 341-350.
4. Detterbeck FC, Lewis SZ, Diekemper R, Addrizzo-Harris D, Alberts WM. Executive summary: diagnosis and management of lung cancer, 3rd ed: American College of Chest Physicians evidence-based clinical practice guidelines. *Chest.* 2013; 143:7S-37S.
5. Detterbeck FC, Postmus PE, Tanoue LT. The stage classification of lung cancer: diagnosis and management of lung cancer, 3rd ed: American College of Chest Physicians evidence-based clinical practice guidelines. *Chest.* 2013;143:e191S-e210S.
6. Gould MK, Donington J, Lynch WR, et al. Evaluation of individuals with pulmonary nodules: when is it lung cancer? Diagnosis and management of lung cancer, 3rd ed: American College of Chest Physicians evidence-based clinical practice guidelines. *Chest.* 2013;143:e93S-e120S.
7. Brunelli A, Kim AW, Berger KI, Addrizzo-Harris DJ. Physiologic evaluation of the patient with lung cancer being considered for resectional surgery: diagnosis and management of lung cancer, 3rd ed: American College of Chest Physicians evidence-based clinical practice guidelines. *Chest.* 2013;143:e166S-e190S.
8. Moyer VA. Screening for lung cancer: U.S. Preventive Services Task Force Recommendation Statement. *Ann Intern Med.* 2014;160:330-338.
9. de Koning H, Meza R, Plevritis S, et al. *Benefits and Harms of Computed Tomography Lung Cancer Screening Programs for High-Risk Populations.* AHRQ Publication No. 13-05196-EF-2. Rockville, MD: Agency for Healthcare Research and Quality; 2013.
10. Aberle DR, Adams AM, Berg CD, et al. Reduced lung-cancer mortality with low-dose computed tomographic screening. *N Engl J Med.* 2011;365:395-409.
11. Kovalchik SA, Tammemagi M, Berg CD, et al. Targeting of low-dose CT screening according to the risk of lung-cancer death. *N Engl J Med.* 2013;369:245-254.
12. Wender R, Fontham ET, Barrera E Jr, et al. American Cancer Society lung cancer screening guidelines. *CA Cancer J Clin.* 2013;63:107-117.
13. Bach PB, Mirkin JN, Oliver TK, et al. Benefits and harms of CT screening for lung cancer: a systematic review. *JAMA.* 2012;307:2418-2429.
14. Tammemägi MC, Katki HA, Hocking WG, et al. Selection criteria for lung-cancer screening. *N Engl J Med.* 2013;368:728-736.

15. Naidich DP, Bankier AA, MacMahon H, et al. Recommendations for the management of subsolid pulmonary nodules detected at CT: a statement from the Fleischner Society. *Radiology.* 2013;266:304-317.
16. MacMahon H, Austin JH, Gamsu G, et al. Guidelines for management of small pulmonary nodules detected on CT scans: a statement from the Fleischner Society. *Radiology.* 2005;237:395-400.
17. McWilliams A, Tammemagi MC, Mayo JR, et al. Probability of cancer in pulmonary nodules detected on first screening CT. *N Engl J Med.* 2013;369:910-919.
18. Cardarella S, Johnson BE. The impact of genomic changes on treatment of lung cancer. *Am J Respir Crit Care Med.* 2013;188:770-775.
19. Jett JR, Carr LL. Targeted therapy for non-small cell lung cancer. *Am J Respir Crit Care Med.* 2013;188:907-912.

Epidemiology of Lung Cancer

Cancer Statistics, 2013
Siegel R, Naishadham D, Jemal A (American Cancer Society, Atlanta, GA)
CA Cancer J Clin 63:11-30, 2013

Each year, the American Cancer Society estimates the numbers of new cancer cases and deaths expected in the United States in the current year and compiles the most recent data on cancer incidence, mortality, and

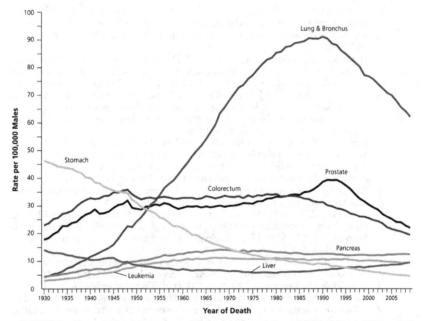

FIGURE 4.—Trends in Death Rates Among Males for Selected Cancers, United States, 1930 to 2009. Rates are age adjusted to the 2000 US standard population. Due to changes in International Classification of Diseases (ICD) coding, numerator information has changed over time. Rates for cancers of the lung and bronchus, colorectum, and liver are affected by these changes. (Reprinted from Siegel R, Naishadham D, Jemal A. Cancer statistics, 2013. *CA Cancer J Clin.* 2013;63:11-30, with permission from CA: A Cancer Journal for Clinicians and John Wiley and Sons, www.interscience.wiley.com.)

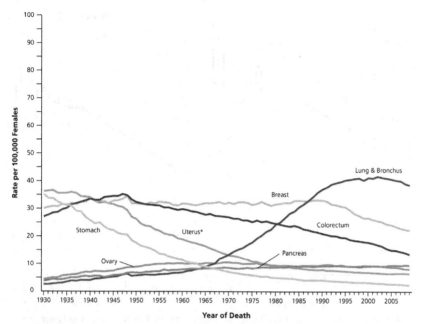

FIGURE 5.—Trends in Death Rates Among Females for Selected Cancers, United States, 1930 to 2009. Rates are age adjusted to the 2000 US standard population. Due to changes in International Classification of Diseases (ICD) coding, numerator information has changed over time. Rates for cancers of the uterus, ovary, lung and bronchus, and colorectum are affected by these changes. *Uterus includes uterine cervix and uterine corpus. (Reprinted from Siegel R, Naishadham D, Jemal A. Cancer statistics, 2013. *CA Cancer J Clin.* 2013;63:11-30, with permission from CA: A Cancer Journal for Clinicians and John Wiley and Sons, www.interscience.wiley.com.)

survival based on incidence data from the National Cancer Institute, the Centers for Disease Control and Prevention, and the North American Association of Central Cancer Registries and mortality data from the National Center for Health Statistics. A total of 1,660,290 new cancer cases and 580,350 cancer deaths are projected to occur in the United States in 2013. During the most recent 5 years for which there are data (2005-2009), delay-adjusted cancer incidence rates declined slightly in men (by 0.6% per year) and were stable in women, while cancer death rates decreased by 1.8% per year in men and by 1.5% per year in women. Overall, cancer death rates have declined 20% from their peak in 1991 (215.1 per 100,000 population) to 2009 (173.1 per 100,000 population). Death rates continue to decline for all 4 major cancer sites (lung, colorectum, breast, and prostate). Over the past 10 years of data (2000-2009), the largest annual declines in death rates were for chronic myeloid leukemia (8.4%), cancers of the stomach (3.1%) and colorectum (3.0%), and non-Hodgkin lymphoma (3.0%). The reduction in overall cancer death rates since 1990 in men and 1991 in women translates to the avoidance of approximately 1.18 million deaths from cancer, with 152,900 of these deaths averted in 2009 alone. Further progress can be accelerated by applying existing cancer control knowledge across all segments of the

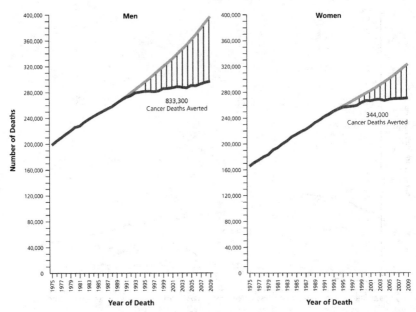

FIGURE 6.—Total Number of Cancer Deaths Averted From 1991 to 2009 in Men and From 1992 to 2009 in Women. The blue line represents the actual number of cancer deaths recorded in each year, and the red line represents the number of cancer deaths that would have been expected if cancer death rates had remained at their peak. For Interpretation of the references to color in this figure legend, the reader is referred to web version of this article. (Reprinted from Siegel R, Naishadham D, Jemal A. Cancer statistics, 2013. *CA Cancer J Clin.* 2013;63:11-30, with permission from CA: A Cancer Journal for Clinicians and John Wiley and Sons, www.interscience.wiley.com.)

population, with an emphasis on those groups in the lowest socioeconomic bracket and other underserved populations (Figs 4-6, Table 12).

▶ Lung cancer is the leading cause of cancer death in both men and women in the United States. In 2013, the American Cancer Society estimated that 87 260 men and 72 220 women died from lung cancer (total deaths 159 480). Lung cancer accounts for 28% of all male cancer deaths and 26% of all female cancer deaths. Although the mortality toll related to lung cancer still exceeds the next 3 leading causes of cancer death (breast, colorectal, and prostate cancers) combined, the good news is that these numbers in both sexes are less than in 2012. As can be seen in Fig 4, the lung cancer death rate in American men has been declining steadily since about 1990. Fig 5 shows that the lung cancer death rate curve in women is finally also bending downward. The 2 figures also point out that death from cancers in general are decreasing, with the total number of cancer deaths averted from 1991 to 2009 demonstrated in Fig 6.

Of all cancers, lung cancer has the largest variation in geographic distribution, which predominantly reflects the differences in smoking prevalence among states. Over the 5-year period from 2005 to 2009, age-adjusted lung cancer death rates in men and women in Kentucky were 128.2 and 55.5 per 100 000, respectively. In contrast, age-adjusted lung cancer death rates in men and women in Utah were 28.1 and 16.1 per 100 000, respectively. Table 12 shows

TABLE 12.—Trends in 5-Year Relative Survival Rates* (%) by Race and Year of Diagnosis, United States, 1975 to 2008

	All Races			White			African American		
	1975 TO 1977	1987 TO 1989	2002 TO 2008	1975 TO 1977	1987 TO 1989	2002 TO 2008	1975 TO 1977	1987 TO 1989	2002 TO 2008
All sites	49	56	68†	50	57	69†	39	43	60†
Brain & other nervous system	22	29	35†	22	28	34†	25	32	41†
Breast (female)	75	84	90†	76	85	92†	62	71	78†
Colon	51	61	65†	51	61	66†	45	53	55†
Esophagus	5	10	19†	6	11	21†	3	7	14†
Hodgkin lymphoma	72	79	87†	72	80	88†	70	72	83†
Kidney & renal pelvis	50	57	72†	50	57	72†	49	55	70†
Larynx	66	66	63†	67	67	65	59	56	51
Leukemia	34	43	58†	35	44	59†	33	35	51†
Liver & intrahepatic bile duct	3	5	16†	3	6	16†	2	3	11†
Lung & bronchus	12	13	17†	12	13	17†	11	11	14†
Melanoma of the skin	82	88	93†	82	88	93†	57‡	79‡	70‡†
Myeloma	25	28	43†	25	27	43†	30	30	43†
Non-Hodgkin lymphoma	47	51	71†	47	52	72†	48	46	63†
Oral cavity & pharynx	53	54	65†	54	56	67†	36	34	45†
Ovary	36	38	43†	35	38	43†	42	34	36
Pancreas	2	4	6†	3	3	6†	2	6	5†
Prostate	68	83	100†	69	85	100†	61	72	98†
Rectum	48	58	68†	48	59	69†	45	52	61†
Stomach	15	20	28†	14	19	27†	16	19	28†
Testis	83	95	96†	83	96	97†	73‡§	88‡	89
Thyroid	92	95	98†	92	94	98†	90	92	96†
Urinary bladder	73	79	80†	74	80	81†	50	63	62†
Uterine cervix	69	70	69	70	73	70	65	57	61
Uterine corpus	87	83	83†	88	84	85†	60	57	63

*Survival rates are adjusted for normal life expectancy and are based on cases diagnosed in the Surveillance, Epidemiology, and End Results (SEER) 9 areas from 1975 to 1977, 1987 to 1989, and 2002 to 2008 and followed through 2009.

†The difference in rates between 1975 to 1977 and 2002 to 2008 is statistically significant (P <.05).

‡The standard error of the survival rate is between 5 and 10 percentage points.

§Survival rate is for 1978 to 1980.

that the overall 5-year survival rate for lung cancer now stands at 17%, which is dismal compared with all sites (overall 5-year survival rate, 68%), in particular compared with the other major causes of cancer death, including breast (5-year survival rate, 90%), colon (5-year survival rate, 65%), and prostate (5-year survival rate, 100%) cancers. Nonetheless, there has been improvement in lung cancer survival, largely related to reduction in tobacco use.[1] In contrast, decreases in death rates for prostate, colorectal, and breast cancers are generally attributed to improvements in early detection and treatment.[2-4] With much attention now focused on screening, we may over the coming years see a change in lung cancer mortality related to early detection for lung cancer as well.[5]

However, clear disparities in outcomes exist and need to be addressed, with African-Americans in particular showing lower 5-year survival rates overall and in lung cancer (5-year survival rate,14%) specifically. With cancer accounting for 23% of all deaths in the United States annually and the leading cause of death among both men and women age 40 to 79 years, much more work is still to be done in primary prevention, early detection, and improving treatment for advanced disease.

L. T. Tanoue, MD

References

1. Jemal A, Thun MJ, Ries LA, et al. Annual report to the nation on the status of cancer, 1975—2005, featuring trends in lung cancer, tobacco use, and tobacco control. *J Natl Cancer Inst.* 2008;100:1672-1694.
2. Berry DA, Cronin KA, Plevritis SK, et al. Effect of screening and adjuvant therapy on mortality from breast cancer. *N Engl J Med.* 2005;353:1784-1792.
3. Etzioni R, Tsodikov A, Mariotto A, et al. Quantifying the role of PSA screening in the US prostate cancer mortality decline. *Cancer Causes Control.* 2008;19:175-181.
4. Edwards BK, Ward E, Kohler BA, et al. Annual report to the nation on the status of cancer, 1975—2006, featuring colorectal cancer trends and impact of interventions (risk factors, screening, and treatment) to reduce future rates. *Cancer.* 2010;116: 544-573.
5. National Lung Screening Trial Research Team, Aberle DR, Adams AM, Berg CD, et al. Reduced lung-cancer mortality with low-dose computed tomographic screening. *N Engl J Med.* 2011;365:395-409.

Epidemic of Lung Cancer in Patients With HIV Infection

Winstone TA, Man SFP, Hull M, et al (Univ of British Columbia, Canada)
Chest 143:305-314, 2013

The survival of patients with HIV infection has improved dramatically over the past 20 years, largely owing to a significant reduction in opportunistic infections and AIDs-defining malignancies, such as lymphoma and Kaposi sarcoma. However, with improved survival, patients with HIV are experiencing morbidity and mortality from other (non-AIDs-defining) complications, such as solid organ malignancies. Of these, the leading cause of mortality in the HIV-infected population is lung cancer, accounting for nearly 30% of all cancer deaths and 10% of all non-HIV-related deaths. Importantly, the average age of onset of lung cancer in the HIV-infected population is 25 to 30 years earlier than that in the general population and at lower exposure to cigarette smoke. This article provides an overview of the epidemiology of lung cancer in the HIV-infected population and discusses some of the important risk factors and pathways that may enhance the risk of lung cancer in this population.

▶ The 2 most frequent AIDS-defining cancers are Kaposi sarcoma and non-Hodgkin's lymphoma. The incidence of both of these malignancies has decreased since the introduction of combination antiretroviral therapies. As in the general population, lung cancer is the most prevalent non—AIDS-defining cancer. Several features highlight why practitioners should be thinking about lung cancer in their patients with AIDS: (1) the risk of lung cancer is approximately 3-fold that of the general population, even with antiretroviral treatment; (2) the age at diagnosis is typically considerably younger than in the general population, on average between 38 and 57 years, and (3) the AIDS population as a group tends to display other characteristics and behaviors increasing the risk of lung cancer. Sixty percent to 80% of persons with HIV in the United States smoke.[1,2] They often have chronic pulmonary inflammation, primarily related to infections and smoking, and they are likely to have impaired immune surveillance, particularly when the CD4 count is low. As is seen in the general population, stage distribution is unfortunately weighted toward diagnosis of advanced disease; what follows inevitably is overall survival tends to be poor, as the stage of tumor is the predominant driver of prognosis.

Survival with HIV in the era of effective antiretroviral therapy has improved dramatically. As a consequence, the number of persons living with HIV and AIDS is growing. Given this, practitioners need to be aware of the increased risk of lung cancer, even in their younger AIDS patients, and should counsel their patients who smoke about the importance of quitting.

L. T. Tanoue, MD

References

1. Engels EA, Brock MV, Chen J, Hooker CM, Gillison M, Moore RD. Elevated incidence of lung cancer among HIV-infected individuals. *J Clin Oncol.* 2006;24: 1383-1388.
2. Giordano TP, Kramer JR. Does HIV infection independently increase the incidence of lung cancer? *Clin Infect Dis.* 2005;40:490-491.

Asbestos, Asbestosis, Smoking, and Lung Cancer. New Findings from the North American Insulator Cohort
Markowitz SB, Levin SM, Miller A, et al (City Univ of New York, Flushing; Mount Sinai School of Medicine, NY)
Am J Respir Crit Care Med 188:90-96, 2013

Rationale.—Asbestos, smoking, and asbestosis increase lung cancer risk in incompletely elucidated ways. Smoking cessation among asbestos-exposed cohorts has been little studied.

Objectives.—To measure the contributions of asbestos exposure, asbestosis, smoking, and their interactions to lung cancer risk in an asbestos-exposed cohort and to describe their reduction in lung cancer risk when they stop smoking.

Methods.—We examined lung cancer mortality obtained through the National Death Index for 1981 to 2008 for 2,377 male North American insulators for whom chest X-ray, spirometric, occupational, and smoking data were collected in 1981 to 1983 and for 54,243 non—asbestos-exposed blue collar male workers from Cancer Prevention Study II for whom occupational and smoking data were collected in 1982.

Measurements and Main Results.—Lung cancer caused 339 (19%) insulator deaths. Lung cancer mortality was increased by asbestos exposure alone among nonsmokers (rate ratio = 3.6 [95% confidence interval (CI), 1.7—7.6]), by asbestosis among nonsmokers (rate ratio = 7.40 [95% CI, 4.0—13.7]), and by smoking without asbestos exposure (rate ratio = 10.3 [95% CI, 8.8—12.2]). The joint effect of smoking and asbestos alone was additive (rate ratio = 14.4 [95% CI, 10.7—19.4]) and with asbestosis, supra-additive (rate ratio = 36.8 [95% CI, 30.1—45.0]). Insulator lung cancer mortality halved within 10 years of smoking cessation and converged with that of never-smokers 30 years after smoking cessation.

Conclusions.—Asbestos increases lung cancer mortality among nonsmokers. Asbestosis further increases the lung cancer risk and, considered jointly with smoking, has a supra-additive effect. Insulators benefit greatly by quitting smoking.

▶ Asbestos exposure with inhalation of asbestos fibers is associated with several categories of lung disease: (1) pneumoconiosis or interstitial lung disease, termed *asbestosis*; (2) pleural plaques; and (3) malignancy, including mesothelioma and bronchogenic carcinoma. Awareness of the health hazards of asbestos exposure dates back at least 100 years, although regulatory interventions to minimize asbestos mining and industrial as well as domestic utilization date back only several decades. Despite widespread public awareness of adverse health consequences, controversy persists about fundamental aspects of asbestos and its relation to lung cancer including (1) the nature, if any, of the risk interaction related to dual exposure to asbestos and cigarette smoking; (2) whether asbestos exposure itself is a lung cancer risk factor or whether only asbestosis, that is, the presence of parenchymal lung disease, is associated with increased risk; and (3) whether asbestos exposure results in increased lung cancer risk in nonsmokers. This article by Markowitz and colleagues and the accompanying editorial by Balmes[1] does not summarily settle these controversies, but the work does bring more clarity to the arguments and is an important contribution to the many other epidemiologic studies evaluating the health effects of asbestos exposure.

This study is a follow-up on data collected between 1981 and 1983 on 2377 North American insulators who had been working in their field for at least 20 years and who were presumably exposed to asbestos during those years. The control group consisted of non—asbestos-exposed blue collar workers in the American Cancer Society Cancer Prevention Study II (CPS II), whose data were collected in 1982. Fig 1 in the original article shows the most important findings. (1) In nonsmoking insulators, asbestos exposure, even without radiographic evidence of asbestosis, was associated with an increased risk of lung cancer compared with the control group. (2) In both smoking and nonsmoking insulators, the presence of asbestosis increased lung cancer mortality risk. (3) In smoking insulators, the combined effect on increased lung cancer risk related to smoking and asbestos exposure without asbestosis was additive, whereas the combined effect of increased risk related to smoking and asbestosis was supra-additive. The study also resulted in one other important conclusion, shown graphically in Fig 3 of the original article, that smoking cessation, even in insulators with asbestosis, resulted in a decrease in lung cancer risk.

L. T. Tanoue, MD

Reference

1. Balmes JR. Asbestos and lung cancer: what we know. *Am J Respir Crit Care Med.* 2013;188:8-9.

Tobacco-related Issues

50-Year Trends in Smoking-Related Mortality in the United States

Thun MJ, Carter BD, Feskanich D, et al (American Cancer Society, Atlanta, GA; Harvard Med School, Boston, MA; et al)
N Engl J Med 368:351-364, 2013

Background.—The disease risks from cigarette smoking increased in the United States over most of the 20th century, first among male smokers and later among female smokers. Whether these risks have continued to increase during the past 20 years is unclear.

Methods.—We measured temporal trends in mortality across three time periods (1959–1965, 1982–1988, and 2000–2010), comparing absolute and relative risks according to sex and self-reported smoking status in two historical cohort studies and in five pooled contemporary cohort studies, among participants who became 55 years of age or older during follow-up.

Results.—For women who were current smokers, as compared with women who had never smoked, the relative risks of death from lung cancer were 2.73, 12.65, and 25.66 in the 1960s, 1980s, and contemporary cohorts, respectively; corresponding relative risks for male current smokers, as compared with men who had never smoked, were 12.22, 23.81, and 24.97. In the contemporary cohorts, male and female current smokers also had similar relative risks for death from chronic obstructive pulmonary disease (COPD) (25.61 for men and 22.35 for women), ischemic heart disease (2.50 for men and 2.86 for women), any type of stroke (1.92 for men and 2.10 for women), and all causes combined (2.80 for men and 2.76 for women). Mortality from COPD among male smokers continued to increase in the contemporary cohorts in nearly all the age groups represented in the study and within each stratum of duration and intensity of smoking. Among men 55 to 74 years of age and women 60 to 74 years of age, all-cause mortality was at least three times as high among current smokers as among those who had never smoked. Smoking cessation at any age dramatically reduced death rates.

Conclusions.—The risk of death from cigarette smoking continues to increase among women and the increased risks are now nearly identical for men and women, as compared with persons who have never smoked. Among men, the risks associated with smoking have plateaued at the high levels seen in the 1980s, except for a continuing, unexplained increase in mortality from COPD.

▶ The first US Surgeon General's report on the health consequences of smoking issued in 1964 suggested that women were less likely than men to suffer from cigarette smoking.[1] The fallacy of that statement was, of course, related to the fact that in 1964 women had not been smoking long enough for those adverse health consequences to have yet become evident. In this report by Thun and colleagues, trends in mortality from 1959 to 2010 were examined in men and women, with specific reference to the influence of cigarette smoking. The authors highlight several points:

- The relative risks of death from the major cigarette-related diseases, including chronic obstructive pulmonary disease (COPD), ischemic heart disease, stroke, and all causes are now essentially equal for both sexes. This reflects the fact that smoking patterns among men and women have converged since the 1960s, when that first Surgeon General's report was published. As demonstrated in Fig 1 of the original article, the rate of death from lung cancer in men has plateaued, whereas in women it is still increasing, and the rate of COPD deaths has increased over time in both sexes.
- The rate of death for men 55 to 74 years and women 60 to 74 years is at least 3 times as high among current smokers compared with never smokers. This observation recapitulates the findings of the newly published US National Health Interview Survey[2] as well as the landmark British Doctors' Study.[3]
- The rate of death from COPD is increasing in both men and women smokers.
- Quitting smoking at any age decreases mortality for all the major smoking-related diseases. As demonstrated in Fig 2 of the original article, smoking cessation before the age of 40 results in a diminution of risk for lung cancer and COPD to nearly that of never smokers.

It is unfortunate that one of the few examples of gender equality resides in the recognition that the risks of the devastating consequences of smoking in women are now equal to those in men.

L. T. Tanoue, MD

References

1. US Public Health Service. *Smoking and health. Report of the Advisory committee to the Surgeon General for the Public Health Service.* Publication No. 1103. Washington, DC: US Department of Health, Education, and Welfare, Public Health Service; 1964.

2. Jha P, Ramasundarahettige C, Landsman V, et al. 21st-century hazards of smoking and benefits of cessation in the United States. *N Engl J Med.* 2013;368:341-350.
3. Doll R, Peto R, Wheatley K, Gray R, Sutherland I. Mortality in relation to smoking: 40 years' observations on male British doctors. *BMJ.* 1994;309:901-911.

The Association Between Smoking Quantity and Lung Cancer in Men and Women

Powell HA, Iyen-Omofoman B, Hubbard RB, et al (Univ of Nottingham, England; et al)

Chest 143:123-129, 2013

Background.—Studies have shown that for the same quantity of cigarettes smoked, women are more likely to develop heart disease than men, but studies in lung cancer have produced conflicting results. We studied the association between smoking quantity and lung cancer in men and women.

Methods.—Using data from The Health Improvement Network (a UK medical research database), we generated a data set comprising 12,121 incident cases of lung cancer and 48,216 age-, sex-, and general practice-matched control subjects. We used conditional logistic regression to calculate ORs for lung cancer according to highest-ever-quantity smoked in men and women separately.

Results.—The odds of lung cancer in women who had ever smoked heavily compared with those who had never smoked were increased 19-fold (OR, 19.10; 95% CI, 16.98-21.49), which was more than for men smoking the same quantity (OR, 12.81; 95% CI, 11.52-14.24). There was strong evidence of a difference in effect of quantity smoked on lung cancer between men and women (interaction $P < .0001$), which remained after adjusting for height (a proxy marker for lung volume).

Conclusions.—Moderate and heavy smoking carry a higher risk of lung cancer in women than in men, and this difference does not seem to be explained by lung volume. The findings suggest that extrapolating risk estimates for lung cancer in men to women will underestimate the adverse impact of smoking in women.

▶ Considerable controversy surrounds the question of whether there is a gender difference in susceptibility to the adverse effects of cigarette smoking. With reference to lung cancer in particular, several studies have found that women develop lung cancer with less smoking exposure than men.[1,2] However, other studies, using data obtained predominantly by questionnaires, have not found any such differences.[3,4] This study by Powell and colleagues is an analysis of the Health Improvement Network based in the United Kingdom, a large database with more than 12 000 lung cancer cases and more than 48 000 matched controls. Forty-one percent of the cases of lung cancer were in women. Of note, as has been previously consistently observed, a higher proportion of women than men who developed lung cancer were never smokers (13% vs 8%). The odds ratios (ORs) for lung cancer in women were equal to or higher than those in men for every level of smoking: light smokers (1–9 cigarettes per day) OR, 1.06 (95% confidence interval [CI], 0.91–1.15); moderate smokers (10–19 cigarettes per day), OR, 1.32 (95% CI, 1.20–1.46); heavy smokers (> 20 cigarettes per day), OR, 1.42 (95% CI, 1.31–1.54).

This study adds evidence to the argument that women are at higher risk for lung cancer than men. The authors used height as a surrogate for lung volume to examine the question of whether the smaller lung volumes in women might explain the difference in lung cancer risk; no correlation was identified. Other factors presumably must contribute; further studies addressing the effects on lung cancer of gender differences in patterns of smoking as well as the influences of hormonal effects on carcinogen metabolism and tumor development are needed.

L. T. Tanoue, MD

References

1. Brownson RC, Chang JC, Davis JR. Gender and histologic type variations in smoking-related risk of lung cancer. *Epidemiology.* 1992;3:61-64.
2. Zang EA, Wynder EL. Differences in lung cancer risk between men and women: examination of the evidence. *J Natl Cancer Inst.* 1996;88:183-192.
3. Freedman ND, Leitzmann MF, Hollenbeck AR, Schatzkin A, Abnet CC. Cigarette smoking and subsequent risk of lung cancer in men and women: analysis of a prospective cohort study. *Lancet Oncol.* 2008;9:649-656.
4. Bain C, Feskanich D, Speizer FE, et al. Lung cancer rates in men and women with comparable histories of smoking. *J Natl Cancer Inst.* 2004;96:826-834.

21st-Century Hazards of Smoking and Benefits of Cessation in the United States
Jha P, Ramasundarahettige C, Landsman V, et al (Ctr for Global Health Res, Toronto, Canada; et al)
N Engl J Med 368:341-350, 2013

Background.—Extrapolation from studies in the 1980s suggests that smoking causes 25% of deaths among women and men 35 to 69 years of age in the United States. Nationally representative measurements of the current risks of smoking and the benefits of cessation at various ages are unavailable.

Methods.—We obtained smoking and smoking-cessation histories from 113,752 women and 88,496 men 25 years of age or older who were interviewed between 1997 and 2004 in the U.S. National Health Interview Survey and related these data to the causes of deaths that occurred by December 31, 2006 (8236 deaths in women and 7479 in men). Hazard ratios for death among current smokers, as compared with those who had never smoked, were adjusted for age, educational level, adiposity, and alcohol consumption.

Results.—For participants who were 25 to 79 years of age, the rate of death from any cause among current smokers was about three times that

TABLE 2.—Adjusted Hazard Ratios for Various Causes of Death among Current Smokers, as Compared with Those Who Never Smoked, among Women and Men 25 to 79 Years of Age*

Cause of Death	Women				Men			
	Never Smoked No. of Deaths	Current Smoker No. of Deaths	Adjusted Hazard Ratio (99% CI)	Deaths Attributable to Smoking among Smokers No. (%)	Never Smoked No. of Deaths	Current Smokers No. of Deaths	Adjusted Hazard Ratio (99% CI)	Deaths Attributable to Smoking among Smokers No. (%)
Lung cancer	61	267	17.8 (11.4–27.8)	252 (94)	44	348	14.6 (9.1–23.4)	324 (93)
Cancers other than lung cancer	544	258	1.7 (1.4–2.1)	106 (41)	280	317	2.2 (1.7–2.8)	173 (55)
All cancers	605	525	3.2 (2.6–3.9)	360 (69)	324	665	3.8 (3.1–4.8)	491 (74)
Ischemic heart disease	382	251	3.5 (2.7–4.6)	179 (72)	285	416	3.2 (2.5–4.1)	288 (69)
Stroke	150	88	3.2 (2.2–4.7)	60 (69)	74	66	1.7 (1.0–2.8)	27 (40)
Other vascular disease	252	137	3.1 (2.2–4.4)	93 (68)	141	161	2.1 (1.5–3.0)	84 (52)
All vascular diseases	784	476	3.2 (2.7–3.9)	328 (69)	500	643	2.6 (2.1–3.2)	395 (61)
Respiratory diseases	119	206	8.5 (6.1–11.8)	182 (88)	45	188	9.0 (5.6–14.4)	167 (89)
Other medical disorders not shown above	581	277	2.2 (1.7–2.8)	151 (55)	295	370	2.2 (1.7–2.9)	205 (55)
All medical disorders	2089	1484	3.0 (2.7–3.3)	986 (66)	1164	1866	2.9 (2.5–3.2)	1211 (65)
Accidents and injuries	101	95	3.9 (2.4–6.2)	0	119	164	2.1 (1.4–3.0)	0
All causes[†]	2190	1579	3.0 (2.7–3.3)	986 (62)	1283	2030	2.8 (2.4–3.1)	1211 (60)

*Hazard ratios were adjusted for age, educational level, alcohol consumption, and body-mass index.
[†]Deaths attributable to smoking were determined with the use of the hazard ratios for all medical causes of death. With the exclusion of the 199 women and 222 men who had quit smoking less than 5 years before their deaths and the exclusion of the 1795 women and 2184 men who reported a history of coronary heart disease, stroke, or cancer, the hazard ratios for all-cause mortality were 3.1 for women and 2.8 for men.

among those who had never smoked (hazard ratio for women, 3.0; 99% confidence interval [CI], 2.7 to 3.3; hazard ratio for men, 2.8; 99% CI, 2.4 to 3.1). Most of the excess mortality among smokers was due to neoplastic, vascular, respiratory, and other diseases that can be caused by smoking. The probability of surviving from 25 to 79 years of age was about twice as great in those who had never smoked as in current smokers (70% vs. 38% among women and 61% vs. 26% among men). Life expectancy was shortened by more than 10 years among the current smokers, as compared with those who had never smoked. Adults who had quit smoking at 25 to 34, 35 to 44, or 45 to 54 years of age gained about 10, 9, and 6 years of life, respectively, as compared with those who continued to smoke.

Conclusions.—Smokers lose at least one decade of life expectancy, as compared with those who have never smoked. Cessation before the age of 40 years reduces the risk of death associated with continued smoking by about 90% (Table 2).

▶ Smoking causes premature death. This indisputable fact is driven home by this study evaluating the impact of smoking and smoking cessation on mortality and survival in 113 752 women and 88 496 men, 25 years or older, who were interviewed as part of the United States National Health Interview Survey between 1997 and 2004. Table 2 shows the adjusted hazard ratios for causes of death among current smokers compared with never smokers. The adjusted hazard ratio for all causes of death in women was 3.0 (95% confidence interval [CI], 2.7–3.3) and in men was 2.8 (95% CI, 2.4–3.1). Simply put, these data indicate that the rate of death from any cause among current smokers was 3-fold that of never smokers. For lung cancer specifically, the adjusted hazard ratio for lung cancer in women was a staggering 17.8 (95% CI, 11.4–27.8) and in men was 14.6 (95% CI, 9.1–23.4).

Smoking cessation has predictable benefit with regard to improving survival. As was demonstrated in previous work by Peto and colleagues,[1] smoking cessation even into the sixth and seventh decades of life is associated with benefit, including reduction in lung cancer risk. Patients may be better able to understand the magnitude of benefit if it is expressed as years of life gained as opposed to probability of survival. As shown in Fig 3 of the original article, the younger one is at the time of smoking cessation, the more life years are gained. Smokers who quit at age 25 to 34 gain, on average, 10 years of life; smokers who quit at age 55 to 64 gain, on average, 4 years of life. It is important to note that there is still benefit even when smoking cessation comes at an older age, that is, it is never too late to quit!

L. T. Tanoue, MD

Reference

1. Peto R, Darby S, Deo H, Silcocks P, Whitley E, Doll R. Smoking, smoking cessation, and lung cancer in the UK since 1950: combination of national statistics with two case-control studies. *BMJ.* 2000;321:323-329.

Electronic cigarettes for smoking cessation: a randomised controlled trial

Bullen C, Howe C, Laugesen M, et al (The Univ of Auckland, New Zealand; Health New Zealand, Lyttelton, Christchurch; et al)

Lancet 382:1629-1637, 2013

Background.—Electronic cigarettes (e-cigarettes) can deliver nicotine and mitigate tobacco withdrawal and are used by many smokers to assist quit attempts. We investigated whether e-cigarettes are more effective than nicotine patches at helping smokers to quit.

Methods.—We did this pragmatic randomised-controlled superiority trial in Auckland, New Zealand, between Sept 6, 2011, and July 5, 2013. Adult (≥18 years) smokers wanting to quit were randomised (with computerised block randomisation, block size nine, stratified by ethnicity [Māori; Pacific; or non-Māori, non-Pacific], sex [men or women], and level of nicotine dependence [>5 or ≤5 Fagerström test for nicotine dependence]) in a 4:4:1 ratio to 16 mg nicotine e-cigarettes, nicotine patches (21 mg patch, one daily), or placebo e-cigarettes (no nicotine), from 1 week before until 12 weeks after quit day, with low intensity behavioural support via voluntary telephone counselling. The primary outcome was biochemically verified continuous abstinence at 6 months (exhaled breath carbon monoxide measurement <10 ppm). Primary analysis was by intention to treat. This trial is registered with the Australian New Zealand Clinical Trials Registry, number ACTRN12610000866000.

Findings.—657 people were randomised (289 to nicotine e-cigarettes, 295 to patches, and 73 to placebo e-cigarettes) and were included in the

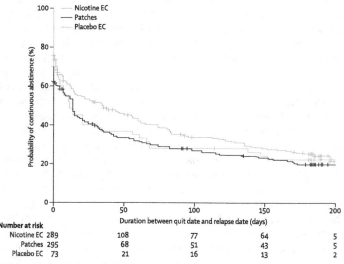

FIGURE 2.—Kaplan-Meier analysis of time to relapse. EC=e-cigarettes. (Reprinted from Bullen C, Howe C, Laugesen M, et al. Electronic cigarettes for smoking cessation: a randomised controlled trial. *Lancet.* 2013;382:1629-1637, Copyright 2013, with permission from Elsevier.)

intention-to-treat analysis. At 6 months, verified abstinence was 7·3% (21 of 289) with nicotine e-cigarettes, 5·8% (17 of 295) with patches, and 4·1% (three of 73) with placebo e-cigarettes (risk difference for nicotine e-cigarette vs patches 1·51 [95% CI −2·49 to 5·51]; for nicotine e-cigarettes vs placebo e-cigarettes 3·16 [95% CI −2·29 to 8·61]). Achievement of abstinence was substantially lower than we anticipated for the power calculation, thus we had insufficient statistical power to conclude superiority of nicotine e-cigarettes to patches or to placebo e-cigarettes. We identified no significant differences in adverse events, with 137 events in the nicotine e-cigarettes group, 119 events in the patches group, and 36 events in the placebo e-cigarettes group. We noted no evidence of an association between adverse events and study product.

Interpretation.—E-cigarettes, with or without nicotine, were modestly effective at helping smokers to quit, with similar achievement of abstinence as with nicotine patches, and few adverse events. Uncertainty exists about the place of e-cigarettes in tobacco control, and more research is urgently needed to clearly establish their overall benefits and harms at both individual and population levels (Fig 2).

▶ Electronic cigarettes (e-cigarettes) appear to be increasingly used as aids to quit smoking. They are obvious alternatives to traditional tobacco cigarettes, but unless they are marketed as smoking cessation devices, regulation by the US Food and Drug Administration is not required. Little rigorous research exists about their effects on health other than as related to smoking cessation, and even for that there have been little data available. This study by Bullen and colleagues compared the effects of e-cigarettes containing nicotine, placebo e-cigarettes without nicotine, and nicotine patches on smoking cessation in subjects who were habitual smokers of at least one-half pack of cigarettes per day. The primary outcome was abstinence from traditional cigarettes. Fig 2 shows the main findings. The use of e-cigarettes containing nicotine for 13 weeks resulted in increased smoking abstinence at 6 months compared with placebo e-cigarettes or nicotine patches, but there was no statistical difference, and the relapse to smoking rates were high in all groups. The authors conclude that nicotine e-cigarettes were at least as effective as nicotine patches.

The e-cigarette literature is full of controversy. The cartridges with which these devices are loaded vary in ingredients. Because they are not regulated, cartridge contents other than nicotine likely vary by manufacturer. Of concern, a number of potential harmful substances, including N-nitrosamines, polycyclic aromatic hydrocarbons, glycerin, and oils, have been identified in these devices, and a number of reports have documented adverse events related to their use.[1-3] It is also clear that some patients may decrease or eliminate traditional cigarette use but then become habitual e-cigarette smokers. It may take years for us to understand the health effects of substituting one smoking habit for another. Nonetheless, the consequences of cigarette smoking are very clear. Given the struggle to get the smoking rate of adult Americans below its current level of approximately

20%, it will be necessary to try to understand the short- and long-term risks as well as benefits of cigarette replacement therapies of all varieties.

L. T. Tanoue, MD

References

1. Avdalovic MV, Murin S. Electronic cigarettes: no such thing as a free lunch...Or puff. *Chest.* 2012;141:1371-1372.
2. Vardavas CI, Anagnostopoulos N, Kougias M, Evangelopoulou V, Connolly GN, Behrakis PK. Short-term pulmonary effects of using an electronic cigarette: impact on respiratory flow resistance, impedance, and exhaled nitric oxide. *Chest.* 2012; 141:1400-1406.
3. McCauley L, Markin C, Hosmer D. An unexpected consequence of electronic cigarette use. *Chest.* 2012;141:1110-1113.

Lung Cancer Screening

Screening for Lung Cancer: U.S. Preventive Services Task Force Recommendation Statement
Moyer VA, on behalf of the U.S. Preventive Services Task Force (U.S. Preventive Services Task Force, Rockville, MD)
Ann Intern Med 2013 [Epub ahead of print]

Description.—Update of the 2004 U.S. Preventive Services Task Force (USPSTF) recommendation on screening for lung cancer.

Methods.—The USPSTF reviewed the evidence on the efficacy of low-dose computed tomography, chest radiography, and sputum cytologic evaluation for lung cancer screening in asymptomatic persons who are at average or high risk for lung cancer (current or former smokers) and the benefits and harms of these screening tests and of surgical resection of early-stage non–small cell lung cancer. The USPSTF also commissioned modeling studies to provide information about the optimum age at which to begin and end screening, the optimum screening interval, and the relative benefits and harms of different screening strategies.

Population.—This recommendation applies to asymptomatic adults aged 55 to 80 years who have a 30 pack-year smoking history and currently smoke or have quit within the past 15 years.

Recommendation.—The USPSTF recommends annual screening for lung cancer with low-dose computed tomography in adults aged 55 to 80 years who have a 30 pack-year smoking history and currently smoke or have quit within the past 15 years. Screening should be discontinued once a person has not smoked for 15 years or develops a health problem that substantially limits life expectancy or the ability or willingness to have curative lung surgery. (B recommendation) (Table)

▶ The United States Preventive Services Task Force (USPSTF) finalized its updated recommendation on screening for lung cancer at the end of 2013. The new recommendation is as follows:

TABLE.—Screening Scenarios From CISNET Models*

| Minimum Pack-Years at Screening, n | Screening Scenario† | | | Benefit | | | Harm‡ | | CT Screens per Lung Cancer Death Averted, n |
	Minimum Age at Which to Begin Screening, y	Time Since Last Cigarette, y	Population Ever Screened, %	Lung Cancer Deaths Averted, %	Lung Cancer Deaths Averted, n	Total CT Screens, n	Radiation-Induced Lung Cancer Deaths, n	Overdiagnosis, %§	
40	60	25	13.0	11.0	410	171 924	17	11.2	437
40	55	25	13.9	12.3	458	221 606	20	11.1	506
30	60	25	18.8	13.3	495	253 095	21	11.9	534
30	**55**	**15**	**19.3**	**14.0**	**521**	**286 813**	**24**	**9.9**	**577**
20	60	25	24.8	15.4	573	327 024	25	9.8	597
30	55	25	20.4	15.8	588	342 880	25	10.0	609
20	55	25	27.4	17.9	664	455 381	31	10.4	719
10	55	25	36.0	19.4	721	561 744	35	9.5	819

CISNET = Cancer Intervention and Surveillance Modeling Network; CT = computed tomography.
*All scenarios model the results of following a cohort of 100 000 persons from age 45 to 90 y or until death from any cause, with a varying number of smokers and former smokers screened on the basis of smoking history, age, and years since stopping smoking. Bold text indicates the screening scenario with a reasonable balance of benefits and harms and that is recommended by the U.S. Preventive Services Task Force.
†In all scenarios, screening is continued through age 80 y.
‡Number of CT screenings is a measure of harm because it relates to the number of patients who will have risk for overdiagnosis and potential consequences from false-positive results.
§Percentage of screen-detected cancer that is overdiagnosis; that is, cancer that would not have been diagnosed in the patient's lifetime without screening.

"The USPSTF recommends annual screening for lung cancer with low-dose computed tomography in adults aged 55 to 80 years who have a 30 pack-year *30 PY* smoking history and currently smoke or have quit within the past 15 years. *15 years* Screening should be discontinued once a person has not smoked for 15 years *(55-80)* or develops a health problem that substantially limits life expectancy or the ability or willingness to have curative lung surgery."

The recommendation was given a B grade, the definition of which is, "The USPSTF recommends the service. There is high certainty that the net benefit is moderate or there is moderate certainty that the net benefit is moderate to substantial." The USPSTF suggestion for practice is "Offer/provide this service." To inform this recommendation, the USPSTF performed a comprehensive systematic evidence review of all relevant screening trials, the largest and most compelling of which was the National Lung Screening Trial.[1] Additionally, modeling studies were performed by the Cancer Intervention and Surveillance Modeling Network (CISNET), which examined the harms and benefits relating to different screening scenarios.[2] CISNET considered scenarios with varying minimum pack-years of smoking, ages at beginning screening, and years since the last cigarette smoked. As is evident in the Table, the number of computed tomography screenings needing to be performed to avert one lung cancer death was lowest in the highest risk group, which had the most intense smoking history and was older at the age of screening initiation. This article also describes the guidelines of several of the major societies and institutions focusing on lung cancer, as these differ from each other as well as from the USPSTF in the specific recommendations relating to the intensity of smoking that would warrant screening, at what ages to start and stop screening, and whether to consider risk factors for lung cancer other than smoking.

The USPSTF recommendation is the most powerful endorsement of lung cancer screening to date. It now seems inevitable that insurance carriers, including Medicare, will cover the service. It is our responsibility to ensure that screening, as it is introduced into the community, is performed appropriately and safely to maximize benefit and minimize harm.

L. T. Tanoue, MD

References

1. National Lung Screening Trial Research Team, Aberle DR, Adams AM, Berg CD, et al. Reduced lung-cancer mortality with low-dose computed tomographic screening. *N Engl J Med.* 2011;365:395-409.
2. de Koning H, Meza R, Plevritis SK, et al. *Benefits and Harms of Computed Tomography Lung Cancer Screening Programs for High-Risk Populations.* AHRQ Publication No. 13—05196-EF-2. Rockville, MD: Agency for Healthcare Research and Quality; 2013.

Benefits and Harms of Computed Tomography Lung Cancer Screening Programs for High-Risk Populations
National Cancer Institute, Cancer Intervention and Surveillance Modeling Network, Lung Cancer Working Group (Erasmus MC, the Netherlands; Univ of Michigan, Ann Arbor; Stanford Univ, CA; et al) 2013

Background.—The National Lung Screening Trial (NLST) demonstrated that three annual computed tomography (CT) screenings reduced lung cancer-specific mortality by 20% compared with annual chest radiography screenings in a volunteer population of current and former smokers ages 55 to 74 years with at least 30 pack-years of cigarette smoking history and no more than 15 years since quitting for former smokers. To inform the updated U.S. Preventive Services Task Force recommendations on lung cancer screening, we assessed the benefits and harms of CT screening programs that varied by age, pack-year, and years since quitting criteria, as well as the frequency of screening.

Methods.—Five independent microsimulation models estimated the long-term harms and benefits of screening as experienced by the U.S. cohort born in 1950. The five models were calibrated to the NLST to predict lung cancer outcomes consistent with the trial's observations. These models were also then calibrated to the lung cancer screening portion of the Prostate, Lung, Colorectal, and Ovarian Cancer Screening Trial. We evaluated 576 scenarios with annual or less frequent screening of individuals between the ages of 45 and 85 years, for a range of minimum smoking exposure (measured in pack-years) and maximum time since quitting. Screening benefits are expressed in terms of the percentage of cancers detected at an early stage (stages I or II), percentage and absolute number of lung cancer deaths prevented, and life-years gained compared with a reference scenario with no screening. Screening harms are expressed as the number of CT screenings required (and percentage of the cohort ever screened), number of followup imaging examinations, and number of overdiagnosed lung cancers and radiation-related lung cancer deaths. We identified consensus strategies that the models identified as efficient, preventing the greatest number of lung cancer deaths for the screening examinations required. Counts and percentages reported are calculated as averages of outcomes from the five models, following a 100,000 person cohort from ages 45 to 90 years.

Results.—The models ranked strategies similarly and identified a consensus set of programs. We focus in this report on 26 efficient screening scenarios that start screening at age 50, 55, or 60 years and stop screening at age 80 or 85 years. Among these 26 programs, triennial screening reduced total lung cancer mortality in the cohort by 5% to 6% compared with biennial programs that reduced mortality by 7% to 10% and annual programs that reduced mortality by 11% to 21%. When we focused on annual programs that began screening at age 55 or 60 years, ended screening at age 80 years, and required between 200,000 to 600,000 screenings per 100,000 persons, a set of seven programs remained. We added a lower-intensity

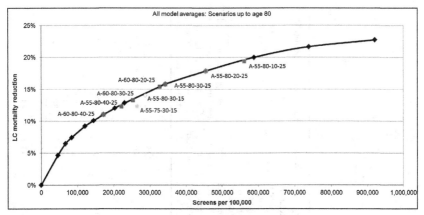

FIGURE 3.—Estimated lung cancer mortality reduction (Average of Five Models) from annual computed tomography screening in the 1950 birth cohort for programs with eligible ages of 55 to 80 years and different smoking eligibility cutoffs*. (Reprinted from National Cancer Institute, Cancer Intervention and Surveillance Modeling Network, Lung Cancer Working Group. Benefits and harms of computed tomography lung cancer screening programs for high-risk populations. 2013.)

reference scenario, for a total of eight programs. These eight programs include a program similar to the NLST criteria except for the stopping age: starting annual screening at age 55 years, ending at age 80 years for ever-smokers with at least 30 pack-years, and no more than 15 years since quitting for former smokers. With this program, 19.3% of the cohort would be screened at least once, requiring 287,000 CT screenings per 100,000 persons, leading to 50% of lung cancers being detected at an early stage and a 14% lung cancer mortality reduction (about 520 lung cancer deaths averted per 100,000 population), resulting in about 5,500 life-years gained per 100,000 population. These benefits must be weighed against the following harms: 330,000 CT examinations per 100,000 persons (screenings and followup CT scans), an estimated 4% overdiagnosis rate (of all lung cancers in the cohort), and 0.8% of lung cancer deaths (24 per 100,000 population) related to radiation exposure (based on two models). Important tradeoffs between the eight programs are discussed.

Conclusions.—Our findings support a range of possible lung cancer screening programs, including annual lung cancer screening of individuals with at least 30 pack-years of smoking who are between the ages of 55 and 80 years, but cannot determine which tradeoff of harms and benefits is "best." Scenarios with an older starting age (60 years) but increased maximum years since quitting (from 15 to 25 years) offer different tradeoffs of benefits and harms (depending on the minimum pack-years). Extending eligibility to individuals with fewer pack-years—although still efficient—leads to additional benefits but more additional harms. Overdiagnosis remained limited for annual screening (Fig 3, Table 2).

▶ The current draft recommendation by the United States Preventive Services Task Force (USPSTF) now supports screening of high-risk individuals with

TABLE 2. —Benefits of 26 Selected Efficient Screening Programs and the Screening Program Most Similar to NLST Eligibility Criteria (Average of Results From Five Models)

Scenario	Percentage Ever Screened	CT Screenings Per 100,000	Percentage of Cases Detected at an Early Stage*	Lung Cancer Mortality Reduction	Average Lung Cancer Deaths Averted Per 100,000**	Life-Years Gained Per 100,000	Life-Years Gained Per Death Averted	Relative Increase in Screenings Compared With Previous Scenario (%)	Relative Increase in Lung Cancer Deaths Averted Compared With Previous Scenario (%)	Screenings Per Life-Year Gained	Screenings Per Lung Cancer Death Averted	Number of Persons Needed to Screen (Ever) Per Lung Cancer Death Averted
Triennial Screening												
T-60-80-40-10	11.2%	45,685	42.0%	4.6%	172	1,823	10.6			25	265	65
T-60-85-40-10	11.3%	48,317	42.6%	5.1%	190	1,894	10.0			26	254	59
T-60-85-40-15	12.0%	55,316	43.3%	5.4%	201	2,000	10.0			28	275	60
T-60-85-40-25	13.0%	66,333	44.1%	6.0%	225	2,252	10.0			29	294	58
Biennial Screening												
B-60-80-40-10	11.2%	67,167	44.0%	6.5%	241	2,526	10.5			27	278	47
B-60-85-40-10	11.3%	69,662	44.3%	6.9%	256	2,665	10.4			26	272	44
B-60-85-40-15	12.0%	79,757	45.3%	7.4%	275	2,882	10.5			28	290	44
B-60-80-40-25	13.0%	90,337	45.5%	7.7%	286	3,017	10.6			30	315	45
B-60-85-40-25	13.0%	95,914	46.3%	8.4%	312	3,045	9.8			32	307	42
B-60-85-30-20	17.9%	127,046	47.5%	9.6%	358	3,451	9.6			37	354	50
Annual Screening												
A-60-80-40-25†	13.0%	171,924	48.1%	11.0%	410	4,211	10.3	ref	ref	41	419	32

Program												
A-60-85-40-25	13.0%	185,451	49.4%	12.1%	449	4,203	9.4			44	413	29
A-55-85-40-20	14.0%	220,505	50.0%	13.0%	485	4,811	9.9			46	454	29
A-55-80-40-25†	13.9%	221,606	49.2%	12.3%	458	4,777	10.4	29%	12%	46	483	30
A-60-80-30-25†	18.8%	253,095	50.4%	13.3%	495	4,940	10.0	14%	8%	51	511	38
A-55-75-30-15‡	19.2%	265,049	48.4%	12.3%	459	5,375	11.7			49	577	42
A-60-85-30-25	18.8%	271,152	52.1%	14.7%	547	5,322	9.7			51	495	34
A-50-85-40-25	14.6%	281,218	51.4%	14.6%	542	5,908	10.9			48	518	27
A-55-80-30-15‡	19.3%	286,813	50.5%	14.0%	521	5,517	10.6	13%	5%	52	550	37
A-60-80-20-25†	24.8%	327,024	51.9%	15.4%	573	5,707	10.0	14%	10%	57	570	43
A-55-80-30-25†	20.4%	342,880	52.1%	15.8%	588	6,321	10.8	5%	3%	54	583	35
A-60-85-20-25	24.8%	348,894	53.7%	16.8%	624	5,934	9.5			59	559	40
A-55-80-20-25†	27.4%	455,381	53.9%	17.9%	664	7,092	10.7	33%	13%	64	685	41
A-55-85-20-25	27.4%	477,334	55.6%	19.1%	712	7,490	10.5			64	670	38
A-55-80-10-25†	36.0%	561,744	55.2%	19.4%	721	7,693	10.7	23%	9%	73	777	50
A-50-80-20-25	29.0%	588,516	55.2%	20.0%	743	8,530	11.5			69	792	39
A-50-85-20-25	29.0%	610,443	56.9%	21.2%	787	8,948	11.4			68	775	37

Note: All counts are cumulative, per a cohort of 100,000 persons age 45 years, followed until age 90 years. Radiation-related lung cancer deaths are not included in lung cancer deaths in Table 2 (see Table 3).

*Percentage of cases detected at an early stage in no screening scenario was 37.4%.

**Average lung cancer deaths in no screening scenario was 3,719 per 100,000 persons.

†Consensus efficient annual programs with a stopping age of 80 years and screening counts between 200,000 and 600,000, plus an 8th program (A60-80-40-25) with just under 200,000 screenings included as a reference program.

‡Denotes eligibility most similar to the NLST.

low-dose computed tomography (CT).[1] This publication by de Koning and colleagues on behalf of the Cancer Intervention and Surveillance Modeling Network (CISNET) was prepared for the Agency for Healthcare Research and Quality. It provides the important analysis leading to the change in the USPSTF recommendation.

Using individual de-identified data from the National Lung Screening Trial (NLST) and the lung cancer screening portion of the Prostate, Lung, Colorectal and Ovarian Cancer Screening Trial, the CISNET group developed 5 independent models estimating the benefits and long-term harms of screening as experienced by the US cohort born in 1950. All 5 models included dose-response information relating to cigarette exposure. Importantly, CISNET conducted the study with the intent of extrapolating the NLST findings to screening programs that could potentially be adopted in the general population. Twenty-six scenarios were examined, with variation in the ages of when screening would start (range, 45–60 years) and end (range, 75–85 years), the frequency of screening (annual, biennial, triennial), and eligibility based on minimum number of pack-years smoked (range, 10–40 pack years) and maximum number of years since quitting (10–25 years). As outlined in Table 2, these scenarios then were applied to yield a series of outcome measurements, including lung cancer mortality reduction, CT screenings, life-years gained, and screenings per lung cancer death averted, with considerable variation in outcomes depending on the screening scenario. In Table 2, the NLST criteria are identified as A55-75-30-15. Expanding the NLST age criteria by 5 years (A55-80-30-15) or extending the beginning and stopping of screening by 5 years and extending the time since quitting to up to 25 years (A60-80-30-25), resulted in the same number of screenings leading to more lung cancer deaths averted than in the NLST. Table 2 also shows that extending the age of screening to 85 also achieves larger lung cancer mortality reductions but at the expense of a substantial increase in the number of screenings. The study group elected to focus on scenarios stopping screening at age 80 because of the increased risk of treatment in older individuals with heavy smoking histories and presumed higher comorbidities. Fig 3 graphically depicts the efficiency (lung cancer mortality reduction vs number of screens per 100 000) for multiple annual lung cancer screening scenarios. As would be anticipated, annual screening in an older population with more intense smoking was more efficient than screening a younger population with less smoking, but benefit was gained even in the latter groups, although at the price of considerably more screening interventions.

The take-home message is that, based on the CISNET modeling, a range of different screening scenarios are possible and arguably valid, with different balances of benefits and harms. The most efficient scenarios offer an efficiency of screening similar to that of the NLST. Extending screening to individuals who are younger or have fewer pack-years of smoking may still be beneficial and efficient but will lead to additional harms. The current USPSTF draft recommendation, which recommends screening for individuals ages 55 to 80, already extends the age of screening by 5 years more than the NLST and, at least in its current format, refrains from dictating the exact number of pack-years or the number of years since quitting. This leaves a fair amount of discretion in the hands of practitioners for whom this work by CISNET should provide some guidance.

L. T. Tanoue, MD

Reference

1. Screening for Lung Cancer: Draft Recommendation Statement. AHRQ Publication No. 13—05196-EF-3, 2013. (Accessed December 9, 2013)

Selection Criteria for Lung-Cancer Screening
Tammemägi MC, Katki HA, Hocking WG, et al (Brock Univ, St. Catharines, Ontario, Canada; Division of Cancer Epidemiology and Genetics, Rockville, MD; Marshfield Clinic Res Foundation, WI; et al)
N Engl J Med 368:728-736, 2013

Background.—The National Lung Screening Trial (NLST) used risk factors for lung cancer (e.g., $\geq$30 pack-years of smoking and <15 years since quitting) as selection criteria for lung-cancer screening. Use of an accurate model that incorporates additional risk factors to select persons for screening may identify more persons who have lung cancer or in whom lung cancer will develop.

Methods.—We modified the 2011 lung-cancer risk-prediction model from our Prostate, Lung, Colorectal, and Ovarian (PLCO) Cancer Screening Trial to ensure applicability to NLST data; risk was the probability of a diagnosis of lung cancer during the 6-year study period. We developed and validated the model ($PLCO_{M2012}$) with data from the 80,375 persons in the PLCO control and intervention groups who had ever smoked. Discrimination (area under the receiver-operating-characteristic curve [AUC]) and calibration were assessed. In the validation data set, 14,144 of 37,332 persons (37.9%) met NLST criteria. For comparison, 14,144 highest-risk persons were considered positive (eligible for screening) according to $PLCO_{M2012}$ criteria. We compared the accuracy of $PLCO_{M2012}$ criteria with NLST criteria to detect lung cancer. Cox models were used to evaluate whether the reduction in mortality among 53,202 persons undergoing low-dose computed tomographic screening in the NLST differed according to risk.

Results.—The AUC was 0.803 in the development data set and 0.797 in the validation data set. As compared with NLST criteria, $PLCO_{M2012}$ criteria had improved sensitivity (83.0% vs. 71.1%, $P < 0.001$) and positive predictive value (4.0% vs. 3.4%, $P = 0.01$), without loss of specificity (62.9% and. 62.7%, respectively; $P = 0.54$); 41.3% fewer lung cancers were missed. The NLST screening effect did not vary according to $PLCO_{M2012}$ risk ($P = 0.61$ for interaction).

TABLE 2.—Modified Logistic-Regression Prediction Model (PLCO$_{M2012}$) of Cancer Risk for 36,286 Control Participants Who Had Ever Smoked*

Variable	Odds Ratio (95% CI)	P Value	Beta Coefficient
Age, per 1–yr increase[†]	1.081 (1.057–1.105)	<0.001	0.0778868
Race or ethnic group[‡]			
White	1.000		Reference group
Black	1.484 (1.083–2.033)	0.01	0.3944778
Hispanic	0.475 (0.195–1.160)	0.10	−0.7434744
Asian	0.627 (0.332–1.185)	0.15	−0.466585
American Indian or Alaskan Native	1		0
Native Hawaiian or Pacific Islander	2.793 (0.992–7.862)	0.05	1.027152
Education, per increase of 1 level[†§]	0.922 (0.874–0.972)	0.003	−0.0812744
Body-mass index, per 1-unit increase[†]	0.973 (0.955–0.991)	0.003	−0.0274194
Chronic obstructive pulmonary disease (yes vs. no)	1.427 (1.162–1.751)	0.001	0.3553063
Personal history of cancer (yes vs. no)	1.582 (1.172–2.128)	0.003	0.4589971
Family history of lung cancer (yes vs. no)	1.799 (1.471–2.200)	<0.001	0.587185
Smoking status (current vs. former)	1.297 (1.047–1.605)	0.02	0.2597431
Smoking intensity[¶]			−1.822606
Duration of smoking, per 1-yr increase[†]	1.032 (1.014–1.051)	0.001	0.0317321
Smoking quit time, per 1-yr increase[†]	0.970 (0.950–0.990)	0.003	−0.0308572
Model constant			−4.532506

*To calculate the 6-year probability of lung cancer in an individual person with the use of categorical variables, multiply the variable or the level beta coefficient of the variable by 1 if the factor is present and by 0 if it is absent. For continuous variables other than smoking intensity, subtract the centering value from the person's value and multiply the difference by the beta coefficient of the variable. For smoking intensity, calculate the contribution of the variable to the model by dividing by 10, exponentiating by the power −1, centering by subtracting 0.4021541613, and multiplying this number by the beta coefficient of the variable. Add together all the previously calculated beta-coefficient products and the model constant. This sum is called the model logit. To obtain the person's 6-year lung-cancer probability, calculate $e^{logit}/(1+e^{logit})$. CI denotes confidence interval.

[†]Age was centered on 62 years, education was centered on level 4, body-mass index was centered on 27, duration of smoking was centered on 27 years, and smoking quit time was centered on 10 years.

[‡]Race or ethnic group was self-reported.

[§]Education was measured in six ordinal levels: less than high-school graduate (level 1), high-school graduate (level 2), some training after high school (level 3), some college (level 4), college graduate (level 5), and postgraduate or professional degree (level 6).

[¶]Smoking intensity (the average number of cigarettes smoked per day) had a nonlinear association with lung cancer, and this variable was transformed. For this reason, the odds ratio is not directly interpretable in a meaningful fashion.

Conclusions.—The use of the PLCO$_{M2012}$ model was more sensitive than the NLST criteria for lung-cancer detection (Tables 2 and 4).

▶ The National Lung Screening Trial (NLST) found a 20% reduction in lung cancer mortality in a population, age 55 to 74 years with a history of at least 30 pack-years of smoking, who were currently smoking or had quit within the previous 15 years, and who were screened with annual low-dose chest computed tomography scan as opposed to chest radiography.[1] In contrast, the Prostate, Lung, Colorectal, and Ovarian (PLCO) Cancer Screening Trial found no reduction in lung cancer mortality when annual chest radiography as the lung cancer screening intervention was compared with no screening.[2] On the basis of these 2 landmark studies, the United States Preventive Services Task Force has issued a draft recommendation change recommending lung cancer screening in persons at high risk based on smoking and age.[3]

The PLCO trial is still ongoing. Initiated in 1993, it has enrolled more than 154 000 subjects in the United States age 55 to 74 years and is designed to

TABLE 4.—Accuracy of Lung-Cancer Classification According to Alternative Criteria in the PLCO Intervention-Group Smokers*

Criteria[†]	Participants with Lung Cancer (N = 678)	Participants without Lung Cancer (N = 36,654)	Total Participants (N = 37,332)	Predictive Value
NLST				
Criteria positive	482 TP (3.4%)	13,662 FP (96.6%)	14,144	PPV, 3.4%
Criteria negative	196 FN (0.8%)	22,992 TN (99.2%)	23,188	NPV, 99.2%
Sensitivity	71.1%			
Specificity		62.7%		
PLCO$_{M2012}$[‡]				
Criteria positive	563 TP (4.0%)	13,581 FP (96%)	14,144	PPV, 4.0%
Criteria negative	115 FN (0.5%)	23,073 TN (99.5%)	23,188	NPV, 99.5%
Sensitivity	83.0%			
Specificity		62.9%		

*FN denotes false negative, FP false positive, NPV negative predictive value, PPV positive predictive value, TN true negative, and TP true positive.
†NLST criteria for study entry included a history of cigarette smoking of at least 30 pack-years and, for former smokers, cessation within the previous 15 years.
‡According to the PLCO$_{M2012}$ criteria, positivity was defined as a probability of lung cancer that was greater than 1.3455% over a period of 6 years.

assess the effect of screening interventions on mortality from 4 different cancers, including lung cancer. Smoking was not a required entry criterion. Although no benefit in lung cancer mortality was seen in the PLCO trial from screening with chest radiography, the PLCO has ongoing tremendous value related to its potential to develop risk-predictive tools for lung cancer.

A previous article by Tammemagi and colleagues in 2011 described 2 lung cancer risk predictive models developed from the PLCO database, one for the general population and one for a population of ever smokers.[4] The current report describes an updated prediction model for the latter population, which the authors named *PLCO$_{M2012}$*. Importantly, the model acknowledges that the selection criteria of the NLST excludes many known risk factors for lung cancer, and limiting screening to individuals meeting the NLST criteria will inevitably result in many persons with lung cancer not ever being identified for screening. Ideally, accurate lung cancer risk prediction models should be better able to identify persons at highest risk, and using such models should result in a reasonable number of persons needing to be screened to save a life that otherwise would be lost. This point was highlighted in a commentary by Bach and Gould pointing out that the number of persons needing to be screened to prevent one lung cancer death varied tremendously depending on the compiled risks of individuals, even within the group meeting the NLST criteria.[5]

In the original PLCO predictive model, significant contributing factors included age, level of education, body mass index (BMI), family history of lung cancer, chronic obstructive pulmonary disease (COPD), chest radiography in the previous 3 years, smoking status, pack-year smoking history, duration of smoking, and quit time. Risks were based on a median follow-up of 9.2 years. The updated model was refined and updated to be directly applicable to NLST data, and then a comparison was made between the NSLT criteria and the revised model in their respective abilities to select the population at risk for lung cancer. The subjects included the 51 033 individuals who participated in the NLST. The comparison sample from the PLCO was identified by applying the NLST criteria to the 73 618 smokers in the PLCO study and adjusting for the NLST follow-up period. Six-year risk was defined as low (<1.0%), intermediate (1.0% to <2.0%), or high (2.0% or more).

The risk of lung cancer in $PLCO_{M2012}$ increased with age, black vs white race, lower socioeconomic status (surrogate = education), lower BMI, self-reported history of COPD, personal history of cancer, family history of lung cancer, current smoking, increased smoking intensity (average cigarettes per day) and duration, and shorter time since quitting (Table 2). The distributions of true- and false-positive and negative results comparing the NLST criteria and the $PLCO_{M2012}$ are shown in Table 4. In comparing the selection of persons who eventually had lung cancer diagnosed by NLST criteria vs the model, the sensitivities were 71.1% vs 83.0%, whereas the specificities were 62.7% vs 62.9%, respectively. The false-positive rates for both approaches remained very high (96.6% and 96%, respectively). Overall, the $PLCO_{M2012}$ model identified 81 more of the 678 lung cancers eventually found in the NLST than did the NLST criteria.

The $PLCO_{M2012}$ clearly performs better than the NLST criteria in identifying a population at risk for lung cancer and represents an important step in what should be a more comprehensive approach to individual risk assessment. It is still imperfect. $PLCO_{M2012}$ excludes persons who have never smoked; for that population, there is no reliable model for lung cancer risk prediction. Considering that 15% of women with lung cancer in the United States are never smokers, this highlights a gaping need. The age of persons who can be examined by the model is limited to 55 to 74 years, which excludes an older population for whom risk is presumably actually increasing because of age. Because the average age at presentation with lung cancer is in the early 70s, this is a significant limitation.

Importantly, when compared with the NLST criteria, the predictive model identifies a higher number of cancers for the number of persons screened. This should result in better cost effectiveness as well as additional saved lives. Use of such models should be incorporated into daily clinical life, with the goal of providing clinicians with tools that can facilitate early detection of lung cancer and decrease the burden of mortality.

L. T. Tanoue, MD

References

1. Aberle DR, Adams AM, Berg CD, et al; National Lung Screening Trial Research Team. Reduced lung-cancer mortality with low-dose computed tomographic screening. *N Engl J Med.* 2011;365:395-409.
2. Oken MM, Hocking WG, Kvale PA, et al. Screening by chest radiograph and lung cancer mortality: the Prostate, Lung, Colorectal, and Ovarian (PLCO) randomized trial. *JAMA.* 2011;306:1865-1873.
3. Screening for Lung Cancer: Draft Recommendation Statement. 2013 [cited 2013 December 9, 2013].
4. Tammemagi CM, Pinsky PF, Caporaso NE, et al. Lung cancer risk prediction: prostate, Lung, Colorectal And Ovarian Cancer Screening Trial models and validation. *J Natl Cancer Inst.* 2011;103:1058-1068.
5. Bach PB, Gould MK. When the average applies to no one: personalized decision making about potential benefits of lung cancer screening. *Ann Intern Med.* 2012;157:571-573.

American Cancer Society Lung Cancer Screening Guidelines
Wender R, Fontham ETH, Barrera E Jr, et al (Thomas Jefferson Univ Med College, Philadelphia, PA; Louisiana State Univ Health Science Ctr, New Orleans; Univ Health System, Evanston, IL; et al)
CA Cancer J Clin 63:107-117, 2013

Findings from the National Cancer Institute's National Lung Screening Trial established that lung cancer mortality in specific high-risk groups can be reduced by annual screening with low-dose computed tomography. These findings indicate that the adoption of lung cancer screening could save many lives. Based on the results of the National Lung Screening Trial, the American Cancer Society is issuing an initial guideline for lung cancer screening. This guideline recommends that clinicians with access to high-volume, high-quality lung cancer screening and treatment centers should initiate a discussion about screening with apparently healthy patients aged 55 years to 74 years who have at least a 30-pack-year smoking history and who currently smoke or have quit within the past 15 years. A process of informed and shared decision-making with a clinician related to the potential benefits, limitations, and harms associated with screening for lung cancer with low-dose computed tomography should occur before any decision is made to initiate lung cancer screening. Smoking cessation counseling remains a high priority for clinical attention in discussions with current smokers, who should be informed of their continuing risk of lung cancer. Screening should not be viewed as an alternative to smoking cessation.

▶ The publication of the National Lung Screening Trial (NLST) prompted the major societies and institutions with an interest in lung cancer to publish new screening guidelines.[1] The American Cancer Society and the American College of Chest Physicians both now recommend that screening be done in asymptomatic persons ages 55 to 74 years with at least a 30 pack-year smoking history who are currently smoking or have quit within the previous 15 years, and that screening be performed within the context of a high-quality, high-volume screening center.[2] These criteria match the entry criteria of the NLST, and it is in this specific population that the mortality benefit from screening was shown. Other guidelines from the National Comprehensive Cancer Network and the American Academy of Thoracic Surgeons recommend screening for broader populations, extending the age of screening to both younger and older persons and in persons with risks for lung cancer other than smoking (eg, family history, underlying lung disease, occupational exposure). These extensions of screening to non-NLST populations are not grounded in evidence but acknowledge our awareness that substantial lung cancer risk exists for groups of individuals who do not exactly fit the NLST criteria. However, rigorous studies of screening for lung cancer in these populations are unlikely to be accomplished, and so it is unlikely that we will ever have the evidence base to precisely answer the question of benefit vs risk of screening for all patients. The decision to screen a person for lung cancer who does not meet NLST criteria resides in an individual discussion between patient and practitioner. For these discussions, an objective lung cancer risk predictive model, such as the one developed by Tammemagi and colleagues out of the Prostate, Lung, Colon, Ovarian Screening Trial, could be clinically very useful.[3]

L. T. Tanoue, MD

References

1. Aberle DR, Adams AM, Berg CD, et al. Reduced lung-cancer mortality with low-dose computed tomographic screening. *N Engl J Med.* 2011;365:395-409.
2. Detterbeck FC, Mazzone PJ, Naidich DP, Bach PB. Screening for lung cancer: diagnosis and management of lung cancer, 3rd ed: American College of Chest Physicians evidence-based clinical practice guidelines. *Chest.* 2013;143:e78S-e92S.
3. Tammemägi MC, Katki HA, Hocking WG, et al. Selection criteria for lung-cancer screening. *N Engl J Med.* 2013;368:728-736.

Interstitial Lung Abnormalities in a CT Lung Cancer Screening Population: Prevalence and Progression Rate

Jin GY, Lynch D, Chawla A, et al (Res Inst of Clinical Medicine, Jeonju, Jeonbuk, South Korea; Natl Jewish Health, Denver, Colorado; Sri Aurobindo Inst of Med Sciences, Indore, India; et al)
Radiology 268:563-571, 2013

Purpose.—To determine the prevalence of interstitial lung abnormalities (ILAs) at initial computed tomography (CT) examination and the rate of progression of ILAs on 2-year follow-up CT images in a National Lung Screening Trial population studied at a single site.

Materials and Methods.—The study was approved by the institutional review board and informed consent was obtained from all participants. Image review for this study was HIPAA compliant. We reviewed the CT images of 884 cigarette smokers who underwent low-dose CT at a single site in the National Lung Screening Trial. CT findings were categorized as having no evidence of ILA, equivocal for ILA, or ILA. We categorized the type of ILA as nonfibrotic (ground-glass opacity, consolidation, mosaic attenuation), or fibrotic (ground glass with reticular pattern, reticular pattern, honeycombing). We evaluated the temporal change of the CT findings (no change, improvement, or progression) of ILA at 2-year follow-up. A χ^2 with Fisher exact test or unpaired t test was used to determine whether smoking parameters were associated with progression of ILA at 2-year follow-up CT.

Results.—The prevalence of ILA was 9.7% (86 of 884 participants; 95% confidence interval: 7.9%, 11.9%), with a further 11.5% (102 of 884 participants) who had findings equivocal for ILA. The pattern was fibrotic in 19 (2.1%), nonfibrotic in 52 (5.9%), and mixed fibrotic and nonfibrotic in 15 (1.7%) of the 86 participants with ILA. The percentage of current smokers ($P = .001$) and mean number of cigarette pack-years ($P = .001$) were significantly higher in those with ILA than those without. At 2-year follow-up of those with ILA ($n = 79$), findings of nonfibrotic ILA improved in 49% of cases and progressed in 11%. Fibrotic ILA improved in 0% and progressed in 37% of cases.

Conclusion.—ILA is common in cigarette smokers. Nonfibrotic ILA improved in about 50% of cases, and fibrotic ILA progressed in about 37%.

▶ As computed tomography (CT) scanning of the chest and abdomen became part of the routine radiologic evaluation for a multitude of symptoms and diseases, incidental pulmonary nodules discovered in the course of such imaging became much more frequent. Pulmonary nodules are even more common when CT scanning is done for lung cancer screening, although in this scenario they would not be considered incidental. However, several nonnodule incidental findings on these scans may herald the presence of other diseases that would otherwise have gone unrecognized. Because screening is targeted to a population of heavy smokers of older age, it is not surprising that other tobacco-related diseases, most prominently chronic obstructive pulmonary disease and cardiovascular disease, would be common in those individuals.[1-3] Screening CT provides an opportunity to identify and perhaps quantitate those illnesses.

This article by Jin and colleagues highlights the observation that interstitial lung disease may also be identified by screening CT. Further, the fact that screening imaging studies are performed serially presents an opportunity to monitor progression (or not) of such abnormalities over time. In this study, a surprising 10% of the study population was found to have fibrotic interstitial lung changes; most of these abnormalities were nonfibrotic, but 2% of study subjects had fibrotic lung disease. The presence of interstitial lung abnormalities was associated with higher levels of cigarette consumption as measured by the median number of pack-years as well as the percentage of current smokers. Of note, none of the subjects with fibrotic interstitial abnormalities had improvement over the 2 years of follow-up, and a third of these patients had worsening of their interstitial findings over that timeframe.

Lung cancer screening with low-dose chest CT has the potential to yield valuable information about diseases other than lung cancer, particularly those associated with cigarette smoking. If this additional information can be harnessed without adding cost, low-dose CT screening may have the potential to increase health care efficiency.

L. T. Tanoue, MD

References

1. Mets OM, de Jong PA, Prokop M. Computed tomographic screening for lung cancer: an opportunity to evaluate other diseases. *JAMA*. 2012;308:1433-1434.
2. Mets OM, Buckens CF, Zanen P, et al. Identification of chronic obstructive pulmonary disease in lung cancer screening computed tomographic scans. *JAMA*. 2011;306:1775-1781.
3. Sverzellati N, Cademartiri F, Bravi F, et al. Relationship and prognostic value of modified coronary artery calcium score, FEV1, and emphysema in lung cancer screening population: the MILD trial. *Radiology*. 2012;262:460-467.

Targeting of Low-Dose CT Screening According to the Risk of Lung-Cancer Death

Kovalchik SA, Tammemagi M, Berg CD, et al (Natl Cancer Inst, Rockville, MD; Brock Univ, St Catharines, Ontario, Canada; et al)
N Engl J Med 369:245-254, 2013

Background.—In the National Lung Screening Trial (NLST), screening with low-dose computed tomography (CT) resulted in a 20% reduction in lung-cancer mortality among participants between the ages of 55 and 74 years with a minimum of 30 pack-years of smoking and no more than 15 years since quitting. It is not known whether the benefits and potential harms of such screening vary according to lung-cancer risk.

Methods.—We assessed the variation in efficacy, the number of false positive results, and the number of lung-cancer deaths prevented among 26,604 participants in the NLST who underwent low-dose CT screening, as compared with the 26,554 participants who underwent chest radiography, according to the quintile of 5-year risk of lung-cancer death (ranging from 0.15 to 0.55% in the lowest-risk group [quintile 1] to more than 2.00% in the highest-risk group [quintile 5]).

Results.—The number of lung-cancer deaths per 10,000 person-years that were prevented in the CT-screening group, as compared with the radiography group, increased according to risk quintile (0.2 in quintile 1, 3.5 in quintile 2, 5.1 in quintile 3, 11.0 in quintile 4, and 12.0 in quintile 5; $P = 0.01$ for trend). Across risk quintiles, there were significant decreasing trends in the number of participants with false positive results per screening-prevented lung-cancer death (1648 in quintile 1, 181 in quintile 2, 147 in quintile 3, 64 in quintile 4, and 65 in quintile 5). The 60% of participants at highest risk for lung-cancer death (quintiles 3 through 5) accounted for 88% of the screening-prevented lung-cancer deaths and for 64% of participants with false positive results. The 20% of participants at lowest risk (quintile 1) accounted for only 1% of prevented lung-cancer deaths.

Conclusions.—Screening with low-dose CT prevented the greatest number of deaths from lung cancer among participants who were at highest risk and prevented very few deaths among those at lowest risk. These findings provide empirical support for risk-based targeting of smokers for such screening. (Funded by the National Cancer Institute.)

▶ The National Lung Screening Trial (NLST) found a 20% reduction in lung cancer mortality in a population of subjects ages 55 to 74 with at least 30 pack-years of smoking, who were currently smoking or had quit within the previous 15 years and who were screened with annual low-dose computed tomography (CT).[1] However, the participants within the NLST varied with regard to age and smoking intensity and so their individual risks for lung cancer.[2] Kovalchik and colleagues developed an absolute risk prediction model for lung cancer mortality based on the data of the NLST and were able to separate the NLST participants into 5 quintiles of predicted 5-year risk of death from lung cancer. They then evaluated the benefit related to screening, measured as number of lung cancer deaths prevented by screening, stratified by quintile. Fig 1B in the original article shows the important finding. The highest risk quintile (Q5) had the highest number of lung cancer deaths prevented by screening, whereas the lowest risk quintile (Q1) had very few prevented or actual deaths.

The findings of this provocative study support individualization of lung cancer screening. Although several current lung cancer screening guidelines recommend low-dose CT screening strictly for patients who meet the NLST criteria, others have expanded those criteria, acknowledging that some patients outside the NLST criteria have sufficient lung cancer risk to warrant screening. The authors state, "Our results confirm that tailoring of low-dose CT screening to a patient's predicted risk of lung cancer death could narrow the NLST-eligible population without a loss in the potential public health benefits of screening or a disproportionate increase in the potential harms." In other words, thoughtful use of risk prediction models potentially could help limit screening of individuals meeting NLST criteria to only those at highest risk, which would result in a reduction of the number needed to screen to spare one lung cancer death as well as a decrease in the number of false-positive results in those at lowest risk. Conversely, utilization of risk prediction could, in the authors' words, "provide a rational, empirical framework for the inclusion of NLST-ineligible smokers at high risk for lung-cancer death." We need to recognize that no evidence base exists to support generalization of the NLST results to non-NLST populations but also acknowledge that such an evidence base may never exist. The difficult question is whether high-risk individuals who do not fit the NLST criteria should be targeted for low-dose CT screening. Ultimately, the decisions for these patients may rely on our incorporating risk prediction models into our practices[3] and accepting that the optimal risk-benefit, cost-effective limitations to lung cancer screening cannot currently, and may not ever, be exactly known.

L. T. Tanoue, MD

References

1. National Lung Screening Trial Research Team, Aberle DR, Adams AM, Berg CD, et al. Reduced lung-cancer mortality with low-dose computed tomographic screening. *N Engl J Med.* 2011;365:395-409.
2. Bach PB, Gould MK. When the average applies to no one: personalized decision making about potential benefits of lung cancer screening. *Ann Intern Med.* 2012;157:571-573.
3. Tammemägi MC, Katki HA, Hocking WG, et al. Selection criteria for lung-cancer screening. *N Engl J Med.* 2013;368:728-736.

Diagnostic Evaluation

Executive Summary: Diagnosis and Management of Lung Cancer, 3rd ed: American College of Chest Physicians Evidence-Based Clinical Practice Guidelines
Detterbeck FC, Lewis SZ, Diekemper R, et al (Yale Univ School of Medicine, New Haven, CT; American College of Chest Physicians, Northbrook, IL; et al)
Chest 143:7S-37S, 2013

Background.—The deaths from lung cancer are expected to increase over the next decades and already equal those related to the next four leading causes of death combined. Many advances have occurred in the approaches to diagnosing and treating lung cancer. The third edition of the American College of Chest Physicians (ACCP) Lung Cancer Guidelines (LC III) offers a systematic, extensive, comprehensive review of relevant literature, a structured interpretation of the data, and recommendations for practical patient management. This document addresses issues related to preventive and screening efforts; evaluations to diagnose lung cancer; assessments in preparation for treatment, which include staging and assessing surgical pathology; and treatment or palliative approaches.

Prevention and Screening.—Biomarkers to identify persons at risk and to facilitate early detection are being sought. Cigarette smoking is still the major risk factor for lung cancer. Screening methods using low-dose computed tomography (LDCT) scanning is being developed. Genetic assessments are seeking mutations that may respond to targeted interventions, which may prove especially useful for patients with non-n-small cell lung cancer (NSCLC). However, none of the factors investigated for chemopreventive efficacy have proved to have any benefit and some are harmful. The focus has shifted from large randomized controlled trials (RCTs) to small studies designed to increase the understanding of relevant biology and to define surrogate end points to build a foundation for future developments. Smoking cessation efforts have been identified that yield the best results in specific situations and reduce tobacco use.

Screening has been identified as a complex interplay of baseline patient risk, the test used for screening, test interpretation, and management of the findings. The management of patients found to have a solitary pulmonary nodule is complex, relying on a multitude of factors such as the size and consistency of the lesion; patient history, values, and preferences; the reliability of the test used; and the risk of malignancy.

Evaluations.—For patients suspected or known to have lung cancer, the delivery of care should be timely and efficient, usually involving a multidisciplinary approach. Among the tests used to assess suspicious lesions or findings, those that are the least invasive and the safest should be chosen first to confirm the diagnosis, with more invasive methods chosen if the initial test does not confirm or rule out lung cancer. When diagnosing a primary tumor, if the initial method produces non-diagnostic results and the suspicion of lung cancer remains, further tests are advisable. Potential candidates for curative surgical resection should be further evaluated by a multidisciplinary team before surgery is undertaken. Patient age should not be viewed as a contraindication to curative resection. Comorbidities must be considered, with the approach chosen varying according to the risks and benefits involved.

Staging is often based on positron emission tomography (PET) imaging, but positive PET results should be confirmed by biopsy in most cases. Patients at greatest risk for distant metastases and those who do not undergo extensive imaging for distant metastases or invasive mediastinal staging are the most likely to benefit from PET imaging. Invasive medistinal staging is advised for most patients who have no distant metastases. Node sampling during mediastinoscopy is usually limited. For patients with NSCLC, staging is usually based on a CT scan of the chest with contrast medium coupled with a thorough clinical evaluation and additional imaging as indicated. The use of extrathoracic staging and mediastinal staging is reserved for patients with specific characteristics. It is important to define the histologic subtype of NSCLC when selecting chemotherapy regimens, with further subtyping also needed to determine biologic behavior and the extent of local therapy.

Treatment and Palliation.—Treatment varies depending on the staging, histologic characteristics, and size of the lesion. Specific recommendations are made based on whether it is a bronchial intraepithelial neoplasm, on its stage and characteristic (infiltrative or not) as a NSCLC lesion, on its involvement of mediastinal nodes, and on its occult node involvement. Adjuvant therapy also varies, but is recommended for patients with resected NSCLC with incidental N2 disease. Treatment can include first-line approaches, maintenance therapy, second-line approaches, and third-line management. Special considerations may also apply to specific patient groups.

For patients with small cell lung cancer (SCLC), PET imaging can be used for upstaging or downstaging lesions. Limited-stage (LS) SCLC concurrent chemoradiotherapy is the best course of treatment, with radiation included early in the clinical course. No major breakthroughs have been documented in the search for better chemotherapeutic agents or treatment combinations.

Complementary therapies and integrative medicine can alleviate physical and emotional symptoms, improve the patient's quality of life (QoL), and improve patient compliance with treatment regimens. Patients often turn to these approaches, so the clinician must be familiar with them. Mind-body modalities such as meditation, mindfulness-based stress reduction, yoga, tai chi, qigong, psychosocial methods, hypnosis, and mind-body relaxation techniques may help to manage chronic pain, chemotherapy-induced nausea and vomiting, fatigue, mood disturbances, and QoL. These complementary strategies are done in combination with standard interventions.

After curative-intent therapy, patients with lung cancer should be followed up using periodic chest CT, a validated health-related QoL instrument, and surveillance bronchoscopy. Tools have now been developed to help manage patients' symptoms, especially those associated with advanced disease. These help to address pain, airway obstruction, cough, and palliation of bone metastasis, brain metastasis, spinal cord compression, superior vena cava syndrome, hemoptysis, airway-esophageal fistulas, malignant pleural effusion, depression, fatigue, anorexia, and insomnia. Although many treatments are effective even for patients with incurable lung cancer, the focus eventually becomes how to manage end-of-life issues. These should be incorporated into management from the outset rather than avoided until death is imminent and should be considered part of the active cancer treatment methods.

Conclusions.—It is difficult to keep up with the vast literature addressing issues related to lung cancer. The evidence-based clinical practice guidelines offered by the American College of Chest Physicians provide detailed recommendations for clinicians dealing with patients who may have lung cancer.

▶ The Third Edition of the American College of Chest Physicians Guidelines for the Diagnosis and Management of Lung Cancer is a comprehensive compilation and discussion of the evidence base available for the field. The guidelines provide a detailed rationale for the recommendations made for all aspects of lung cancer, from epidemiology to staging and treatment, and also make clear where those recommendations are solidly based in evidence and where they rely on expert opinion. They are intentionally written to be useful for practicing clinicians. There are 24 articles in the complete guidelines:

1 Executive Summary
2 Methodology for Development of Guidelines for Lung Cancer
3 Epidemiology of Lung Cancer
4 Molecular Biology of Lung Cancer
5 Chemoprevention of Lung Cancer
6 Treatment of Tobacco Use in Lung Cancer
7 Screening for Lung Cancer
8 Evaluation of Individuals with Pulmonary Nodules: When Is It Lung Cancer?
9 Clinical and Organizational Factors in the Initial Evaluation of Patients with Lung Cancer
10 Establishing the Diagnosis of Lung Cancer
11 Physiologic Evaluation of the Patient with Lung Cancer Being Considered for Resectional Surgery
12 The Stage Classification of Lung Cancer
13 Methods of Staging for Non-small Cell Lung Cancer
14 Diagnostic Surgical Pathology in Lung Cancer
15 Diagnosis and Treatment of Bronchial Intraepithelial Neoplasia and Early Lung Cancer of the Central Airways
16 Treatment of Stage I and II Non-small Cell Lung Cancer
17 Treatment of Stage III Non-small Cell Lung Cancer

18 Treatment of Stage IV Non-small Cell Lung Cancer

19 Special Treatment Issues in NSCLC

20 Treatment of Small Cell Lung Cancer

21 Complementary Therapies and Integrative Medicine in Lung Cancer

22 Follow-up and Surveillance of the Patient with Lung Cancer After Curative-Intent Therapy

23 Symptom Management in Patients with Lung Cancer

24 Palliative and End-of-Life Care in Lung Cancer

Although each of these articles is noteworthy, only a few could be discussed in more detail in this section. The Executive Summary provides a concise synopsis with the full set of recommendations and remarks for each article. As a quick guide for each topic, the summary is a remarkable work. The reader seeking more in-depth and detailed discussion of a specific topic is referred to the individual articles.

L. T. Tanoue, MD

Evaluation of Individuals With Pulmonary Nodules: When Is It Lung Cancer? Diagnosis and Management of Lung Cancer, 3rd ed: American College of Chest Physicians Evidence-Based Clinical Practice Guidelines

Gould MK, Donington J, Lynch WR, et al (Kaiser Permanente Southern California, Pasadena; NYU School of Medicine, NY; Univ of Michigan, Ann Arbor; et al)

Chest 143:e93S-120S, 2013

Objectives.—The objective of this article is to update previous evidence-based recommendations for evaluation and management of individuals with solid pulmonary nodules and to generate new recommendations for those with nonsolid nodules.

Methods.—We updated prior literature reviews, synthesized evidence, and formulated recommendations by using the methods described in the "Methodology for Development of Guidelines for Lung Cancer" in the American College of Chest Physicians Lung Cancer Guidelines, 3rd ed.

Results.—We formulated recommendations for evaluating solid pulmonary nodules that measure >8 mm in diameter, solid nodules that measure ≤8 mm in diameter, and subsolid nodules. The recommendations stress the value of assessing the probability of malignancy, the utility of imaging tests, the need to weigh the benefits and harms of different management strategies (nonsurgical biopsy, surgical resection, and surveillance with chest CT imaging), and the importance of eliciting patient preferences.

Conclusions.—Individuals with pulmonary nodules should be evaluated and managed by estimating the probability of malignancy, performing imaging tests to better characterize the lesions, evaluating the risks associated

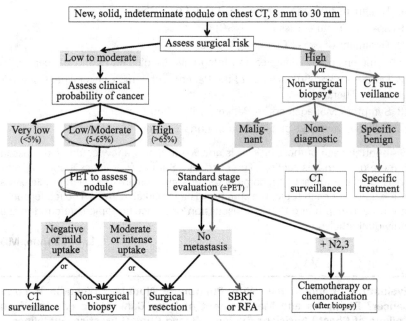

FIGURE 1.—[Sections 4.0, 4.3] Management algorithm for individuals with solid nodules measuring 8 to 30 mm in diameter. Branches indicate steps in the algorithm following nonsurgical biopsy. *Among individuals at high risk for surgical complications, we recommend either CT scan surveillance (when the clinical probability of malignancy is low to moderate) or nonsurgical biopsy (when the clinical probability of malignancy is moderate to high). RFA = radiofrequency ablation; SBRT = stereotactic body radiotherapy. (*Reprinted from* Gould MK, Donington J, Lynch WR, et al. Evaluation of individuals with pulmonary nodules: when is it lung cancer? Diagnosis and management of lung cancer, 3rd ed: American College of Chest Physicians evidence-based clinical practice guidelines. *Chest.* 2013;143:e93S-120S, Copyright 2013, with permission from American College of Chest Physicians.)

with various management alternatives, and eliciting their preferences for management Figs 1 and 6.

▶ Pulmonary nodules are defined as small, focal, rounded radiographic opacities up to 30 mm in diameter; lung masses are pulmonary nodules that measure more than 30 mm in diameter. This comprehensive article in the American College of Chest Physician (ACCP) Guidelines on the Diagnosis and Management of Lung Cancer discusses an evidence-based approach to the entire spectrum of pulmonary nodules. It provides recommendations for evaluation and management of pulmonary nodules according to size and density, grouped as solid nodules measuring 8 to 30 mm in diameter, solid nodules measuring less than 8 mm in diameter, and subsolid nodules. Every pulmonologist should review this article.

Fig 1 is the recommended management algorithm for individuals with solid nodules measuring 8 to 30 mm in diameter. The first major decision point in this algorithm addresses surgical risk. A minority of patients will be deemed at high surgical risk or will voluntarily decline invasive evaluation. For patients

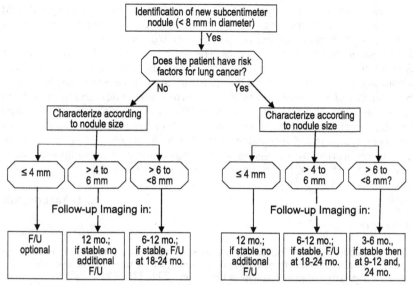

FIGURE 6.—[Section 5.2] Management algorithm for individuals with solid nodules measuring <8 mm in diameter. F/U = follow-up. (*Reprinted from* Gould MK, Donington J, Lynch WR, et al. Evaluation of individuals with pulmonary nodules: when is it lung cancer? Diagnosis and management of lung cancer, 3rd ed: American College of Chest Physicians evidence-based clinical practice guidelines. *Chest.* 2013;143:e93S-120S, Copyright 2013, with permission from American College of Chest Physicians.)

willing to undergo further evaluation and in whom surgical risk is low to moderate, the next major decision point is the assessment of the pretest probability of lung cancer. The decision to watchfully monitor, perform further noninvasive assessment, proceed to biopsy, or elect surgical resection is guided by that pretest probability. Validated models for predicting the likelihood of a nodule being malignant are readily available, but it should be recognized that, in this particular task, seasoned clinicians perform as well as the models.[1-4]

Fig 6 outlines the recommended management algorithm for individuals with solid nodules less than 8 mm in diameter. This algorithm parallels the recommendations of the Fleischner Society for solid nodules less than 8 mm in diameter discovered incidentally on computed tomography (CT) imaging studies.[5] These recommendations are largely based on expert opinion and should be applied to asymptomatic persons without a history of extrathoracic malignancy. The first major decision factor in this algorithm is the assessment of whether the patient has risk factors for lung cancer. The second decision factor is the size of the nodule. As is evident in the algorithm, the recommended interval for radiographic follow-up is determined by those 2 factors. Stability at 24 months of follow-up is felt to be of sufficient duration to obviate the need for continued serial imaging, whereas growth of a nodule should trigger more assessment.

The ACCP guidelines for subsolid nodules were published before the release of recommendations for subsolid nodules by the Fleischner Society.[6] The ACCP defines subsolid nodules as "nonsolid" (pure ground glass) or "part-solid" (>50% ground glass but with a solid component). Accurate linear measurement of these nodules can be challenging. It is increasingly clear that these subsolid nodules have a high prevalence of premalignant and malignant disease. Recognizing this, the duration of follow-up necessary to determine stability and obviate further serial imaging is controversial. The ACCP guidelines, like the Fleischner Society recommendations, recommend surveillance for at least 3 years but acknowledge that these nodules may have very slow growth rates and long doubling times and may be indolent lung cancers that are not destined to cause harm (overdiagnosis). The differences between the ACCP guideline recommendations and the Fleischer Society recommendations for the management of subsolid nodules are detailed in the discussion of the article in this chapter by Naidich and colleagues on Recommendations for the Management of Subsolid Pulmonary Nodules Detected at CT: A Statement from the Fleischner Society, published in the journal *Radiology*.[6]

L. T. Tanoue, MD

References

1. Herder GJ, van Tinteren H, Golding RP, et al. Clinical prediction model to characterize pulmonary nodules: validation and added value of 18F-fluorodeoxyglucose positron emission tomography. *Chest.* 2005;128:2490-2496.
2. Isbell JM, Deppen S, Putnam JB Jr, et al. Existing general population models inaccurately predict lung cancer risk in patients referred for surgical evaluation. *Ann Thorac Surg.* 2011;91:227-233 [discussion: 33].
3. Schultz EM, Sanders GD, Trotter PR, et al. Validation of two models to estimate the probability of malignancy in patients with solitary pulmonary nodules. *Thorax.* 2008;63:335-341.
4. Tammemagi MC, Freedman MT, Pinsky PF, et al. Prediction of true positive lung cancers in individuals with abnormal suspicious chest radiographs: a prostate, lung, colorectal, and ovarian cancer screening trial study. *J Thorac Oncol.* 2009; 4:710-721.
5. MacMahon H, Austin JH, Gamsu G, et al. Guidelines for management of small pulmonary nodules detected on CT scans: a statement from the Fleischner Society. *Radiology.* 2005;237:395-400.
6. Naidich DP, Bankier AA, MacMahon H, et al. Recommendations for the management of subsolid pulmonary nodules detected at CT: a statement from the Fleischner Society. *Radiology.* 2013;266:304-317.

Recommendations for the Management of Subsolid Pulmonary Nodules Detected at CT: A Statement from the Fleischner Society
Naidich DP, Bankier AA, MacMahon H, et al (New York Univ Med Ctr; Harvard Med School, Boston, MA; Univ of Chicago Med Ctr, IL; et al)
Radiology 266:304-317, 2013

This report is to complement the original Fleischner Society recommendations for incidentally detected solid nodules by proposing a set of recommendations specifically aimed at subsolid nodules. The development of a standardized approach to the interpretation and management of subsolid nodules remains critically important given that peripheral adenocarcinomas represent the most common type of lung cancer, with evidence of

TABLE.—Recommendations for the Management of Subsolid Pulmonary Nodules Detected at CT: A Statement from the Fleischner Society

Nodule Type	Management Recommendations	Additional Remarks
Solitary pure GGNs		
≤5 mm	No CT follow-up required	Obtain contiguous 1-mm-thick sections to confirm that nodule is truly a pure GGN
>5 mm	Initial follow-up CT at 3 months to confirm persistence then annual surveillance CT for a minimum of 3 years	FDG PET is of limited value, potentially misleading, and therefore not recommended
Solitary part-solid nodules	Initial follow-up CT at 3 months to confirm persistence. If persistent and solid component ≤5 mm, then yearly surveillance CT for a minimum of 3 years. If persistent and solid component ≤5 mm, then biopsy or surgical resection	Consider PET/CT for part-solid nodules >10 mm
Multiple subsolid nodules		
Pure GGNs ≤5 mm	Obtain follow-up CT at 2 and 4 years	Consider alternate causes for multiple GGNs ≤5 mm
Pure GGNs >5 mm without a dominant lesion(s)	Initial follow-up CT at 3 months to confirm persistence and then annual surveillance CT for a minimum of 3 years	FDG PET is of limited value, potentially misleading, and therefore not recommended
Dominant nodule(s) with part-solid or solid component	Initial follow-up CT at 3 months to confirm persistence. If persistent, biopsy or surgical resection is recommended, especially for lesions with >5 mm solid component	Consider lung-sparing surgery for patients with dominant lesion(s) suspicious for lung cancer

Note.—These guidelines assume meticulous evaluation, optimally with contiguous thin sections (1 mm) reconstructed with narrow and/or mediastinal windows to evaluate the solid component and wide and/or lung windows to evaluate the nonsolid component of nodules, if indicated. When electronic calipers are used, bidimensional measurements of both the solid and ground-glass components of lesions should be obtained as necessary. The use of a consistent low-dose technique is recommended, especially in cases for which prolonged follow-up is recommended, particularly in younger patients. With serial scans, always compare with the original baseline study to detect subtle indolent growth.

increasing frequency. Following an initial consideration of appropriate terminology to describe subsolid nodules and a brief review of the new classification system for peripheral lung adenocarcinomas sponsored by the International Association for the Study of Lung Cancer (IASLC), American Thoracic Society (ATS), and European Respiratory Society (ERS), six specific recommendations were made, three with regard to solitary subsolid nodules and three with regard to multiple subsolid nodules. Each recommendation is followed first by the rationales underlying the recommendation and then by specific pertinent remarks. Finally, issues for which future research is needed are discussed. The recommendations are the result of careful review of the literature now available regarding subsolid nodules. Given the complexity of these lesions, the current recommendations are more varied than the original Fleischner Society guidelines for solid nodules. It cannot be overemphasized that these guidelines must be interpreted in light of an individual's clinical history. Given the frequency with which subsolid nodules are encountered in daily clinical practice, and notwithstanding continuing controversy on many of these issues, it is anticipated that further refinements and modifications to these recommendations will be forthcoming as information continues to emerge from ongoing research (Table).

▶ In 2005, the Fleischner Society of the Radiologic Society of North America published recommendations for the management of small (< 8 mm diameter) solid pulmonary nodules identified incidentally by computed tomography (CT) imaging.[1] These recommendations have been enormously helpful in clinical practice, given widespread utilization of CT scanning, and in particular as more small nodules are identified with the advent of lung cancer screening. Nonetheless, these recommendations are not all inclusive, and substantive limitations in clinical application have been clear. Specifically, the 2005 statement does not address subsolid pulmonary nodules, either solitary or multiple, which are common and often challenging findings. This new report is intended to fill that void. The 2 statements are meant to be complementary and together provide a framework to approach both small solid nodules as well as nonsolid nodules of varying size.

We commonly use the terms *ground glass opacity (GGO)* or *ground glass nodule (GGN)* to describe focal nodular areas of increased lung attenuation, with the characteristic feature being that normal parenchymal structures, including airways and vessels, are still identifiable within those areas.[2,3] Subsolid pulmonary nodules as defined by the Fleischner Society include 2 categories: (1) those that are pure GGO or GGN and (2) those that are part solid, composed of areas that are ground glass as well as areas that are solid.

The recommendations of the Fleischner Society for management of subsolid pulmonary nodules are outlined in the Table. Notably, there is no distinction of management of subsolid nodules based on smoking history or any other known lung cancer risk factor. This reflects an appreciation that the epidemiology of malignant subsolid lesions appears to differ in many respects from typical lung cancers and are often observed occurring in younger individuals with less or no smoking exposure.

It is important to note that the American College of Chest Physicians (ACCP) Guidelines on the Diagnosis and Management of Lung Cancer, published in 2013 before the release of the Fleischner Society statement, also include new recommendations for the management of subsolid lung nodules.[4] The Fleischner Society and the ACCP recommendations essentially agree on the management of pure ground glass nodules. However, they differ in recommendations for the management of part-solid nodules as follows:

- Fleischner Society recommendations for the management of solitary part-solid nodules:
  - Initial follow-up CT at 3 months to confirm persistence
  - If persistent and the solid component is less than 5 mm, then yearly surveillance CT for a minimum of 3 years
  - If persistent and the solid component is greater than 5 mm, then biopsy or surgical resection
  - Remarks: Consider positron emission tomography (PET)/CT for part-solid nodules greater than 10 mm.

- ACCP recommendations for the management of part-solid nodules:
  - For a part-solid nodule measuring less than 8 mm in diameter, CT surveillance at approximately 3, 12, and 24 months, followed by annual CT surveillance for an additional 1 to 3 years
  - For a part-solid nodule measuring greater than 8 mm in diameter, repeat chest CT at 3 months, followed by further evaluation with PET, nonsurgical biopsy, or surgical resection for nodules that persist
  - Remarks:
    - Part-solid nodules that grow or develop a solid component are often malignant and should prompt further evaluation or consideration of resection
    - PET should not be used to characterize part-solid lesions in which the solid component measures less than 8 mm
    - Part-solid nodules measuring greater than 15 mm in diameter should proceed directly to further evaluation with PET, nonsurgical biopsy, or surgical resection

Because the evidence base for the 2 sets of recommendations is relatively small, they should be recognized as being predominantly based on expert opinion. The differences in the recommendations for subsolid nodules inevitably reflect the consensus of the physicians who wrote them; both groups are highly respected and equally engaged in providing the medical community with as unbiased and useful recommendations as possible.

L. T. Tanoue, MD

References

1. MacMahon H, Austin JH, Gamsu G, et al. Guidelines for management of small pulmonary nodules detected on CT scans: a statement from the Fleischner Society. *Radiology.* 2005;237:395-400.
2. Hansell DM, Bankier AA, MacMahon H, McLoud TC, Müller NL, Remy J. Fleischner Society: glossary of terms for thoracic imaging. *Radiology.* 2008;246: 697-722.
3. Austin JH, Müller NL, Friedman PJ, et al. Glossary of terms for CT of the lungs: recommendations of the Nomenclature Committee of the Fleischner Society. *Radiology.* 1996;200:327-331.
4. Gould MK, Donington J, Lynch WR, et al. Evaluation of individuals with pulmonary nodules: when is it lung cancer? Diagnosis and management of lung cancer, 3rd ed: American College of Chest Physicians evidence-based clinical practice guidelines. *Chest.* 2013;143:e93S-120S.

Radiation and Chest CT Scan Examinations: What Do We Know?
Sarma A, Heilbrun ME, Conner KE, et al (Intermountain Med Ctr, Murray, UT; Univ of Utah School of Medicine, Salt Lake City)
Chest 142:750-760, 2012

In the past 3 decades, the total number of CT scans performed has grown exponentially. In 2007, >70 million CT scans were performed in the United States. CT scan studies of the chest comprise a large portion of the CT scans performed today because the technology has transformed the management of common chest diseases, including pulmonary embolism and coronary artery disease. As the number of studies performed yearly increases, a growing fraction of the population is exposed to low-dose ionizing radiation from CT scan. Data extrapolated from atomic bomb survivors and other populations exposed to low-dose ionizing radiation suggest that CT scan-associated radiation may increase an individual's lifetime risk of developing cancer. This finding, however, is not incontrovertible. Because this topic has recently attracted the attention of both the scientific community and the general public, it has become increasingly important for physicians to understand the cancer risk associated with CT scan and be capable of engaging in productive dialogue with patients. This article reviews the current literature on the public health debate surrounding CT scan and cancer risk, quantifies radiation doses associated with specific studies, and describes efforts to reduce population-wide CT scan-associated radiation exposure. CT scan examinations of the chest, including CT scan pulmonary and coronary angiography, high-resolution CT scan, low-dose lung cancer screening, and triple rule-out CT scan, are specifically considered Table 4.

▶ Advances in imaging technology, particularly in computed tomography (CT), over the last several decades have been immeasurably beneficial in improving our ability to diagnose and manage any number of diseases. It is difficult to remember a time when the precise anatomic information provided by CT imaging was not easily at our disposal. However, practitioners and patients are increasingly aware of the downsides of imaging, in particular the risks related to cumulative medical radiation exposure. In the United States, more than 85 million CT scans are performed annually, a number that continues to climb.[1] New modalities such as positron emission tomography (PET) and CT screening for lung cancer will inevitably add more radiation exposure, as they are broadly adopted into routine clinical practice.

Over the last 30 years, radiation exposure related to medical imaging has increased approximately 7-fold, with CT being the largest contributor to that increase. In discussions with patients relating to the risks of diagnostic evaluation, radiation related to a single imaging study may not be a factor, but cumulative radiation related to many imaging studies is an increasing and reasonable public health concern. Quantification of radiation-induced cancer risk to a large extent has been based on indirect evidence in atomic bomb survivors, but there is direct evidence of small but significant increased cancer risk based on medical imaging radiation exposure, particularly in children.[2,3] An exception to this is that, in atomic bomb survivors, older age at the time of exposure correlated with increased lung cancer risk.[4] This and the known synergistic carcinogenic effect of radiation and smoking raise inevitable and real concerns that serial chest CT imaging as a screening intervention may actually be associated with carcinogenesis related to the imaging studies themselves.[5]

The authors of this report and the accompanying editorial by Brenner point out 3 key areas—quality control, training, and overuse—that need attention to

TABLE 4.—Current Measured or Estimated Radiation Exposure for Chest Imaging Procedures[a]

Study Type	Equivalent Dose Range, mSv	Mean Equivalent Dose, mSv	Organ Dose Breast, mGy or mSv	Organ Dose Lung, mGy or mSv	Equivalent Time for Background Radiation Exposure	Equivalent Number of PA Chest Radiographs (0.02 mSv)
PA/lateral chest radiograph	0.05-0.25			0.01-0.15	10 d	
Screening mammogram	0.1-0.6	0.4	3-4.7		42 d	
Routine chest CT scan	4-27.0	7.5-8	22	24	3 y	400
Chest HRCT scan	0.2-0.98 (3.1-15)[b]	0.8-0.9 (3.8)[b]	3.4	3.5	89 d (1 y)[b]	43 (190)[b]
Lung cancer screening CT scan	0.6-1.1	0.65	5.7	2.5-9.0	68 d	33
CTPA	1.4-40	15	20-60	N/A	4.3 y	750
Coronary calcium scoring	1.0-12	3	4.3-18	2.6-10.3	312 d	150
CTCA	1.0-32	8.7-16	4.8-44.0	3.9-37.6	3.5 y	435
TROCT scan	4-31.8	7.5-19.4	91	80	3.8 y	672
V̇/Q̇ lung scan		1.2	0.28		164 d	60
Pulmonary arteriogram[c]		7.1			2.4 y	355
FDG-PET/CT scan[c]	8.5-26.4	13.5-18.85			5.4 y	809

Data from References 5,12,18,21,34,56-74. CTCA = CT scan coronary angiography; CTPA = CT scan pulmonary angiography; FDG = flurodeoxyglucose; HRCT = high-resolution CT; N/A = not applicable; PA = posteroanterior; TROCT = triple rule-out CT; V̇/Q̇ = ventilation and perfusion. Effective end-organ doses vary based on patient factors such as age and sex. Equivalent number of chest radiographs and time for background radiation exposure are calculated from mean effective dose.

[a]Values with ranges are based on variations in technique and dose reduction strategies.

[b]When performed with volumetric CT scan.

[c]Full-body FDG-PET can be subdivided into low-dose and high-dose CT scan. Note that FDG-PET/CT can be subdivided into low-dose and high-dose CT scan.

minimize risks related to medical imaging.[1] Wide variations in the amount of radiation exposure for the same imaging study are well documented and should be eliminated.[6] Ordering practitioners should be aware of what radiation dose their patients will receive as a consequence of a given study; if that information is not readily available, it should be demanded. Radiologists should be held accountable for standards of practice and the assurance of quality control. Practitioners should also be held accountable that imaging studies, when ordered, are actually appropriate. Campaigns to increase awareness about radiation exposure, such as the Image Wisely effort by the American College of Radiology or algorithmic decision support tools and computerized appropriateness criteria, may help inform us in more judicious use of CT imaging.[7,8]

Finally, we require a language with which we can communicate the magnitude of exposure and risk to our patients. Table 4 outlines several different methods of expressing radiation exposure for different chest imaging procedures. Physicians might understand the meaning of dose range given in millisieverts. Patients might better understand radiation dose if given in units of equivalent time of background radiation exposure acquired in ordinary daily life from cosmic radiation and environmental radon. What we don't understand is how much diagnostic radiation is too much or when a patient crosses a threshold at which the risk of a radiation-associated cancer is in excess of the benefit of the information to be obtained by a given study. Until we have better information to answer these questions, what we can do is be cognizant and honest about the risk incurred by the radiation associated with imaging studies, particularly CT scans; order studies judiciously; educate ourselves and our patients about the potential risks of those studies; and ensure that our patients are having imaging performed at facilities that we are confident are attentive to quality control.

L. T. Tanoue, MD

References

1. Brenner DJ. Radiation and chest CT scans: are there problems? What should we do? *Chest.* 2012;142:549-550.
2. Pearce MS, Salotti JA, Little MP, et al. Radiation exposure from CT scans in childhood and subsequent risk of leukaemia and brain tumours: a retrospective cohort study. *Lancet.* 2012;380:499-505.
3. Brenner DJ, Hall EJ. Computed tomography—an increasing source of radiation exposure. *N Engl J Med.* 2007;357:2277-2284.
4. Preston DL, Ron E, Tokuoka S, et al. Solid cancer incidence in atomic bomb survivors: 1958–1998. *Radiat Res.* 2007;168:1-64.
5. Brenner DJ. Radiation risks potentially associated with low-dose CT screening of adult smokers for lung cancer. *Radiology.* 2004;231:440-445.
6. Smith-Bindman R, Lipson J, Marcus, et al. Radiation dose associated with common computed tomography examinations and the associated lifetime attributable risk of cancer. *Arch Intern Med.* 2009;169:2078-2086.
7. Brink JA, Amis ES Jr. Image Wisely: a campaign to increase awareness about adult radiation protection. *Radiology.* 2010;257:601-602.
8. Sistrom CL, Dang PA, Weilburg JB, Dreyer KJ, Rosenthal DI, Thrall JH. Effect of computerized order entry with integrated decision support on the growth of outpatient procedure volumes: seven-year time series analysis. *Radiology.* 2009;251: 147-155.

What Do You Mean, a Spot? A Qualitative Analysis of Patients' Reactions to Discussions With Their Physicians About Pulmonary Nodules

Wiener RS, Gould MK, Woloshin S, et al (Boston Univ School of Medicine, MA; Kaiser Permanente Southern California, Pasadena, CA; Dept of Veterans Affairs Med Ctr, White River Junction, VT; et al)

Chest 143:672-677, 2013

Background.—More than 150,000 Americans each year are found to have a pulmonary nodule. Even more will be affected following the publication of the National Lung Screening Trial. Patient-doctor communication about pulmonary nodules can be challenging. Although most nodules are benign, it may take 2 to 3 years to rule out cancer. We sought to characterize patients' perceptions of communication with their providers about pulmonary nodules.

Methods.—We conducted four focus groups at two sites with 22 adults with an indeterminate pulmonary nodule. Transcripts were analyzed using principles of grounded theory.

Results.—Patients described conversations with 53 different providers about the pulmonary nodule. Almost all patients immediately assumed that they had cancer when first told about the nodule. Some whose providers did not discuss the actual cancer risk or explain the evaluation plan experienced confusion and distress that sometimes lasted for months. Patients were frustrated when their providers did not address their concerns about cancer or potential adverse effects of surveillance (eg, prolonged uncertainty, radiation exposure), which in some cases led to poor adherence to evaluation plans. Patients found it helpful when physicians used lay terms, showed the CT image, and quantified cancer risk. By contrast, patients resented medical jargon and dismissive language.

Conclusions.—Patients commonly assume that a pulmonary nodule means cancer. What providers tell (or do not tell) patients about their cancer risk and the evaluation plan can strongly influence patients' perceptions of the nodule and related distress. We describe simple communication strategies that may help patients to come to terms with an indeterminate pulmonary nodule.

▶ This article addresses, in a very practical way, the reality that discussions with patients about their pulmonary nodules are rarely simple. The thoughtful editorial that accompanies it is well worth reading.[1] We all recognize that, when a patient is told he or she has an abnormality on a chest computed tomography (CT) scan, typically his or her immediate concern will be whether that abnormality is cancer. We are aware that most small pulmonary nodules, whether found incidentally on chest or abdominal CT scans done for other purposes or on dedicated chest CT screening examinations, are benign, but patients by and large don't know that. Moreover, we are often referred these patients after they have been informed of the abnormality by another provider, and by then a period of uncertainty and worry may have transpired. This scenario will become more common as lung cancer screening is incorporated into primary care practice. Alleviating a patient's concerns when reassurance is appropriate takes time. As this article points out, these discussions are best facilitated by using simple and direct language, presenting in understandable terms evidence supporting a recommendation to watchfully monitor or to intervene and engaging the patient in the decision-making process (Table 2 in the original article).

L. T. Tanoue, MD

Reference

1. Silvestri GA. Lumps, bumps, spots, and shadows: the scary world of the solitary pulmonary nodule. *Chest.* 2013;143:592-594.

The Stage Classification of Lung Cancer: Diagnosis and Management of Lung Cancer, 3rd ed: American College of Chest Physicians Evidence-Based Clinical Practice Guidelines

Detterbeck FC, Postmus PE, Tanoue LT (Yale Univ School of Medicine, New Haven, CT; VU Univ Med Ctr, Amsterdam, The Netherlands; Yale School of Medicine, New Haven, CT)
Chest 143:e191S-e210S, 2013

Background.—Stage classification systems are designed to provide a consistent description of the anatomic extent of disease. Clinical stage and pathologic stage are both determined in the TNM system, with clinical stage identified before treatment and pathologic stage determined after resection. A major revamping of the stage classification of lung cancer was done based on extensive statistical analysis.

TNM Changes.—Subgroups were defined for T1 (T1a and T1b) and T2 (T2a and T2b), reflecting significant survival differences in each size subgroup. The traditional definitions of invasion were retained. Invasion beyond the pleura's elastic layer is T2, with T3 adding invasion into the parietal or mediastinal pleura or the parietal pericardium, and T4 adding invasion of the visceral pericardial surface, intrapericardial pulmonary artery, and pulmonary veins. Pancoast tumor is also classified as T4. For the N descriptor, the traditional definitions of N0, N1, N2, and N3 were retained, but a new node map was developed to address ambiguities in previous node maps. The number of involved nodal zones seemed to have prognostic significance. The MX term was discontinued. M1 remains subdivided into M1a and M1b, with clarification of M1a's definition.

Other Considerations.—An online tool is now available to manage the complexity of the stage group definitions and assist in immediately defining a tumor's stage. Categories of patients with additional tumor nodules and multiple primary lung cancers were evaluated, and annotations were suggested for ambiguous cases. Clarification in cases of newly found lung cancer accompanied by a small nodule detected on imaging and those with advanced primary cancer with several pulmonary nodules or nodules elsewhere that appear to represent distant metastases should be referred to an expert panel for a consensus diagnosis. The pathologist has been singled out as the person responsible for identifying second primary lung cancers. Because of confusing rules regarding stage classification, second primary lung cancers can be defined by an experienced multidisciplinary team, with a careful evaluation for distant and mediastinal metastases. Additional descriptors that are more clearly defined include the certainty or C factor, completeness of resection, and minimal disease. The point was also made that the new edition of the Lung Cancer Stage Classification is applicable to all major types of primary lung cancer despite its development based on non-n-small cell lung cancer.

Conclusions.—The International Association for the Study of Lung Cancer (IASLC) staging classification document offers a relatively unique approach among cancer staging systems. The size of the database used, the broad international spectrum considered, the detailed analysis, and the internal and external validation applied to its development provide a more complex approach, but there is also increased ability to incorporate granular details. The fundamental definitions are supplemented by suggestions to minimize ambiguity.

▶ Staging is a critical process in the evaluation of every patient known or suspected to have lung cancer. The current international staging classification for lung cancer applies to both non—small-cell and small-cell lung cancers and was the culmination of 12 years of international collaboration and work by the International Association for the Study of Lung Cancer, informed by a case database of more than 100 000 patients.[1-3] This article by Detterbeck and colleagues discusses in detail the Tumor, Node, and Metastasis (TNM) descriptors, including the changes made with the recent reclassification as well as areas of controversy or limitation. These descriptors are outlined in Fig 1 of the original article. Different combinations of T, N, and M identify stage, with the determinant of stage being prognosis. Inherent in this is that anatomically different cancers are grouped together because of similar survival. This is demonstrated in Fig 5 of the original article, which is also a useful tool for determining stage based on the TNM descriptors. It is important to remember that the stage classification is not an algorithm for treatment, as other factors including performance status, other medical comorbidities, and patient preference influence therapeutic decisions. Furthermore, the stage classification, even in its more robust recent iteration, does not include molecular information relating to analysis of potentially targetable tumor mutations, which increasingly factors into therapeutic decisions and clinical outcomes. Accepting these caveats, every clinician should be proficient in staging, as the consistent and accurate description of the extent of anatomic disease is vital to the care of patients with lung cancer.

L. T. Tanoue, MD

References

1. Rami-Porta R, Ball D, Crowley J, et al. The IASLC Lung Cancer Staging Project: proposals for the revision of the T descriptors in the forthcoming (seventh) edition of the TNM classification for lung cancer. *J Thorac Oncol.* 2007;2:593-602.

2. Goldstraw P, Crowley J, Chansky K, et al. The IASLC Lung Cancer Staging Project: proposals for the revision of the TNM stage groupings in the forthcoming (seventh) edition of the TNM Classification of malignant tumours. *J Thorac Oncol.* 2007;2:706-714.

3. Rusch VW, Asamura H, Watanabe H, Giroux DJ, Rami-Porta R, Goldstraw P. The IASLC lung cancer staging project: a proposal for a new international lymph node map in the forthcoming seventh edition of the TNM classification for lung cancer. *J Thorac Oncol.* 2009;4:568-577.

Probability of Cancer in Pulmonary Nodules Detected on First Screening CT

McWilliams A, Tammemagi MC, Mayo JR, et al (Vancouver General Hosp, British Columbia, Canada; Univ, St Catharines, Ontario, Canada; et al)

N Engl J Med 369:910-919, 2013

Background.—Major issues in the implementation of screening for lung cancer by means of low-dose computed tomography (CT) are the definition of a positive result and the management of lung nodules detected on the scans. We conducted a population-based prospective study to determine factors predicting the probability that lung nodules detected on the first screening low-dose CT scans are malignant or will be found to be malignant on follow-up.

Methods.—We analyzed data from two cohorts of participants undergoing low-dose CT screening. The development data set included participants in the Pan-Canadian Early Detection of Lung Cancer Study (PanCan). The validation data set included participants involved in chemoprevention trials at the British Columbia Cancer Agency (BCCA), sponsored by the U.S. National Cancer Institute. The final outcomes of all nodules of any size that were detected on baseline low-dose CT scans were tracked. Parsimonious and fuller multivariable logistic-regression models were prepared to estimate the probability of lung cancer.

Results.—In the PanCan data set, 1871 persons had 7008 nodules, of which 102 were malignant, and in the BCCA data set, 1090 persons had 5021 nodules, of which 42 were malignant. Among persons with nodules, the rates of cancer in the two data sets were 5.5% and 3.7%, respectively. Predictors of cancer in the model included older age, female sex, family history of lung cancer, emphysema, larger nodule size, location of the nodule in the upper lobe, part-solid nodule type, lower nodule count, and spiculation. Our final parsimonious and full models showed excellent discrimination and calibration, with areas under the receiver-operating-characteristic curve of more than 0.90, even for nodules that were 10 mm or smaller in the validation set.

Conclusions.—Predictive tools based on patient and nodule characteristics can be used to accurately estimate the probability that lung nodules detected on baseline screening low-dose CT scans are malignant. (Funded

TABLE 2.—Prediction Models for the Probability of Lung Cancer in Pulmonary Nodules*

Predictor Variables	Model 1a: Parsimonious Model, No Spiculation			Model 2a: Full Model, No Spiculation		
	Odds Ratio (95% CI)	P Value	Beta Coefficient	Odds Ratio (95% CI)	P Value	Beta Coefficient
Age, per yr				1.03 (0.99–1.07)	0.11	0.0321
Sex, female vs. male	1.79 (1.13–2.82)	0.01	0.5806	1.76 (1.09–2.83)	0.02	0.5635
Family history of lung cancer, yes vs. no				1.35 (0.84–2.16)	0.21	0.3013
Emphysema, yes vs. no				1.41 (0.82–2.42)	0.21	0.3462
Nodule size		<0.001†	−5.8616		<0.001†	−5.6693
Nodule type						
Nonsolid or with ground-glass opacity				0.74 (0.40–1.35)	0.33	−0.3005
Part-solid				1.40 (0.72–2.74)	0.32	0.3395
Solid				Reference		Reference
Nodule location, upper vs. middle or lower lobe	1.90 (1.78–3.08)	0.009	0.6439	2.04 (1.22–3.41)	0.007	0.7116
Nodule count per scan, per each additional nodule				0.92 (0.85–1.00)	0.05	−0.0803
Model constant			−6.5929			−6.8071

Predictor Variables	Model 1b: Parsimonious Model, with Spiculation			Model 2b: Full Model, with Spiculation		
	Odds Ratio (95% CI)	P Value	Beta Coefficient	Odds Ratio (95% CI)	P Value	Beta Coefficient
Age, per yr				1.03 (0.99–1.07)	0.16	0.0287
Sex, female vs. male	1.91 (1.19–3.07)	0.008	0.6467	1.82 (1.12–2.97)	0.02	0.6011
Family history of lung cancer, yes vs. no				1.34 (0.83–2.17)	0.23	0.2961
Emphysema, yes vs. no				1.34 (0.78–2.33)	0.29	0.2953
Nodule size		<0.001†	−5.5537		<0.001†	−5.3854
Nodule type						
Nonsolid or with ground-glass opacity				0.88 (0.48–1.62)	0.68	−0.1276
Part-solid				1.46 (0.74–2.88)	0.28	0.3770
Solid				Reference		Reference
Nodule location, upper vs. middle or lower lobe	1.82 (1.12–2.98)	0.02	0.6009	1.93 (1.14–3.27)	0.02	0.6581
Nodule count per scan, per each additional nodule				0.92 (0.85–1.00)	0.049	−0.0824
Spiculation, yes vs. no	2.54 (1.45–4.43)	0.001	0.9309	2.17 (1.16–4.05)	0.02	0.7729
Model constant			−6.6144			−6.7892

*Models 1a and 1b are parsimonious prediction models, and Models 2a and 2b are full logistic-regression prediction models. Age is centered on the mean of 62 years, nodule size is centered on 4 mm, and nodule count is centered on 4 (i.e., 62 is subtracted from the actual age, 4 mm is subtracted from the actual nodule size, and 4 is subtracted from the actual number of nodules).

†Nodule size had a nonlinear relationship with lung cancer and is transformed in this model. The odds ratio of the transformed variable has no direct interpretation without back-transformation. Nodule-size transformation, which is based on multiple fractional polynomial analyses, was performed with the following calculation: $((Nodulesize10) − 0.5) −1.58113883$; nodule size was measured in millimeters.

by the Terry Fox Research Institute and others; ClinicalTrials.gov number, NCT00751660) (Table 2).

▶ Pulmonary nodules are common findings on computed tomography (CT) scans in general. They are very common findings on low-dose CT scans done for lung cancer screening in particular. In the National Lung Screening Trial (NLST), approximately 27% of study subjects had at least one nodule identified on the baseline screening CT, and more nodules were identified in those same subjects over the subsequent 2 years of screening.[1] In the Mayo Clinic lung cancer screening study, which performed annual low-dose screening over 5 years, more than 70% of subjects eventually had at least one nodule identified.[2]

Our approach to evaluating the likelihood of a pulmonary nodule being cancer has largely been focused on addressing nodules incidentally discovered on CT scans done for reasons other than screening, and algorithms such as those proposed by the Fleischner Society and the American College of Chest Physicians by and large address these nodules.[3,4] This article by McWilliams and colleagues specifically addresses the probability of cancer in pulmonary nodules found on a baseline low-dose screening chest CT. As screening becomes incorporated into routine clinical practice, this issue will become increasingly common. The models described by this group for assessing the likelihood of cancer were developed in subjects in the Pan-Canadian Early Detection of Lung Cancer Study (PanCan) and validated in subjects participating in chemoprevention trials at the British Columbia Cancer Agency (BCCA). The PanCan subjects included 1871 persons who were current and former smokers between 50 and 75 years of age without a history of lung cancer and who had a 3-year risk of lung cancer of at least 2% based on risk-prediction models developed in the Prostate, Lung, Colorectal, and Ovarian Screening Trial.[5] BCCA subjects included individuals who were current and former smokers of at least 30 pack-years between 50 and 74 years of age without a history of lung cancer. The demographics of these 2 study groups are similar but not identical to the entry criteria for the NLST. As with the NLST, the prevalence of lung nodules was high. A total of 5.5% of subjects over a median follow-up of 3.1 years in the PanCan study and 3.7% of subjects over a median follow-up of 8.6 years in the BCCA group were found to have lung cancer.

The prediction models developed for the probability of lung cancer in pulmonary nodules identified on the baseline screening CT are outlined in Table 2. Both parsimonious and full models are outlined as well as models with and without description of spiculation, as the BCCA database did not include that information on all patients. Of note, approximately 80% of the nodules described in the 2 studies were solid. In the full model with spiculation information (model 2b, Table 2), the factors contributing significantly to increasing lung cancer risk included older age, female vs male sex, a positive family history of lung cancer, increasing nodule size, the density of the nodule (with highest risk associated with solid density, followed by part-solid density, and with ground glass density being associated with the least risk), upper vs lower lung location, solitary versus multiple nodules, and the presence of spiculation.

Clinicians historically have performed well when compared with multivariable models in terms of ability to predict the probability of lung cancer in incidentally discovered pulmonary nodules. Whether we will do as well with nodules identified on screening CT examinations is unknown. Objective predictive tools such as the models proposed by McWilliams and colleagues should be incorporated into clinical practice, and the authors have facilitated this by making their models available as spreadsheet calculators, accessible at www.brocku.ca/cancerpredictionresearch.

L. T. Tanoue, MD

References

1. National Lung Screening Trial Research Team, Aberle DR, Adams AM, Berg CD, et al. Reduced lung-cancer mortality with low-dose computed tomographic screening. *N Engl J Med*. 2011;365:395-409.
2. Swensen SJ, Jett JR, Hartman TE, et al. CT screening for lung cancer: five-year prospective experience. *Radiology*. 2005;235:259-265.
3. MacMahon H, Austin JH, Gamsu G, et al. Guidelines for management of small pulmonary nodules detected on CT scans: a statement from the Fleischner Society. *Radiology*. 2005;237:395-400.
4. Gould MK, Donington J, Lynch WR, et al. Evaluation of individuals with pulmonary nodules: when is it lung cancer? Diagnosis and management of lung cancer, 3rd ed: American College of Chest Physicians evidence-based clinical practice guidelines. *Chest*. 2013;143:e93S-120S.
5. Tammemagi CM, Pinsky PF, Caporaso NE, et al. Lung cancer risk prediction: Prostate, Lung, Colorectal And Ovarian Cancer Screening Trial models and validation. *J Natl Cancer Inst*. 2011;103:1058-1068.

Endobronchial Ultrasound-Guided Transbronchial Needle Aspiration for Differentiating N0 Versus N1 Lung Cancer

Yasufuku K, Nakajima T, Waddell T, et al (Univ of Toronto, Ontario, Canada; Chiba Univ, Chiba, Japan)
Ann Thorac Surg 96:1756-1760, 2013

Background.—The aim of this study was to assess the value of endobronchial ultrasound-guided transbronchial needle aspiration (EBUS-TBNA) for differentiating cN0 versus cN1 non-small cell lung cancer.

Methods.—A retrospective review of EBUS-TBNA results in patients with potentially resectable clinical N0 or N1 non-small cell lung cancer based on computed tomography and positron emission tomography was performed. Systematic mediastinal and hilar lymph node sampling was performed by EBUS-TBNA. Lymph nodes larger than 5 mm in short axis or suspicious nodes were targeted. In the absence of N2 or N3 disease, patients underwent resection with lymph node dissection.

Results.—A total of 981 patients underwent EBUSTBNA during the study period, of which 163 patients met the study criteria. There were 94 cN0 and 69 cN1 patients. A total of 453 lymph nodes (338 mediastinal and 115 N1 lymph nodes, average 2.8 nodes/patient) were sampled. Endobronchial ultrasound upstaged 9 (5.5%) patients to N2 disease, but was

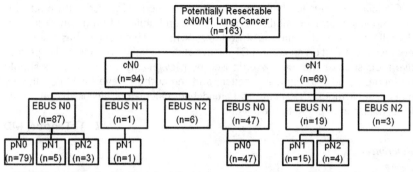

FIGURE 1.—Flow chart showing the 163 patients enrolled in this study. Clinical N0 and N1 were based on preoperative computed tomography and positron emission tomography scans. Patients found to have N2 disease on endobronchial ultrasound (EBUS) did not undergo surgical resection. (Reprinted from Yasufuku K, Nakajima T, Waddell T, et al. Endobronchial ultrasound-guided transbronchial needle aspiration for differentiating N0 versus N1 lung cancer. *Ann Thorac Surg.* 2013;96:1756-1760, Copyright 2013, with permission from The Society of Thoracic Surgeons.)

falsely negative in the mediastinum in 7 (4.3%) patients. In cN0 patients, EBUS confirmed N0 in 87 (53.4%) and upstaged in 7 (4.3%, N1 in 1, N2 in 6). In cN1 patients, EBUS confirmed N1 in 19 (11.7%), downstaged in 47 (28.8%), and upstaged in 3 (1.8%). The sensitivity, specificity, diagnostic accuracy, and negative predictive value of EBUS-TBNA to accurately differentiate between N0 and N1 disease was 76.2%, 100%, 96.6%, and 96.2%, respectively. The accuracy of mediastinal staging was 95.7%.

Conclusions.—Endobronchial ultrasound-guided transbronchial needle aspiration can accurately access the hilar and interlobar lymph nodes in patients with potentially resectable lung cancer. Accurate assessment of cN0 versus cN1 by EBUS-TBNA may be used to guide induction therapy before surgery (Fig 1).

▶ The diagnostic utility of endobronchial ultrasonography (EBUS) continues to expand. This retrospective review by Yasufuku and colleagues specifically evaluates the ability of EBUS to assess the hilar and interlobar nodes (nodal stations 10, 11, and 12) in patients with potentially resectable clinical stage I and II lung cancer. The main findings are shown in Fig 1. As in other studies looking at EBUS, the likelihood of finding hilar or mediastinal cancer in patients with no radiographic evidence of nodal involvement (cN0) was low although present. EBUS missed 5% of cancers found to be pN1 and 3% of cancers found to be pN2 at resection The more interesting finding of this study relates to the group of patients with radiographically abnormal N1 nodes (cN1). In those 69 patients, 47 were found to have N0 by EBUS and all 47 were confirmed to have pN0 at resection. As a diagnostic modality, the role of EBUS was initially felt to be in confirming cancer in radiographically abnormal nodes. In this particular study, the other end of the spectrum also appears to be valid, that EBUS is accurate enough to exclude cancer in radiographically abnormal nodes.

Radiographically abnormal N2 nodes should be biopsy-confirmed before assuming they are malignant, as the consequences of falsely assuming a patient has stage III or higher disease are significant.[1] Any number of staging modalities can be used to provide biopsy confirmation of N2 disease.[2] Assessment of N1 nodes has been more difficult. The clinical situation in which this becomes most relevant is the patient for whom limited, highly localized therapy (sublobar resection, stereotactic body radiotherapy, radiofrequency ablation) for the primary tumor is preferred because of pulmonary physiologic limitations or other comorbidities, but where there is a question of malignant involvement of the hilar nodes. This study suggests that EBUS may be highly accurate in assessing the N1 nodes in these cases and may identify more candidates for definitive treatment.

L. T. Tanoue, MD

References

1. Silvestri GA, Gonzalez AV, Jantz MA, et al. Methods for staging non-small cell lung cancer: Diagnosis and management of lung cancer, 3rd ed: American College of Chest Physicians evidence-based clinical practice guidelines. *Chest.* 2013;143: e211S-e250S.
2. Detterbeck FC, Jantz MA, Wallace M, et al. Invasive mediastinal staging of lung cancer: ACCP evidence-based clinical practice guidelines (2nd edition). *Chest.* 2007;132:202S-220S.

Lung Cancer Treatment

Physiologic Evaluation of the Patient With Lung Cancer Being Considered for Resectional Surgery: Diagnosis and Management of Lung Cancer, 3rd ed: American College of Chest Physicians Evidence-Based Clinical Practice Guidelines
Brunelli A, Kim AW, Berger KI, et al (OspedaliRiuniti, Ancona, Italy; Yale Univ School of Medicine, New Haven, CT; New York Univ School of Medicine)
Chest 143:e166S-e190S, 2013

Background.—This section of the guidelines is intended to provide an evidence-based approach to the preoperative physiologic assessment of a patient being considered for surgical resection of lung cancer.

Methods.—The current guidelines and medical literature applicable to this issue were identified by computerized search and were evaluated using standardized methods. Recommendations were framed using the approach described by the Guidelines Oversight Committee.

Results.—The preoperative physiologic assessment should begin with a cardiovascular evaluation and spirometry to measure the FEV_1 and the diffusing capacity for carbon monoxide (D_{LCO}). Predicted postoperative (PPO) lung functions should be calculated. If the % PPO FEV_1 and % PPO D_{LCO} values are both >60%, the patient is considered at low risk of anatomic lung resection, and no further tests are indicated. If either the % PPO FEV_1 or % PPO D_{LCO} are within 60% and 30% predicted, a low technology exercise test should be performed as a screening test. If performance on the low technology exercise test is satisfactory (stair climbing altitude >22 m or shuttle walk distance >400 m), patients are regarded as at

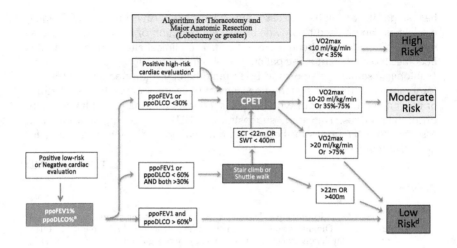

FIGURE 2.—[Section 4.0] Physiologic evaluation resection algorithm. (a) For pneumonectomy candidates, we suggest to use Q scan to calculate predicted postoperative values of FEV1 or DLCO (PPO values = preoperative values × (1 − fraction of total perfusion for the resected lung), where the preoperative values are taken as the best measured postbronchodilator values. For lobectomy patients, segmental counting is indicated to calculate predicted postoperative values of FEV1 or DLCO (PPO values = preoperative values × (1 − y/z), where the preoperative values are taken as the best measured postbronchodilator value and the number of functional or unobstructed lung segments to be removed is y and the total number of functional segments is z. (b) PpoFEV1 or ppoDLCO cut off values of 60% predicted values has been chosen based on indirect evidences and expert consensus opinion. (c) For patients with a positive high-risk cardiac evaluation deemed to be stable to proceed to surgery we suggest to perform both pulmonary function tests and cardiopulmonary exercise test for a more precise definition of risk. (d) Definition of risk: Low risk: The expected risk of mortality is below 1%. Major anatomic resections can be safely performed in this group. Moderate risk: Morbidity and mortality rates may vary according to the values of split lung functions, exercise tolerance and extent of resection. Risks and benefits of the operation should be thoroughly discussed with the patient. High risk: The risk of mortality after standard major anatomic resections may be higher than 10%. Considerable risk of severe cardiopulmonary morbidity and residual functional loss is expected. Patients should be counseled about alternative surgical (minor resections or minimally invasive surgery) or nonsurgical options. ppoDLCO = predicted postoperative diffusing capacity for carbon mon oxide; ppoDLCO% = percent predicted postoperative diffusing capacity for carbon monoxide; ppoFEV1 = predicted postoperative FEV1; ppoFEV1% = percent predicted postoperative FEV1; SCT = stair climb test; SWT = shuttle walk test; VO2max = maximal oxygen consumption. See Figure 1 legend for expansion of other abbreviations. (Reprinted from Brunelli A, Kim AW, Berger KI, et al. Physiologic evaluation of the patient with lung cancer being considered for resectional surgery: diagnosis and management of lung cancer, 3rd ed: American College of Chest Physicians evidence-based clinical practice guidelines. *Chest.* 2013;143:e166S-e190S, with permission from American College of Chest Physicians.)

low risk of anatomic resection. A cardiopulmonary exercise test is indicated when the PPO FEV$_1$ or PPO D$_{LCO}$ (or both) are <30% or when the performance of the stair-climbing test or the shuttle walk test is not satisfactory. A peak oxygen consumption (VO$_2$peak) <10 mL/kg/min or 35% predicted indicates a high risk of mortality and long-term disability for major anatomic resection. Conversely, a $\dot{V}O_2$peak >20 mL/kg/min or 75% predicted indicates a low risk.

Conclusions.—A careful preoperative physiologic assessment is useful for identifying those patients at increased risk with standard lung cancer resection and for enabling an informed decision by the patient about the appropriate therapeutic approach to treating his or her lung cancer. This preoperative risk assessment must be placed in the context that surgery for early-stage lung cancer is the most effective currently available treatment of this disease (Fig 2).

▶ Preoperative physiologic assessment of the patient being considered for lung cancer resection is a bread-and-butter challenge in pulmonary medicine and thoracic surgery. Many patients with lung cancer have underlying comorbidities, particularly cardiovascular disease. The challenge, however, is often related to whether they will be able to withstand resection with preservation of pulmonary function and quality of life, typically because of concern related to concurrent chronic obstructive pulmonary disease, interstitial lung disease, or other lung disease. This article discusses in detail the evidence behind the algorithm (Fig 2) proposed to guide physiologic evaluation before major anatomic lung resection (lobectomy or greater).

The algorithm assumes an exclusion of cardiac issues precluding surgery and begins with the calculation of predicted postoperative (PPO) forced expiratory volume in 1 second (FEV_1) and diffusing capacity for carbon monoxide (D_{LCO}). For pneumonectomy candidates, a perfusion scan is recommended, to inform the calculation: PPO values for FEV_1 and D_{LCO} = preoperative values × (1 − fraction of total perfusion for the resected lung). For lobectomy patients, the algorithm recommends that segmental counting is adequate, using the calculation: PPO values of FEV_1 and D_{LCO} = preoperative values × (1 − y/z), where y is the number of functional lung segments to be removed and z is the total number of functional segments. Of note, the authors suggest that, for patients with PPO FEV_1 and D_{LCO} less than 60% but greater than 30%, low technology tests such as stair climb or shuttle walk may be sufficient. In contrast, patients with worse pulmonary function (PPO FEV_1 or PPO D_{LCO} < 30%) or whose low technology test results are poor should undergo formal cardiopulmonary exercise testing to assess their risk for significant postresection impairment or increased mortality.

Surgery is still the best therapy for patients with early-stage lung cancer.[1] Patients with impaired pulmonary function should undergo a thoughtful objective physiologic assessment as an essential part of informing any decision to consider or recommend a nonsurgical approach.

L. T. Tanoue, MD

Reference

1. Howington JA, Blum MG, Chang AC, Balekian AA, Murthy SC. Treatment of stage I and II non-small cell lung cancer: Diagnosis and management of lung cancer, 3rd ed: American College of Chest Physicians evidence-based clinical practice guidelines. *Chest.* 2013;143:e278S-e313S.

Mechanism of Action of Conventional and Targeted Anticancer Therapies: Reinstating Immunosurveillance

Zitvogel L, Galluzzi L, Smyth MJ, et al (INSERM, Villejuif, France; Université Paris Descartes/Paris V, France; Queensland Inst of Med Res, Herston, Australia; et al)
Immunity 39:74-88, 2013

Conventional chemotherapeutics and targeted antineoplastic agents have been developed based on the simplistic notion that cancer constitutes a cell-autonomous genetic or epigenetic disease. However, it is becoming clear that many of the available anticancer drugs that have collectively saved millions of life-years mediate therapeutic effects by eliciting de novo or reactivating pre-existing tumor-specific immune responses. Here, we discuss the capacity of both conventional and targeted anticancer therapies to enhance the immunogenic properties of malignant cells and to stimulate immune effector cells, either directly or by subverting the immunosuppressive circuitries that preclude antitumor immune responses in cancer patients. Accumulating evidence indicates that the therapeutic efficacy of several antineoplastic agents relies on their capacity to influence the tumor-host interaction, tipping the balance toward the activation of an immune response specific for malignant cells. We surmise that the development of successful anticancer therapies will be improved and accelerated by the immunological characterization of candidate agents.

▶ Substantive progress in treatment of advanced-stage non–small-cell lung cancer (NSCLC) has been made over the last several years. Previously, standard first-line treatment for advanced-stage disease had been a one-size-fits-all approach with platinum-based combination chemotherapy. In the last several years, this has been dramatically influenced by the identification of driver mutations, particularly epidermal growth factor receptor mutations and anaplastic lymphoma kinase rearrangements.[1-3] For patients with these identifiable genetic abnormalities, first-line treatment with targeted agents may be as, or more, effective and less toxic than standard combination chemotherapy. More recently, an antitumor effect in NSCLC was observed using inhibitors of the immune checkpoint receptor, programmed death receptor-1.[4,5] This latter discovery as well as the benefit of the anti–CTLA-4 antibody, ipilimumab, in advanced melanoma has rekindled interest in the concept that the immune system can be targeted or harnessed for antitumor effects. Although immunotherapy has historically been ineffective in the treatment of advanced solid tumors, a protective endogenous anticancer immune response is generally held to exist and is presumably bypassed or suppressed by tumors through several mechanisms. Therapeutic antineoplastic immunomodulatory approaches include interventions to increase endogenous immunosurveillance or mitigate immunosubversion by tumor cells. Cancer vaccines, immunomodulators, and immune checkpoint blockers are all potential avenues for research in this field. As it becomes increasingly possible to understand the biology milieu of individual tumors, the choice of treatment should be increasingly specific to their biologic weak points.

L. T. Tanoue, MD

References

1. Kwak EL, Bang YJ, Camidge DR, et al. Anaplastic lymphoma kinase inhibition in non-small-cell lung cancer. *N Engl J Med.* 2010;363:1693-1703.
2. Pao W, Girard N. New driver mutations in non-small-cell lung cancer. *Lancet Oncol.* 2011;12:175-180.
3. Maemondo M, Inoue A, Kobayashi K, et al. Gefitinib or chemotherapy for non-small-cell lung cancer with mutated EGFR. *N Engl J Med.* 2010;362:2380-2388.
4. Brahmer JR, Tykodi SS, Chow LQ, et al. Safety and activity of anti-PD-L1 antibody in patients with advanced cancer. *N Engl J Med.* 2012;366:2455-2465.
5. Topalian SL, Hodi FS, Brahmer JR, et al. Safety, activity, and immune correlates of anti-PD-1 antibody in cancer. *N Engl J Med.* 2012;366:2443-2454.

American College of Chest Physicians and Society of Thoracic Surgeons Consensus Statement for Evaluation and Management for High-Risk Patients With Stage I Non-small Cell Lung Cancer

Donington J, for the Thoracic Oncology Network of American College of Chest Physicians, Workforce on Evidence-Based Surgery of Society of Thoracic Surgeons (NYU School of Medicine; et al)

Chest 142:1620-1635, 2012

Background.—The standard treatment of stage I non-small cell lung cancer (NSCLC) is lobectomy with systematic mediastinal lymph node evaluation. Unfortunately, up to 25% of patients with stage I NSCLC are not candidates for lobectomy because of severe medical comorbidity.

Methods.—A panel of experts was convened through the Thoracic Oncology Network of the American College of Chest Physicians and the Workforce on Evidence-Based Surgery of the Society of Thoracic Surgeons. Following a literature review, the panel developed 13 suggestions for evaluation and treatment through iterative discussion and debate until unanimous agreement was achieved.

Results.—Pretreatment evaluation should focus primarily on measures of cardiopulmonary physiology, as respiratory failure represents the greatest interventional risk. Alternative treatment options to lobectomy for high-risk patients include sublobar resection with or without brachytherapy, stereotactic body radiation therapy, and radiofrequency ablation. Each is associated with decreased procedural morbidity and mortality but increased risk for involved lobe and regional recurrence compared with lobectomy, but direct comparisons between modalities are lacking.

Conclusions.—Therapeutic options for the treatment of high-risk patients are evolving quickly. Improved radiographic staging and the diagnosis of smaller and more indolent tumors push the risk-benefit decision toward parenchymal-sparing or nonoperative therapies in high-risk patients. Unbiased assessment of treatment options requires uniform reporting of treatment populations and outcomes in clinical series, which has been lacking to date.

▶ Surgical resection is the optimal treatment for patients with stage I non−small-cell lung cancer (NSCLC). However, patients with lung cancer often have concomitant comorbidities related to cigarette smoking, particularly chronic obstructive pulmonary disease, and also tend to be older. In situations in which the standard approach with lobectomy and mediastinal lymphadenectomy is precluded because of unacceptably high risks of morbidity and mortality, alternative approaches include anatomic segmentectomy or wedge resection, stereotactic body radiotherapy (SBRT), conventional external beam radiation therapy, or radiofrequency ablation (RFA). There is little rigorous study comparing these options, and what evidence does exist tends to be retrospective. Compared with lobectomy, these more limited approaches to treatment do appear to decrease the risk of respiratory failure, pulmonary disability, and death, but whether survival outcome is equivalent to that of lobectomy is not clear.

Based on the available medical literature and expert opinion, the consensus recommendations include the following:

- Segmentectomy or extended wedge resection with margins greater than 1 cm or equal to the tumor diameter with hilar and mediastinal nodal evaluation is suggested as a safe and effective alternative to lobectomy in high-risk patients with stage I NSCLC.
- In patients with stage I NSCLC who are older than 75 years, segmentectomy or extended wedge resection is suggested as an effective and potentially beneficial alternative to lobectomy.
- Anatomic segmentectomy is preferred, when possible, to wedge resection in patients who undergo sublobar resection for stage I NSCLC.
- Conventionally fractionated radiation therapy with definitive intent and sufficient dose intensity is a reasonable treatment option for high-risk stage I NSCLC, but, for tumors greater than 5 cm, in which normal tissue dose constraints can be respected, SBRT is preferred over conventionally fractionated radiation therapy for definitive treatment of high-risk stage I NSCLC.
- RFA is a reasonable treatment option in high-risk patients with stage I NSCLC with peripheral lesions less than 3 cm, but reduced primary tumor control limits enthusiasm for its use to those patients who are not candidates for SBRT or sublobar resection.

A discussion of the medical literature informing these recommendations is provided in the text.

Anticipating lung cancer screening will increase the numbers of patients diagnosed with early stage lung cancer, decisions of how best to treat patients with stage I NSCLC who are not optimal lobectomy candidates because of comorbid conditions will become more common. Given the options that are available, these decisions should ideally be made using a multidisciplinary approach. More study is required to compare the benefits and limitations of each modality.

L. T. Tanoue, MD

Molecular Approach to Lung Cancer

Targeted Therapy for Non—Small Cell Lung Cancer

Jett JR, Carr LL (Natl Jewish Health, Denver, CO)
Am J Respir Crit Care Med 188:907-912, 2013

Background.—Treatment for stage IV non-n-small cell lung cancer (NSCLC) before 2005 relied on platinum-based doublet chemotherapy for all subtypes of this disease. Sensitizing mutations (driver mutations) in the epidermal growth factor receptor (EGFR) tyrosine kinase (TK) domain were discovered in 2004. The two sensitizing EGFR driver mutations occur predominantly in lung adenocarcinomas. A transforming echinoderm microtubule-associated protein like (EML)4-anaplastic lymphoma kinase (ALK) gene fusion that functions as a driver mutation was also found and similarly occurs mainly in lung adenocarcinomas. Research to identify the optimal therapy for tumors with these driver mutations has yielded erlotinib and gefitinib for EGFR-TK mutations and crizotinib for ALK-TK mutations. Gefitinib is unavailable in the United States but widely used in other areas of the world and has characteristics similar to those of erlotinib.

Erlotinib.—Erlotinib is an orally administered small molecule that competes with adenosine triphosphate (ATP) and inhibits receptor autophosphorylation and downstream proliferation. The dose is usually 150 mg once a day until disease progression. Erlotinib is best absorbed on a full stomach. Metabolism is hepatic, with excretion mainly in feces. If toxicity develops, dose adjustments are made in 50-mg increments; a short cessation of therapy may be required to recover from toxic effects. Doses as low as 50 and 25 mg/day have yielded clinical responses.

Factors that alter effectiveness include concomitant use of cytochrome (CYP)3A4 inhibitors, CYP3A4 inducers, and smoking. No adjustment in dose is usually required for patients with impaired renal function or moderately impaired hepatic function, but a total bilirubin three times the upper limit of normal is a contraindication. Erlotinib can benefit selected patients with central nervous system (CNS) metastases and patients with malignant pleural effusions. The combination of platinum-based doublet chemotherapy and erlotinib for patients with EGFR-TK mutations may improve progression-free survival and response rates compared to single-agent TK inhibitor (TKI) treatment. Adverse effects with erlotinib are mainly dermatologic and gastrointestinal but also include pulmonary toxicity for patients with pretreatment interstitial lung disease (ILD).

Erlotinib is approved for use as a second-line treatment for NSCLC. Cost analysis indicates erlotinib treatment for previously treated NSCLC is marginally cost effective.

Crizotinib.—Crizotinib is an orally administered small-molecule ATP competitive inhibitor of ALK and c-MET that inhibits TK domain phosphorylation and blocks signals in cell pathways essential to growth and survival. The usual dose is 250 mg twice a day with or without food. Metabolism is mainly hepatic, with excretion largely in feces but 20% in urine. The most common treatment-related adverse effects are visual disturbances, nausea, diarrhea, vomiting, and constipation. Toxic effects can be managed by reducing the dose to 200 mg orally twice a day, then 250 mg once a day as needed. CYP3A4 inhibitors increase the risk of toxicity and inducers decrease drug effectiveness. Mild to moderate renal impairment requires no dose adjustment, but data are incomplete for more severe renal disease and for hepatic impairment. Cerebrospinal fluid penetration is usually poor. Standard doses are ineffective for CNS metastases.

Crizotinib is approved for use only in patients whose NSCLC is positive on fluorescence in situ hybridization (FISH) for ALK fusion. Although a cost analysis is not available for crizotinib, the average wholesale price for this agent in the United States is $12,400 per month. This agent has not been tested in combination with other chemotherapeutic drugs.

Conclusions.—Therapy for advanced NSCLC is determined by the results of histologic and molecular testing done preferably before beginning treatment and targeting EGFR mutations and ALK fusion. Patients with untreated metastatic NSCLC and sensitizing EGFR mutation should be given erlotinib or gefitinib. Patients with untreated metastatic NSCLC and ALK fusion should receive single-agent crizotinib. If patients received chemotherapy before identifying a sensitizing EGFR mutation or ALK fusion, erlotinib/gelitinib for the former and crizotinib for the latter should be considered. Disease progression should trigger the switch, but definitive timing is unclear. Underlying ILD predisposes to pulmonary toxicity and is a relative contraindication to using a TK inhibitor. Otherwise, ILD occurs in a small percentage of patients taking TK inhibitors.

▶ In 2004, lung cancer treatment was revolutionized by the description of epidermal growth factor receptor gene (EGFR) mutations in non–small-cell lung cancers that were associated with responsiveness of those tumors to inhibitors of the EGFR pathway.[1,2] This discovery has led to the recognition of a number of driver mutations that are integral to tumorigenesis in some lung adenocarcinomas. The elegant understanding of the EGFR in the context of lung cancer has been instrumental in the pursuit of other such signaling pathways in lung cancer (Fig 1 in the original article). A growing percentage of lung adenocarcinomas appear to harbor these potentially targetable mutations, and these discoveries are now informing the development of entirely new lines of treatment.

In this article, Jett and Carr discuss the successful therapies targeted to EGFR mutations and the echinoderm microtubule-associated protein like-4 (EML4) anaplastic lymphoma kinase (ALK) gene fusion. Not all mutations predict response to inhibition of the signaling pathways related to these genes. For EGFR, the presence of either exon 19 deletion or exon 21 mutation, but not other mutations, predicts response to treatment with the tyrosine kinase inhibitors erlotinib and gefitinib. Conversely, the presence or development of a second mutation in T790M is associated with the development of resistance to those therapies.[3,4] Crizotinib, another tyrosine kinase inhibitor, is effective in blocking signaling in tumors expressing the EML4-ALK fusion gene.[5,6]

Appreciating the importance of identifying potentially targetable mutations places a responsibility on physicians involved in procuring tissue that will determine a diagnosis and pathologists analyzing diagnostic material. Mutational analysis should ideally be included in the diagnostic algorithm for all patients with lung cancers.

L. T. Tanoue, MD

References

1. Pao W, Miller V, Zakowski M, et al. EGF receptor gene mutations are common in lung cancers from "never smokers" and are associated with sensitivity of tumors to gefitinib and erlotinib. *Proc Natl Acad Sci U S A.* 2004;101:13306-13311.
2. Lynch TJ, Bell DW, Sordella R, et al. Activating mutations in the epidermal growth factor receptor underlying responsiveness of non-small-cell lung cancer to gefitinib. *N Engl J Med.* 2004;350:2129-2139.
3. Yu HA, Arcila ME, Rekhtman N, et al. Analysis of tumor specimens at the time of acquired resistance to EGFR-TKI therapy in 155 patients with EGFR-mutant lung cancers. *Clin Cancer Res.* 2013;19:2240-2247.
4. Sequist LV, Waltman BA, Dias-Santagata D, et al. Genotypic and histological evolution of lung cancers acquiring resistance to EGFR inhibitors. *Sci Transl Med.* 2011;3:75ra26.
5. Kwak EL, Bang YJ, Camidge DR, et al. Anaplastic lymphoma kinase inhibition in non-small-cell lung cancer. *N Engl J Med.* 2010;363:1693-1703.
6. Choi YL, Soda M, Yamashita Y, et al. EML4-ALK mutations in lung cancer that confer resistance to ALK inhibitors. *N Engl J Med.* 2010;363:1734-1739.

The Impact of Genomic Changes on Treatment of Lung Cancer
Cardarella S, Johnson BE (Dana-Farber Cancer Inst, Boston, MA; Brigham and Women's Hosp and Harvard Med School, Boston, MA)
Am J Respir Crit Care Med 188:770-775, 2013

The remarkable success of epidermal growth factor receptor (EGFR) and anaplastic lymphoma kinase (ALK) tyrosine kinase inhibitors in patients with *EGFR* mutations and *ALK* rearrangements, respectively, introduced the era of targeted therapy in advanced non-small cell lung cancer (NSCLC), shifting treatment from platinum-based combination chemotherapy to molecularly tailored therapy. Recent genomic studies in lung adenocarcinoma identified other potential therapeutic targets, including *ROS1* rearrangements, *RET* fusions, *MET* amplification, and activating mutations in *BRAF*, *HER2*, and *KRAS* in frequencies exceeding 1%. Lung cancers that harbor these genomic changes can potentially be targeted with agents approved for other indications or under clinical development. The need to generate increasing amounts of genomic information should prompt health-care providers to be mindful of the amounts of tissue needed for these assays when planning diagnostic procedures. In this review, we summarize oncogenic drivers in NSCLC that can be currently detected, highlight their potential therapeutic implications, and discuss practical considerations for successful application of tumor genotyping in clinical decision making.

▶ The recognition of genetic mutations that drive tumors has energized lung cancer therapeutic innovation over the last 2 decades. The development of agents targeted to these mutations has been of particular impact in the group of patients with advanced disease who account for most patients with lung cancer. Building on the success of tyrosine kinase inhibition for treatment of tumors expressing genetic abnormalities in the epidermal growth factor receptor (EGFR) and anaplastic lymphoma kinase (ALK) genes,[1-3] genomic analyses of lung tumors have identified many other mutations in cellular pathways that may contribute to carcinogenesis. This review is a comprehensive look at the oncogenic driver mutations that are currently identified and of potential interest in developing agents for treatment. Fig 1 in the original article shows that most of adenocarcinomas and squamous cell carcinomas of the lung have demonstrable genetic mutations, all of which are theoretically targetable. These scientific discoveries are rapidly being translated into the development of agents for clinical treatment trials. The importance of a targetable site makes imperative the commitment of physicians obtaining and analyzing diagnostic specimens to obtain mutational analysis for their lung cancer patients, particularly those with disease not amenable to surgical resection.

L. T. Tanoue, MD

References

1. Jett JR, Carr LL. Targeted therapy for non-small cell lung cancer. *Am J Respir Crit Care Med.* 2013;188:907-912.
2. Lynch TJ, Bell DW, Sordella R, et al. Activating mutations in the epidermal growth factor receptor underlying responsiveness of non-small-cell lung cancer to gefitinib. *N Engl J Med.* 2004;350:2129-2139.
3. Kwak EL, Bang YJ, Camidge DR, et al. Anaplastic lymphoma kinase inhibition in non-small-cell lung cancer. *N Engl J Med.* 2010;363:1693-1703.

4 Pleural, Interstitial Lung, and Pulmonary Vascular Disease

Introduction

For this edition of the YEAR BOOK, a broad range of publications was reviewed pertaining to interstitial lung disease, pleural disease, and pulmonary vascular disease. This chapter begins with a couple of impressive studies looking at molecular markers of prognosis in usual interstitial pneumonitis. Echocardiographic and hemodynamic findings are also linked to prognosis in the third paper. In the next, morbidity and mortality of open lung biopsy is assessed. The role of ambulatory oxygen supplementation in fibrosis is also investigated. The section finishes with a review of diagnosis and treatment of connective tissue disease-related interstitial lung disease (CTD-ILD), as well as an assessment of mycophenolate mofetil for treatment of CTD-ILD.

The pleural disease section starts with a look at the association between pleural plaques and development of mesothelioma. The next two papers address surgical treatment of empyema. This is followed by an assessment of tunneled pleural catheter placement verses talc poudrage at time of VATS. An assessment of infection rates and outcomes associated with tunneled pleural catheters completes the section.

This year there was considerable activity in the realm of pulmonary vascular disease in the literature. The section begins with validation of a clinical worsening definition for pulmonary arterial hypertension (PAH). The next paper looks at the disparity between the guidelines and actual treatment at time of death in this disease. A novel channelopathy is then identified as a potential cause of familial PAH. An elegant study follows that evaluates the potential role of a novel agent in counteracting the effect of mutations in familial disease. Next, a catheter-based ablative procedure is proposed as a potential treatment of PAH in a pilot study. Results of two studies of the first in a new class of drug, the guanylate cyclase stimulator riociguat, are presented next. The first looks at the agent in patients with chronic thromboembolic disease, making it the first FDA-approved medical therapy for this indication. The next assesses its efficacy in PAH.

The section and chapter end with a clinical trial investigating the long-term efficacy of macitentan in PAH.

Christopher D. Spradley, MD, FCCP

Interstitial Lung Disease

The Toll-like Receptor 3 L412F Polymorphism and Disease Progression in Idiopathic Pulmonary Fibrosis

O'Dwyer DN, Armstrong ME, Trujillo G, et al (Univ College Dublin, Belfield, Ireland; Univ of Michigan Med School, Ann Arbor; et al)
Am J Respir Crit Care Med 188:1442-1450, 2013

Rationale.—Idiopathic pulmonary fibrosis (IPF) is a fatal progressive interstitial pneumonia. The innate immune system provides a crucial function in the recognition of tissue injury and infection. Toll-like receptor 3 (TLR3) is an innate immune system receptor. We investigated the role of a functional *TLR3* single-nucleotide polymorphism in IPF.

Objectives.—To characterize the effects of the *TLR3* Leu412Phe polymorphism in primary pulmonary fibroblasts from patients with IPF and disease progression in two independent IPF patient cohorts. To investigate the role of TLR3 in a murine model of pulmonary fibrosis.

Methods.—TLR3-mediated cytokine, type 1 IFN, and fibroproliferative responses were examined in TLR3 wild-type (Leu/Leu), heterozygote (Leu/Phe), and homozygote (Phe/Phe) primary IPF pulmonary fibroblasts by ELISA, real-time polymerase chain reaction, and proliferation assays. A murine model of bleomycin-induced pulmonary fibrosis was used in TLR3 wild-type ($tlr3^{+/+}$) and TLR3 knockout mice ($tlr3^{-/-}$). A genotyping approach was used to investigate the role of the TLR3 L412F polymorphism in disease progression in IPF using survival analysis and longitudinal decline in FVC.

Measurements and Main Results.—Activation of TLR3 in primary lung fibroblasts from *TLR3* L412F-variant patients with IPF resulted in defective cytokine, type I IFN, and fibroproliferative responses. We demonstrate increased collagen and profibrotic cytokines in TLR3 knockout mice ($tlr3^{-/-}$) compared with wild-type mice ($tlr3^{+/+}$). TLR3 L412F was also associated with a significantly greater risk of mortality and an accelerated decline in FVC in patients with IPF.

Conclusions.—This study reveals the crucial role of defective TLR3 function in promoting progressive IPF.

▶ In this compelling study by O'Dwyer et al published in the *Blue Journal*, the authors conduct a series of well-designed investigations to identify and elaborate on the role of the toll-like receptor 3 (TLR3) L412F polymorphism in rapid progression of idiopathic pulmonary fibrosis (IPF). The polymorphism has been shown to confer protection against age-related macular degeneration and is implicated in increased risk for cardiomyopathy after viral myocarditis.

The authors investigated 2 large cohorts of human subjects with IPF (the UK IPF cohort and subjects from the INSPIRE IPF trial) and a murine model for the polymorphism using a bleomycin-induced lung injury model.

The findings pose a strong case for the role of TLR3 L412F polymorphism in rapidly progressive IPF. These findings pave the way toward a better understanding of the pathogenesis of IPF. This polymorphism may also serve as a marker for patients with more aggressive disease and may eventually provide a therapeutic target for severe, rapidly progressive IPF.

C. D. Spradley, MD

Patients with Idiopathic Pulmonary Fibrosis with Antibodies to Heat Shock Protein 70 Have Poor Prognoses
Kahloon RA, Xue J, Bhargava A, et al (Univ of Pittsburgh, PA; et al)
Am J Respir Crit Care Med 187:768-775, 2013

Rationale.—Diverse autoantibodies are present in most patients with idiopathic pulmonary fibrosis (IPF). We hypothesized that specific autoantibodies may associate with IPF manifestations.

Objectives.—To identify clinically relevant, antigen-specific immune responses in patients with IPF.

Methods.—Autoantibodies were detected by immunoblots and ELISA. Intrapulmonary immune processes were evaluated by immunohistochemistry. Anti–heat shock protein 70 (HSP70) IgG was isolated from plasma by immunoaffinity. Flow cytometry was used for leukocyte functional studies.

Measurements and Main Results.—HSP70 was identified as a potential IPF autoantigen in discovery assays. Anti-HSP70 IgG autoantibodies were detected by immunoblots in 3% of 60 control subjects versus 25% of a cross-sectional IPF cohort (n = 122) ($P = 0.0004$), one-half the patients with IPF who died ($P = 0.008$), and 70% of those with acute exacerbations ($P = 0.0005$). Anti-HSP70 autoantibodies in patients with IPF were significantly associated with HLA allele biases, greater subsequent FVC reductions ($P = 0.0004$), and lesser 1-year survival (40 ± 10% vs. 80 ± 5%; hazard ratio = 4.2; 95% confidence interval, 2.0–8.6; $P < 0.0001$). HSP70 protein, antigen–antibody complexes, and complement were prevalent in IPF lungs. HSP70 protein was an autoantigen for IPF CD4 T cells, inducing lymphocyte proliferation ($P = 0.004$) and IL-4 production ($P = 0.01$). IPF anti-HSP70 autoantibodies activated monocytes ($P = 0.009$) and increased monocyte IL-8 production ($P = 0.049$). ELISA confirmed the association between anti-HSP70 autoreactivity and IPF outcome. Anti-HSP70 autoantibodies were also found in patients with other interstitial lung diseases but were not associated with their clinical progression.

Conclusions.—Patients with IPF with anti-HSP70 autoantibodies have more near-term lung function deterioration and mortality. These findings suggest antigen-specific immunoassays could provide useful clinical information in individual patients with IPF and may have implications for understanding IPF progression.

▶ Through diligent investigation and deductive reasoning, Kahloon et al identified heat shock protein 70 (HSP70) as a potential auto-antigen with prognostic value in idiopathic pulmonary fibrosis (IPF). The authors then showed CD4T cell activation and elaboration of IL 4 in IPF patients in response to HSP70. This was not observed in non-IPF controls. Anti-HSP70 autoantibodies were also found to activate monocytes and drive production of interleukin 8.

IPF patients with anti-HSP70 positivity were found to have more reduction in forced vital capacity, and survival was decreased. Anti-HSP70 was also present in two-thirds of patients presenting with acute exacerbations of IPF and 75% of those who showed exacerbation within 1 year. Mortality associated with exacerbation at 6 months was 100% in anti-HSP70 subjects verses 33% in auto-antibody-negative patients. Mortality associated with anti-HSP70 was also assessed in a post-hoc analysis of nontransplanted patients, and the survival difference was apparent. Comparison of autoantibody positive and negative groups is provided in Fig 4 of the original article. In addition, a specific human leukocyte antigen class II allele, DRB1*11, was found to be protective, whereas DRB1*15 conferred risk of autoantibody positivity.

The authors also investigated another heat shock protein with similar weight and autoantigenicity in IPF and detected no meaningful clinical difference between antibody-positive and antibody-negative subjects.

The finding of a specific autoantibody that confers greater risk in IPF patients may prove helpful in prognostication and planning for transplantation. It may also pave the way for future targeted therapies in this disease, which currently evades effective treatment.

C. D. Spradley, MD

Echocardiographic and Hemodynamic Predictors of Mortality in Idiopathic Pulmonary Fibrosis

Rivera-Lebron BN, Forfia PR, Kreider M, et al (Univ of Pennsylvania, Philadelphia)
Chest 144:564-570, 2013

Background.—Idiopathic pulmonary fibrosis (IPF) can lead to the development of pulmonary hypertension, which is associated with an increased risk of death. In pulmonary arterial hypertension, survival is directly related to the capacity of the right ventricle to adapt to elevated pulmonary vascular load. The relative importance of right ventricular function in IPF is not well understood. Our objective was to evaluate right ventricular echocardiographic and hemodynamic predictors of mortality in a cohort of patients with IPF referred for lung transplant evaluation.

Methods.—We performed a retrospective cohort study of 135 patients who met 2011 American Thoracic Society/European Respiratory Society criteria for IPF and who were evaluated for lung transplantation at the Hospital of the University of Pennsylvania.

Results.—Right ventricle:left ventricle diameter ratio (hazard ratio [HR], 4.5; 95% CI, 1.7-11.9), moderate to severe right atrial and right ventricular dilation (HR, 2.9; 95% CI, 1.4-5.9; and HR, 2.7; 95% CI, 1.4-5.4, respectively) and right ventricular dysfunction (HR, 5.5; 95% CI, 2.6-11.5) were associated with an increased risk of death. Higher pulmonary vascular resistance was also associated with increased mortality (HR per 1 Wood unit, 1.3; 95% CI, 1.1-1.5). These risk factors were independent of age, sex, race, height, weight, FVC, and lung transplantation status. Other hemodynamic indices, such as mean pulmonary artery pressure and cardiac index, were not associated with outcome.

Conclusions.—Right-sided heart size and right ventricular dysfunction measured by echocardiography and higher pulmonary vascular resistance by invasive hemodynamic assessment predict mortality in patients with IPF evaluated for lung transplantation.

▶ Patients with pulmonary hypertension in the setting of idiopathic pulmonary fibrosis (PH-IPF) have a 3-fold risk of death compared with patients with IPF without PH. In this retrospective cohort study, Rivera-Lebron et al set out to identify the role of echocardiographic and hemodynamic parameters in outcomes of patients with IPF.

The study evaluated patients referred for transplant to a single facility between 2005 and 2010. Of the 787 patients in the cohort, 153 met American Thoracic Society 2011 criteria for the diagnosis of IPF, and 18 of these lacked the requisite echocardiographic or hemodynamic data, leaving 135 subjects for analysis.

The authors worked to ensure the validity of their clinical data by over-reading and correlating all echo results. They also over-read the right heart catheterization data for those studies with available waveforms.

In the end, the team found that right ventricle to left ventricle diameter ratio (RV:LV), moderate to severe right ventricular and right atrial dilation, and right ventricular dysfunction measured by tricuspid annular plane systolic excursion (TAPSE) correlated with increased mortality on echo. They also correlated elevated pulmonary vascular resistance with mortality. An increase of 1 WU was associated with a 25% increased risk of death. Survival curves for TAPSE and RV:LV were presented in Figs 1 and 2 of the original article.

Additionally, the team found that 29% of the cohort had PH-IPF based on mean pulmonary artery pressure ≥25 mm Hg and pulmonary capillary wedge pressure ≤15 mm Hg. When censored for transplantation, these patients had higher risk of death. They also found that RV systolic pressure was unmeasurable in more than 25% of the cohort. Interestingly, classic hemodynamic measures of RV dysfunction, namely stroke volume, cardiac output, and right atrial pressure, did not correlate with mortality. Mean pulmonary artery pressure was also not predictive.

Although this retrospective cohort study needs validation, it does point out potential markers for poor outcome that can only be derived by echocardiography and right heart catheterization.

C. D. Spradley, MD

Morbidity and mortality in patients with usual interstitial pneumonia (UIP) pattern undergoing surgery for lung biopsy
Plönes T, Osei-Agyemang T, Elze M, et al (Univ Med Ctr Freiburg, Germany)
Respir Med 107:629-632, 2013

Background.—Previous studies revealed that surgical lung biopsy in usual interstitial pneumonia (UIP) patients is accompanied with higher morbidity and mortality. The aim of this retrospective analysis was to assess morbidity and mortality of patients with suspected UIP undergoing surgical lung biopsy.

Methods.—We conducted a retrospective study of 45 patients with suspected UIP pattern undergoing surgical biopsy for diffuse pulmonary infiltrates in our department. Data concerning medical history, histology, and survival status were extracted from the medical database of the University Medical Center Freiburg.

Results.—UIP was diagnosed by experienced pneumo-pathologists according to the criteria of American Thoracic Society/European Respiratory Society (ATS/ERS) consensus classification. Due to adhesions the surgeon decided in two patients to perform wedge resection via open surgery. In 43 patients lung biopsy was performed via Video-assisted thoracoscopy (VATS). No intraoperative complications were observed. Postoperative complications consisted of bradyarrhythmia ($n = 1$), gastrointestinal bleeding ($n = 1$), bacterial pneumonia ($n = 1$), candida pneumonia ($n = 1$) and acute exacerbation ($n = 1$). There was no 30-day mortality, but one patient was lost in follow-up and therefore censored. The intraoperative placed thoracic drain was removed at the first postoperative day in most cases (mean day of removal 1.9, ±2.6). The mean length of hospital stay was 8.1 days (±6.8).

Conclusions.—We conclude that surgical biopsy can be safely performed in patients with suspected UIP.

▶ In the era of computed tomography—based diagnosis, need for open lung biopsy in the evaluation of interstitial lung disease has declined. Still, it is occasionally necessary to make firm diagnoses and guide appropriate treatment. The decision to proceed with biopsy is often difficult to make because of studies that suggest mortality rates of 5.3% to 14%.

This retrospective review of 45 consecutive cases at a single German center by Plönes et al contradicts the findings of earlier studies. Although one patient was lost to follow-up, the remainder were alive at 30 days. There were no intraoperative complications. Postoperative complications, each occurring in 1 patient, were bradyarrhythmia, gastrointestinal bleeding, bacterial pneumonia,

Candida pneumonia, and undefined adverse event. There was no need for re-intubation or noninvasive ventilation. Chest drains were removed by the second postoperative day, and the mean length of stay was 8 days.

Based on American Society of Anesthesiology (ASA) class, the patients had a high severity of illness, and pulmonary function testing showed significant impairment. The retrospective nature of this study does leave the sample open to selection bias. Regardless, the authors have shown an impressive success rate obtaining a safe tissue diagnosis in a sick patient population.

C. D. Spradley, MD

Effect of ambulatory oxygen on exertional dyspnea in IPF patients without resting hypoxemia
Nishiyama O, Miyajima H, Fukai Y, et al (Kinki Univ, Osaka, Japan)
Respir Med 107:1241-1246, 2013

Background and Objective.—The effects of ambulatory oxygen for idiopathic pulmonary fibrosis (IPF) patients without resting hypoxemia have not been elucidated. The purpose of this study was to assess the effect of ambulatory oxygen on dyspnea in IPF patients without resting hypoxemia but with desaturation on exertion.

Methods.—This was a double-blind, placebo-controlled, randomized crossover trial of ambulatory oxygen versus ambulatory air. Patients with IPF who had a partial pressure of arterial oxygen (PaO_2) between 60 mm Hg and 80 mm Hg at rest, and desaturation of 88% or less in a room-air 6-min walk test were eligible. Patients underwent a standardized

TABLE 2.—Ordinary 6-min Walk Test Results with Ambulatory Oxygen and Placebo Air

Variables	Oxygen n = 20	Placebo Air n = 20	P Value
Walk distance, m	400 (80)	387 (80)	0.61
Immediately after test			
O_2 saturation, %	84 (5)	80 (6)	0.02
Heart rate, bpm	116 (15)	110 (13)	0.24
Dyspnea	5.8 (2.2)	6.2 (2.2)	0.57
Leg fatigue	3.4 (2.5)	3.6 (2.5)	0.73
One minute after test			
O_2 saturation, %	90 (6)	83 (6)	0.0005
Heart rate, bpm	105 (15)	104 (12)	0.93
Dyspnea	3.9 (2.4)	4.2 (2.2)	0.66
Leg fatigue	2.4 (2.3)	2.0 (2.2)	0.65
Two minutes after test			
O_2 saturation, %	96 (3)	91 (4)	0.0002
Heart rate, bpm	96 (14)	95 (12)	0.69
Dyspnea	2.3 (1.8)	2.8 (2.1)	0.42
Leg fatigue	1.4 (1.9)	1.3 (1.9)	0.87

bpm: beats per minute.
Dyspnea and leg fatigue were assessed with the modified Borg scale.

6-min walk test and a 6-min free walk test under each ambulatory gas. Oxygen and air were provided at 4 L/min intranasally. Dyspnea was evaluated immediately, 1, and 2 min after the tests.

Results.—Twenty patients (16 men), with a mean age of 73.5 (SD 4.1) years, % predicted forced vital capacity (FVC) of 71.0 (13.3) %, % predicted diffusion capacity for carbon monoxide (DLco) of 57.0 (13.3) %, and PaO_2 of 72.5 (5.4) mm Hg were recruited. No significant differences in dyspnea were observed between ambulatory oxygen and air at each time point. However, some patients showed improvement in dyspnea with oxygen on an individual basis.

Conclusions.—Since oxygen provides no additional benefit over air in terms of exertional dyspnea for IPF patients without resting hypoxemia, routine prescription of ambulatory oxygen is not recommended. However, assessment on an individual basis is necessary.

Trial registration.—UMIN Clinical Trial Registry; No.:UMIN000005098; URL:http://www.umin.ac.jp/ctr/ (Table 2).

▶ In this elegant little (n = 20) double-blind, placebo-controlled crossover study by Nishiyama et al published in *Respiratory Medicine*, the authors pose an interesting question: Does oxygen provide benefit in patients with idiopathic pulmonary fibrosis (IPF) who have desaturation during a walk test? The authors randomly assigned their subjects to receive either O_2 or medical air at 4 L/min on day one and then crossed the subjects over and repeated the study on day 2. Results are illustrated in Table 2.

The only statistically significant difference identified was oxygen saturation. Neither intervention improved baseline performance, although there was a small subset of patients with improved Borg dyspnea scores with supplemental oxygen. The authors point out the complexity of dyspnea in this patient population as a possible contributor. They also point out that long-term oxygen therapy was proven beneficial in chronic obstructive pulmonary disease but has never been found to be helpful in IPF. The reality of increased cost in the setting of no clear benefit is also mentioned.

The authors point out 2 limitations of the study. The mild to moderate severity of illness of the group limits extrapolation to patients with more severe disease. They also acknowledge the small size of the study (although it is adequately powered). I would add an additional factor. The modern medical consumer is data-driven. Many IPF patients have their own oximeters, and they know what *abnormal* is. The study subjects were blinded to their oxygen saturation. Our patients are not.

Another word of caution that I can pass on to people with lung disease from the United States who travel to Japan: medical air in Japan is in dark green cylinders. Oxygen tanks are black.

C. D. Spradley, MD

Diagnosis and Treatment of Connective Tissue Disease-Associated Interstitial Lung Disease

Vij R, Strek ME (The Univ of Chicago, IL)
Chest 143:814-824, 2013

Interstitial lung disease (ILD) is one of the most serious pulmonary complications associated with connective tissue diseases (CTDs), resulting in significant morbidity and mortality. Although the various CTDs associated

TABLE 1.—Clinical Approach to Evaluating Patients With ILD for CTDs

Clinical Evaluation	Approach
Key elements of history	Presence of:
	Rashes
	Raynaud phenomenon
	Constitutional symptoms
	Arthralgias
	Sicca symptoms
	Dysphagia
	Proximal muscle weakness
Physical examination	Evaluate for:
	Rashes
	Mechanic's hands
	Gottron papules
	Sclerodactyly
	Digital ulcers
	Synovitis
	Oral ulcers
	Proximal muscle weakness
Laboratory	Antinuclear antibody
	Anti-double-stranded DNA
	Anti-ribonucleoprotein antibody
	Anti-Smith antibody
	Anti-Scl-70
	Anti-Ro (SSA)
	Anti-La (SSB)
	Rheumatoid factor
	Anticyclic citrullinated peptide
	Anti-Jo-1 antibody
	Creatine kinase
	Aldolase
	Erythrocyte sedimentation rate
	C-reactive protein
Pulmonary function testing, 6-min walk test	Perform at diagnosis and for serial monitoring:
	Total lung capacity
	FVC
	D$_{LCO}$
	6-min walk distance and oxygen saturation
Radiographic	All patients should undergo HRCT scan
	NSIP pattern seen most often in CTD-ILD
Pathologic	Utility of surgical lung biopsy specimen in established CTD-ILD unclear
	Biopsy samples from upper, middle, and lower lung fields
	OP and cellular NSIP more likely to respond to immunosuppressive treatment

Anti-Jo-1 = antihistidyl transfer RNA synthetase; anti-Scl-70 = autoantibodies targeted against type I topoisomerase; CTD = connective tissue disease; D$_{LCO}$ = diffusing capacity of lung for carbon monoxide; HRCT = high-resolution CT; ILD = interstitial lung disease, NSIP = nonspecific interstitial pneumonia; OP = organizing pneumonia; SSA = Sjögren syndrome antigen A; SSB = Sjögren syndrome antigen B.

TABLE 3.—Clinical Pearls for CTD-ILD

CTD	Diagnosis	Management
Systemic sclerosis	Esophageal dilation on HRCT scan increases clinical suspicion.	Esophageal dysfunction and gastroesophageal reflux are common. Annual screening for pulmonary hypertension is recommended by the WHO.
Rheumatoid arthritis	Consider drug-induced pneumonitis for new or worsening ILD.	Radiographic and histopathologic findings of UIP portend a worse prognosis. Tobacco cessation is strongly recommended.
Dermatomyositis and polymyositis	Myositis may be subtle and present after ILD. Myositis-associated and -specific antibodies aid in diagnosis.	Early treatment with prednisone and additional immunosuppressive agents may improve outcomes.
Sjögren syndrome	Cysts on HRCT scan increase clinical suspicion.	Severe ILD, with UIP on HRCT scan and pathology, has been reported. LIP may be less common than other histopathologic patterns.
Autoimmune-featured ILD	Comprehensive and systematic evaluation will identify these patients. Seen in patients with UIP on HRCT scan and pathology.	Patients with ANA titer ≥ 1:1,280 may have improved survival.

ANA = antinuclear antibody; LIP = lymphocytic interstitial pneumonia; UIP = usual interstitial pneumonia; WHO = World Health Organization. See Table 1 and 2 legends for expansion of other abbreviations.

with ILD often are considered together because of their shared autoimmune nature, there are substantial differences in the clinical presentations and management of ILD in each specific CTD. This heterogeneity and the cross-disciplinary nature of care have complicated the conduct of prospective multicenter treatment trials and hindered our understanding of the development of ILD in patients with CTD. In this update, we present new information regarding the diagnosis and treatment of patients with ILD secondary to systemic sclerosis, rheumatoid arthritis, dermatomyositis and polymyositis, and Sjögren syndrome. We review information on risk factors for the development of ILD in the setting of CTD. Diagnostic criteria for CTD are presented as well as elements of the clinical evaluation that increase suspicion for CTD-ILD. We review the use of medications in the treatment of CTD-ILD. Although a large, randomized study has examined the impact of immunosuppressive therapy for ILD secondary to systemic sclerosis, additional studies are needed to determine optimal treatment strategies for each distinct form of CTD-ILD. Finally, we review new information regarding the subgroup of patients with ILD who meet some, but not all, diagnostic criteria for a CTD. A careful and systematic approach to diagnosis in patients with ILD may reveal an unrecognized

CTD or evidence of autoimmunity in those previously believed to have idiopathic ILD (Tables 1 and 3).

▶ In this excellent, concise review of connective tissue disease—associated interstitial lung disease, Vij and Strek provide a helpful overview of diagnosis and treatment for these patients. The review focuses on systemic sclerosis, rheumatoid arthritis, dermatomyositis/polymyositis, and Sjögren's syndrome. A logical approach to evaluation is outlined in Table 1 and a summary of clinical pearls is provided in Table 3. Additionally, the authors provide an appendix that summarizes diagnostic criteria for the connective tissue diseases discussed.

The authors also discuss autoimmune-featured interstitial lung disease (AIF ILD), which Vij et al[1] described in an earlier paper in *CHEST* in 2011. These patients have autoimmune features but do not meet classic criteria for a firm diagnosis. These patients have a better prognosis if they present with an antinuclear antibody titer of ≥1:1280. This finding helps reinforce the underlying theme of this review, namely, that it is important to identify these patients because treatment options and prognoses differ between this population and those with idiopathic disease. Indeed, as a group they appear to have better outcomes.

C. D. Spradley, MD

Reference

1. Vij R, Noth I, Strek ME. Autoimmune-featured interstitial lung disease: a distinct entity. *Chest.* 2011;140:1292-1299.

Mycophenolate Mofetil Improves Lung Function in Connective Tissue Disease-associated Interstitial Lung Disease

Fischer A, Brown KK, Du Bois RM, et al (Natl Jewish Health, Denver, CO; Imperial College, London, UK)
J Rheumatol 40:640-646, 2013

Objective.—Small series suggest mycophenolate mofetil (MMF) is well tolerated and may be an effective therapy for connective tissue disease-associated interstitial lung disease (CTD-ILD). We examined the tolerability and longitudinal changes in pulmonary physiology in a large and diverse cohort of patients with CTD-ILD treated with MMF.

Methods.—We identified consecutive patients evaluated at our center between January 2008 and January 2011 and prescribed MMF for CTD-ILD. We assessed safety and tolerability of MMF and used longitudinal data analyses to examine changes in pulmonary physiology over time, before and after initiation of MMF.

Results.—We identified 125 subjects treated with MMF for a median 897 days. MMF was discontinued in 13 subjects. MMF was associated with significant improvements in estimated percentage of predicted forced vital capacity (FVC%) from MMF initiation to 52, 104, and 156 weeks

(4.9% ± 1.9%, $p = 0.01$; 6.1% ± 1.8%, $p = 0.0008$; and 7.3% ± 2.6%, $p = 0.004$, respectively); and in estimated percentage predicted diffusing capacity (DLCO%) from MMF initiation to 52 and 104 weeks (6.3% ± 2.8%, $p = 0.02$; 7.1% ± 2.8%, $p = 0.01$). In the subgroup without usual interstitial pneumonia (UIP)-pattern injury, MMF significantly improved FVC% and DLCO%, and in the subgroup with UIP-pattern injury, MMF was associated with stability in FVC% and DLCO%.

Conclusion.—In a large diverse cohort of CTD-ILD, MMF was well tolerated and had a low rate of discontinuation. Treatment with MMF was associated with either stable or improved pulmonary physiology over a median 2.5 years of followup. MMF appears to be a promising therapy for the spectrum of CTD-ILD.

▶ In this study published in the *Journal of Rheumatology*, Fischer and colleagues present retrospective data describing a 4-year experience treating 125 patients with mycophenolate mofetil (MMF) for connective tissue disease—associated interstitial lung disease (CTD ILD). In the run up to the conclusion of the Scleroderma Lung Study II, the experience may give some early insight into the results.

The group describes average duration of treatment of almost 900 days and follows up with patients for 3 years. Drug was well tolerated and discontinued in only 10% of subjects. In 29%, MMF replaced cyclophosphamide, and in 15% it replaced azathioprine. Median daily prednisone dose decreased from 20 mg at initiation to 5 mg at 9 to 12 months (Fig 2 in the original article). Patients also showed a statistically significant improvement in forced vital capacity and diffusion capacity (Fig 3 in the original article).

As identified by the authors, the study suffers from its retrospective nature and the potential for referral bias. It is also not entirely clear how clinically significant the statistically significant improvements in lung function are. MMF appears to be an attractive option for the treatment of CTD ILD.

C. D. Spradley, MD

Pleural Disease

Pleural Plaques and the Risk of Pleural Mesothelioma
Pairon J-C, Laurent F, Rinaldo M, et al (Université Paris-Est Créteil, France; Centre cardiothoracique INSERM 1045, Bordeaux, France; Centre INSERM 897, Bordeaux, France; et al)
J Natl Cancer Inst 105:293-301, 2013

Background.—The association between pleural plaques and pleural mesothelioma remains controversial. The present study was designed to examine the association between pleural plaques on computed tomography (CT) scan and the risk of pleural mesothelioma in a follow-up study of asbestos-exposed workers.

Methods.—Retired or unemployed workers previously occupationally exposed to asbestos were invited to participate in a screening program

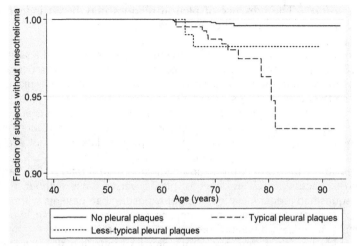

FIGURE 2.—Proportion of subjects without pleural mesothelioma at any given age according to the presence of pleural plaques on computed tomography (CT) scan (Kaplan—Meier survival curve, log-rank test $P < .0001$). N = 34 091 subject-years. At-risk subjects at different ages were as follows for the different groups: subjects with no plaques on CT scan: 1870 at 65 years, 1646 at 70 years, 353 at 75 years, 113 at 80 years, and 23 at 85 years; subjects with typical parietal or diaphragmatic pleural plaques on CT scan: 297 at 65 years, 353 at 70 years, 146 at 75 years, 63 at 80 years, and 22 at 85 years; subjects with other less typical plaques on CT scan: 108 at 65 years, 134 at 70 years, 43 at 75 years, 22 at 80 years, and 8 at 85 years. Parietal pleural plaques were considered to be typical when they were bilateral, thicker than 2 mm, and with an extent greater than 1 cm, regardless of whether they were calcified. (Reprinted from Pairon J-C, Laurent F, Rinaldo M, et al. Pleural plaques and the risk of pleural mesothelioma. *J Natl Cancer Inst.* 2013;105:293-301, by permission of Oxford University Press.)

for asbestos-related diseases, including CT scan, organized between October 2003 and December 2005 in four regions in France. Randomized, independent, double reading of CT scans by a panel of seven chest radiologists focused on benign asbestos-related abnormalities. A 7-year follow-up study was conducted in the 5287 male subjects for whom chest CT scan was available. Annual determination of the number of subjects eligible for free medical care because of pleural mesothelioma was carried out. Diagnosis certification was obtained from the French mesothelioma panel of pathologists. Survival regression based on the Cox model was used to estimate the risk of pleural mesothelioma associated with pleural plaques, with age as the main time variable and time-varying exposure variables, namely duration of exposure, time since first exposure, and cumulative exposure index to asbestos. All statistical tests were two-sided.

Results.—A total of 17 incident cases of pleural mesothelioma were diagnosed. A statistically significant association was observed between mesothelioma and pleural plaques (unadjusted hazard ratio (HR) = 8.9, 95% confidence interval [CI] = 3.0 to 26.5; adjusted HR = 6.8, 95% CI = 2.2 to 21.4 after adjustment for time since first exposure and cumulative exposure index to asbestos).

Conclusion.—The presence of pleural plaques may be an independent risk factor for pleural mesothelioma (Fig 2).

▶ In this French study by Pairon et al, the investigators evaluated a large sample (5287 subjects) of men with prior occupational exposure to asbestos. The aim was to evaluate the relationship between presence of pleural plaques on computed tomography (CT) scan and risk for mesothelioma. Prior studies evaluating the link based on chest radiograph did not show a relationship.

The study relied on a cumulative exposure index based on duration and intensity of exposure, as quantitative fiber exposure data were not available. The study also censored female subjects.

In this study, the authors found an unadjusted hazard ratio of 8.9 for those exposed subjects with CT evidence of plaque verses those without. Patients with plaques had longer mean duration of exposure than patients without plaques. Fig 2, illustrating a fraction of subjects without mesothelioma, shows the statistically significant difference between the groups ($P < .0001$).

The study benefited from strong standards surrounding the definition of pleural plaques, double over-reading of scans with triple reading in the case of disagreement, and reliance on an expert panel of pathologists for confirmation of mesothelioma diagnosis in all but 3 of the 17 incident cases.

Based on this study, it does appear that pleural plaques are a marker for both increased exposure and increased risk of mesothelioma. These patients, therefore, will benefit from closer surveillance than exposed patients without evidence of pleural plaques on CT scan.

C. D. Spradley, MD

Surgical decortication as the first-line treatment for pleural empyema
Shin JA, Chang YS, Kim TH, et al (Yonsei Univ College of Medicine, Seoul, Korea)
J Thorac Cardiovasc Surg 145:933-939.e1, 2013

Objective.—The study objective was to evaluate the clinical outcomes of surgical decortication as the first line of treatment for pleural empyema.

Methods.—We analyzed the medical records of 111 patients who presented with empyema and were treated with simple drainage or surgical decortication as the first line of treatment at Gangnam Severance Hospital, a tertiary referral medical center in Seoul, Korea.

Results.—Of 111 patients with empyema, 27 underwent surgical decortication as the first intervention. Surgical decortication showed a better treatment success rate in all study subjects (96.3%, 26/27 patients) compared with simple drainage (58.3%, 49/84 patients; $P < .0001$ for method comparison). After propensity-scored matching, decortication resulted in a better outcome (95.0%, 19/20 patients) versus drainage (56.7%, 17/30 patients; $P = .003$). Surgical decortication as the first line of treatment for empyema was the best predictor of treatment success after adjustment

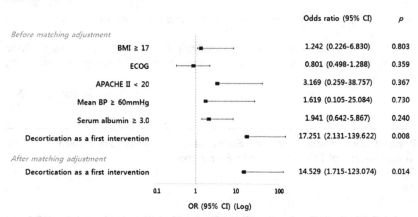

FIGURE 1.—Multivariate analysis of overall treatment success. Odds ratios (95% confidence intervals) of overall treatment success with BMI of 17 kg/m² or greater, ECOG score, APACHE II score less than 20, mean arterial pressure 60 mm Hg or greater, serum albumin 3.0 g/dL or greater, and decortications as a first treatment were analyzed using logistic regression in stepwise manner. After propensity-scored matching adjustment, decortication as a first intervention remained the most important predictive factor of a successful treatment outcome. *APACHE II*, Acute Physiology and Chronic Health Evaluation II; *BMI*, body mass index; *CI*, confidence interval; *ECOG*, Eastern Cooperative Oncology Group; *OR*, odds ratio. (Reprinted from the Journal of Thoracic and Cardiovascular Surgery. Shin JA, Chang YS, Kim TH, et al. Surgical decortication as the first-line treatment for pleural empyema. *J Thorac Cardiovasc Surg.* 2013;145:933-939.e1, Copyright 2013, with permission from The American Association for Thoracic Surgery.)

for compounding factors (odds ratio, 14.529; 95% confidence interval, 1.715-123.074; P =.014).

Conclusions.—The first treatment choice for pleural empyema is a critical determinant of ultimate therapeutic success. After adjusting for confounding variables, surgical decortication is the optimal first treatment choice for advanced empyema (Fig 1).

▶ In this single-center, retrospective study published in *The Journal of Thoracic and Cardiovascular Surgery* by Shin and colleagues, the authors compare primary surgical therapy with decortication to simple pleural drainage for empyema.

The authors define empyema radiographically by septation on computed tomography scan and by appearance of gross puss or microbiologic positivity. The 2 groups studied differed in terms of Eastern Cooperative Oncology Group score, Charleston comorbidity index, and Acute Physiology and Chronic Health Evaluation (APACHE) II score with sicker patients being more common in the simple drainage group. Before propensity matching, body mass index ≥17, APACHE II score less than 20, mean blood pressure ≥60, and serum albumin ≥3.0 were predictors of superior outcome (Fig 1).

To correct for the difference, the authors used propensity matching. They excluded 61 of the original 111 patients and after matching, primary decortication remained the only significant predictor of success (P = .003). Treatment failure correlated with culture positivity after matching (P < .001).

Author-identified weaknesses of this study included the retrospective nature, the potential for selection bias (proven by the difference in the nonmatched populations), and the inclusion of tuberculous effusions with other forms of empyema.

Although this study does have flaws, as noted above, it supports the growing consensus that surgical intervention is the treatment of choice for loculated empyema.

C. D. Spradley, MD

Preoperative Predictors of Successful Surgical Treatment in the Management of Parapneumonic Empyema

Stefani A, Aramini B, della Casa G, et al (Univ of Modena and Reggio Emilia, Italy)
Ann Thorac Surg 96:1812-1819, 2013

Background.—Video-assisted thoracoscopic surgery (VATS) and thoracotomy are the main surgical options for treating parapneumonic empyema. The choice of either operation depends on many preoperative features, including the patient's condition, clinical and radiologic findings, and pleural fluid characteristics. The identification of the combination of those preoperative findings that will allow surgeons to select the appropriate approach for a successful operation (VATS or thoracotomy) could be of great interest in clinical settings.

Methods.—We retrospectively reviewed a series of 97 patients who had undergone successful VATS or thoracotomy for parapneumonic empyema; in all cases, the operation had begun through VATS and was changed to a thoracotomy if a complete decortication was needed. Preoperative clinical, radiologic, and laboratory features were compared between the two groups to search for differences that might serve as predictive factors for either operation. Perioperative findings were also analyzed.

Results.—The operation was accomplished by VATS in 40 patients (41%), and conversion to thoracotomy was necessary in 57 (59%). Significant predictive factors for conversion were a prolonged delay from diagnosis to operation, the presence of fever and of pleural thickness on computed tomography (CT) images. The 25 patients who presented with these three features were cured by thoracotomy. The operative time

TABLE 3.—Multivariate Analysis of Independent Predictors of Thoracotomy

Risk Factor	OR (95% CI)[a]	p Value
Delay in operation	1.97 (1.12–3.48)	0.018
Fever: yes	28.17 (4.75–166.91)	0.000
C-creative protein	0.96 (0.56–1.65)	0.904
Bacteriology: positive	3.28 (0.69–15.52)	0.133
Type of effusion: loculated	1.05 (0.26–4.24)	0.945
Pleural thickening: yes	3.32 (1.01–10.79)	0.046

CI = confidence interval; OR = odds ratio.
[a]An OR >1 indicates a risk factor for thoracotomy.

and postoperative complication rate were significantly higher for the thoracotomy patients.

Conclusions.—Some preoperative features can help the surgeon to better select patients for the appropriate operation. Delayed operation, fever, and pleural thickness can be used to predict the likelihood of conversion to thoracotomy (Table 3).

▶ In this retrospective, single-center study published by Stefani and colleagues in the *Annals of Thoracic Surgery*, the authors address the question of clinical predictors of need for conversion to open thoracotomy in the management of parapneumonic empyema. The authors point out that the current ACCP guideline does not state a preference for video-assisted thoracoscopic surgery (VATS) verses open procedure.[1]

The team excluded patients with lung abscess and tuberculous effusions. All patients initially received VATS and were converted to thoracotomy if results were inadequate or if the pleural space was inaccessible. Ninety-seven of 100 consecutive patients were included in the analysis, of which 57 (59%) were converted to thoracotomy.

Univariate predictors of thoracotomy included longer delay to operation, presence of fever, positive pleural fluid bacteriology, pleural fluid loculation, and pleural thickening greater than 2 mm. Multivariate factors were limited to delay to operation, presence of fever, and pleural thickening (Table 3). Complications were more common in the thoracotomy, and bleeding and air leak were most frequent as expected.

The authors point out the retrospective nature of the study as a weakness and also discuss the high conversion rate, which they base on their standard approach of starting all cases as VATS cases.

Despite its shortcomings, this study does achieve its goal of identifying preoperative factors that predict need for thoracotomy verses VATS. This should assist in preoperative planning and counseling in the management of complex empyema.

C. D. Spradley, MD

Reference

1. Colice GL, Curtis A, Deslauriers J. Medical and surgical treatment of parapneumonic effusions: an evidence-based guideline. *Chest.* 2000;118:1158-1171.

A Propensity-Matched Comparison of Pleurodesis or Tunneled Pleural Catheter in Patients Undergoing Diagnostic Thoracoscopy for Malignancy
Freeman RK, Ascioti AJ, Mahidhara RS (St Vincent Hosp, Indianapolis, IN)
Ann Thorac Surg 96:259-264, 2013

Background.—Patients with a suspected malignant pleural effusion occasionally require thoracoscopy to achieve a diagnosis. It is unclear whether chemical pleurodesis or the placement of a tunneled pleural catheter (TPC) that can be used for intermittent pleural drainage produces superior palliation, a shorter hospital stay, and less morbidity. This investigation compares these 2 treatment groups.

Methods.—Patients with a recurrent, symptomatic, pleural effusion suspected of having a malignant etiology who underwent a thoracoscopic exploration after at least 2 nondiagnostic thoracenteses were identified. Two patient groups were formed, comprised of patients who received either talc pleurodesis or a TPC at the conclusion of the procedure, using propensity matching. Patient demographics, length of stay, interval until the initiation of systemic therapy, need for further intervention for the pleural effusion, and procedural morbidity and mortality were collected and compared.

Results.—Over a 6-year period, 60 patients undergoing treatment were identified and propensity matched. No significant differences in mean age or palliation from their effusion were identified. However, the group treated with TPC realized a significantly shorter hospital stay and interval to systemic therapy for their malignancy as well as a lower rate of operative morbidity than patients undergoing talc pleurodesis.

Conclusions.—This investigation found that a TPC provided palliation of patients' malignant pleural effusions and freedom from reintervention equal to that of talc pleurodesis after thoracoscopy while resulting in a shorter mean length of hospital stay and interval to the initiation of systemic therapy. Lower rates of operative morbidity were also seen in the TPC treatment group. This method of palliation of a malignant pleural effusion should be considered when diagnostic thoracoscopy reveals a malignant pleural effusion.

▶ In this single-center, retrospective cohort comparison by Freeman and colleagues published in the *Annals of Thoracic Surgery*, the authors used propensity matching to compare 30 patients undergoing tunneled plueral catheter placement at time of diagnostic video-assisted thoracic surgery (VATS) to a similar group of patients undergoing conventional talc poudrage. The authors found no difference between the 2 groups when comparing performance status or reintervention rate. They did, however, identify a difference between hospital length of stay (owing to prolonged pleural drainage in the poudrage group) and morbidity (owing to respiratory issues in the poudrage group).

The author-identified weaknesses in the study included the retrospective single-center design. Source of funding was also not disclosed.

The premise of the study does make logical sense, as prolonged in-hospital chest tube drainage is necessitated by the talc poudrage technique, and complications have been well described. Additionally, cost analyses have been performed as recently as last year and likely favor tunneled pleural catheters because of the decreased need for hospitalization despite the cost of proprietary drainage systems[1] (see last year's edition of this publication).

This study makes a strong argument for consideration of placement of a tunneled pleural catheter at the conclusion of diagnostic VATS for suspected malignant effusion. A prospective randomized trial would better answer the question posed but, as was pointed out by the authors, would prove difficult to implement.

C. D. Spradley, MD

Reference

1. Puri V, Pyrdeck TL, Crabtree TD, et al. Treatment of malignant pleural effusion: a cost-effectiveness analysis. *Ann Thorac Surg.* 2012;94:374-380.

Clinical Outcomes of Indwelling Pleural Catheter-Related Pleural Infections: An International Multicenter Study

Fysh ETH, Tremblay A, Feller-Kopman D, et al (Sir Charles Gairdner Hosp, Perth, Western Australia, Australia; Univ of Calgary, Alberta, Canada; Johns Hopkins Hosp, Baltimore, MD)
Chest 144:1597-1602, 2013

Background.—Indwelling pleural catheters (IPCs) offer effective control of malignant pleural effusions (MPEs). IPC-related infection is uncommon but remains a major concern. Individual IPC centers see few infections, and previous reports lack sufficient numbers and detail. This study combined the experience of 11 centers from North America, Europe, and Australia to describe the incidence, microbiology, management, and clinical outcomes of IPC-related pleural infection.

Methods.—This was a multicenter retrospective review of 1,021 patients with IPCs. All had confirmed MPE.

Results.—Only 50 patients (4.9%) developed an IPC-related pleural infection; most (94%) were successfully controlled with antibiotics (62% IV). One death (2%) directly resulted from the infection, whereas two patients (4%) had ongoing infectious symptoms when they died of cancer progression. *Staphylococcus aureus* was the causative organism in 48% of cases. Infections from gram-negative organisms were associated with an increased need for continuous antibiotics or death (60% vs 15% in gram-positive and 25% mixed infections, $P = .02$). The infections in the majority (54%) of cases were managed successfully without removing the IPC. Postinfection pleurodesis developed in 31 patients (62%), especially those infected with staphylococci (79% vs 45% with nonstaphylococcal infections, $P = .04$).

Conclusions.—The incidence of IPC-related pleural infection was low. The overall mortality risk from pleural infection in patients treated with IPC was only 0.29%. Antibiotics should cover *S aureus* and gram-negative organisms until microbiology is confirmed. Postinfection pleurodesis is common and often allows removal of IPC. Heterogeneity in management is common, and future studies to define the optimal treatment strategies are needed.

▶ In this study published in *CHEST* by Fysh and colleagues, the authors attempt to define the infection rate in tunneled indwelling pleural catheters (IPC) used for management of malignant pleural effusion. This international, multicenter, retrospective study includes 1021 subjects, making it the largest published study to date on the topic. The rationale was to address understandable concerns surrounding infection risk in the vulnerable population treated with these devices.

The authors defined pleural infection by the presence of positive bacteriology or puss, signs and symptoms of pleural infection, and need for antibiotics. Rate of infection was 4.9%. Thirty-eight subjects had complete resolution, and 9 were on antibiotics at time of death. Mortality rate associated with infection for the entire sample was 0.29% and 6% for the infected subgroup. Bacteriology is summarized in Fig 1 of the original article. Most patients were treated without catheter removal.

Regular drainage was cited as the likely explanation of low mortality associated with infection (verses the 15%–20% mortality rate associated with non–IPC-associated infection.) The authors recommended that broad-spectrum coverage be used because of the variety of causative agents. They also call for consensus on treatment methodology.

The author-identified shortcomings of the study include its retrospective nature as well as the fact that infection rate may be skewed secondary to the experience of operators at the included centers. The information provided in this study should provide a valuable tool in assessing the risk and educating patients concerning the use of IPCs for malignant effusion.

C. D. Spradley, MD

Pulmonary Vascular Disease

Evaluation of the Predictive Value of a Clinical Worsening Definition Using 2-Year Outcomes in Patients With Pulmonary Arterial Hypertension: A REVEAL Registry Analysis

Frost AE, Badesch DB, Miller DP, et al (Baylor College of Medicine, Houston, TX; Univ of Colorado Health Sciences Ctr, Denver; ICON Late Phase & Outcomes Res, San Francisco, CA; et al)
Chest 144:1521-1529, 2013

Background.—Time to clinical worsening has been proposed as a primary end point in clinical trials of pulmonary arterial hypertension (PAH); however, neither standardized nor validated definitions of clinical worsening across PAH trials exist. This study aims to evaluate a proposed definition of clinical worsening within a large prospective, observational registry of patients with PAH with respect to its value as a predictor of proximate (within 1 year) risk for subsequent major events (ie, death, transplantation, or atrial septostomy).

Methods.—We assessed overall 2-year survival and survival free from major events to determine the relationship between clinical worsening and major events among adults with hemodynamically defined PAH (N = 3,001). Freedom from clinical worsening was defined as freedom from worsening functional class (FC), a $\geq 15\%$ reduction in 6-min walk distance (6MWD), all-cause hospitalization, or the introduction of parenteral prostacyclin analog therapy.

Results.—In the 2 years of follow-up, 583 patients died. Four hundred twenty-six died after a documented clinical worsening event, including FC worsening (n = 128), a ≥ 15% reduction in 6MWD (n = 118), all-cause hospitalization (n = 370), or introduction of a prostacyclin analog (n = 91). Patients who experienced clinical worsening had significantly poorer subsequent 1-year survival postworsening than patients who did not worsen (*P* < .001).

Conclusions.—Clinical worsening was highly predictive of subsequent proximate mortality in this analysis from an observational study. These results validate the use of clinical worsening as a meaningful prognostic tool in clinical practice and as a primary end point in clinical trial design.

Trial Registry.—ClinicalTrials.gov; No.: NCT00370214; URL: www.clinicaltrials.gov.

▶ Selection of an appropriate clinical endpoint is important not only to trial design but also to clinical practice. Frost and colleagues evaluated a definition of clinical worsening over a 1-year period based on the patient population with hemodynamically defined pulmonary arterial hypertension (PAH) from the REVEAL registry.

Six-minute walk distance (6mwd) has long been chosen as the primary endpoint in clinical trials in PAH. There is growing controversy as to the appropriateness of this marker. In their clinical worsening assessment, the authors select a 6mwd decrease of ≤15% as 1 of 4 potential markers of clinical worsening. When these 4 were applied to the patients in the REVEAL registry, they proved to be strong predictors of outcome (death, transplant, atrial septostomy).

The clinical worsening definition held up in composite, incident, and prevalent cases (Fig 3 in the original article). In the words of the authors, the components of "their definition of clinical worsening are both likely to occur in a clinical trial and are highly predictive of a significant decrease in survival."

C. D. Spradley, MD

Treatment of patients with pulmonary arterial hypertension at the time of death or deterioration to functional class IV: Insights from the REVEAL Registry

Farber HW, Miller DP, Meltzer LA, et al (Boston Univ School of Medicine, MA; ICON Late Phase & Outcomes Res, San Francisco, CA; Actelion Pharmaceuticals US Inc, South San Francisco, CA; et al)
J Heart Lung Transplant 32:1114-1122, 2013

Background.—Current guidelines recommend intravenous prostacyclin as first-line therapy for patients with pulmonary arterial hypertension (PAH) in New York Heart Association/World Health Organization functional class (FC) IV, or combination therapy for patients in any FC who do not respond to monotherapy. We investigated the aggressiveness of therapy in patients enrolled in the REVEAL (Registry to Evaluate Early and

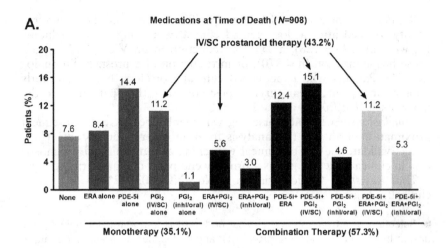

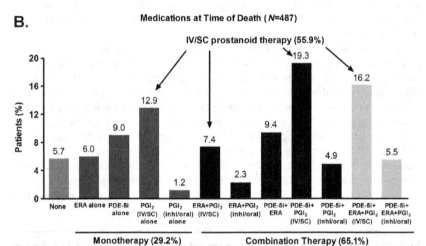

FIGURE 2.—Medication use at time of death—overall. Pulmonary arterial hypertension (PAH)-specific therapy at time of death in (A) the all-cause death cohort ($n = 908$) and (B) the PAH-related death cohort ($n = 487$). The percentages of patients taking monotherapy plus those receiving no therapy almost total the percentage of patients taking prostanoid therapy in the all-cause death cohort, where as a comparatively greater percentage of patients were taking prostanoid therapy in the PAH-related death cohort. Red, no therapy; grey, monotherapy; blue, dual therapy; and orange, triple therapy. ERA, endothelin receptor antagonist; inh, inhaled; IV/SC, intravenous/subcutaneous; PDE-5i, phosphodiesterase type-5inhibitor; PGI_2, prostacyclin. For Interpretation of the references to color in this figure legend, the reader is referred to web version of this article. (Reprinted from The Journal of Heart and Lung Transplantation. Farber HW, Miller DP, Meltzer LA, et al. Treatment of patients with pulmonary arterial hypertension at the time of death or deterioration to functional class IV: insights from the REVEAL Registry. *J Heart Lung Transplant.* 2013;32:1114-1122, Copyright 2013, with permission from International Society for Heart and Lung Transplantation.)

Long-Term PAH Disease Management) Registry who deteriorated to FC IV or died.

Methods.—Among 3,515 patients (age ≥ 18 years) in REVEAL with a mean pulmonary artery pressure ≥ 25 mm Hg and pulmonary capillary wedge pressure ≤ 15 mm Hg, we examined three sub-sets: the 487 patients who had a PAH-related death, the larger set of 908 patients who died from any cause (PAH-related, not PAH-related, or unknown), and the 294 patients who were FC I, II, or III at enrollment and later assessed as FC IV.

Results.—Among patients who died, 56% ($n = 272$ of 487) and 43% ($n = 391$ of 908) were receiving intravenous prostacyclin before death in the PAH-related death and all-cause death cohorts, respectively. In the PAH-related death cohort, 60% and 16% of patients were most recently assessed as FC III and IV, respectively; among those assessed as FC IV within 6 months of death, 57.7% ($n = 15$ of 26) had received intravenous prostacyclin. Because many patients died without an observed assessment of worsening to FC IV, we also evaluated medication use among the cohort of patients who worsened to FC IV during the study. One day before worsening to FC IV, 150 of 294 patients were not receiving intravenous prostacyclin and 70 were receiving only PAH-specific monotherapy; of these, 61% and 67%, respectively, received no additional therapy 90 days later.

Conclusions.—Intravenous prostacyclin and combination therapy are not consistently used in the most seriously ill patients enrolled in REVEAL after being assessed as FC IV or at the time of death (Fig 2).

▶ In this descriptive report published in the *Journal of Heart and Lung Transplantation*, Farber and colleagues query the REVEAL registry with an important question: How are we treating the sickest patients who have pulmonary arterial hypertension (PAH)? The answer is somewhat disturbing and invites a host of additional questions.

Current guidelines recommend combination therapy in moderate to severe PAH and hold up intravenous prostacyclin-based therapy as the gold standard for treatment in this cohort of patients because of its proven track record in severe disease and salvage therapy.

The authors found, rather astoundingly, that of all patients who died (all cause) in the REVEAL registry, only 43% were on intravenous prostacyclin (Fig 2). Of the patients whose deaths were related to PAH, only 56% were on these life-sustaining therapies. There are many potential explanations for the disparity between the guidelines and reality.

Some of this may stem from failure of providers to recognize disease severity, from lack of comfort with advanced therapy, and from patient factors. In my own experience, many patients and their families are reluctant to take the step to transition to pump therapy. Occasionally, when support structure or goals of care are part of the decision process, withholding advanced therapy may be appropriate. In most cases, however, we need to be doing a better job.

C. D. Spradley, MD

A Novel Channelopathy in Pulmonary Arterial Hypertension

Ma L, Roman-Campos D, Austin ED, et al (Columbia Univ Med Ctr, NY; Vanderbilt Univ Med Ctr, Nashville, TN; et al)
N Engl J Med 369:351-361, 2013

Background.—Pulmonary arterial hypertension is a devastating disease with high mortality. Familial cases of pulmonary arterial hypertension are usually characterized by autosomal dominant transmission with reduced penetrance, and some familial cases have unknown genetic causes.

Methods.—We studied a family in which multiple members had pulmonary arterial hypertension without identifiable mutations in any of the genes known to be associated with the disease, including *BMPR2, ALK1, ENG, SMAD9,* and *CAV1.* Three family members were studied with whole-exome sequencing. Additional patients with familial or idiopathic pulmonary arterial hypertension were screened for the mutations in the gene that was identified on whole-exome sequencing. All variants were expressed in COS-7 cells, and channel function was studied by means of patch-clamp analysis.

Results.—We identified a novel heterozygous missense variant c.608 G→A (G203D) in *KCNK3* (the gene encoding potassium channel subfamily K, member 3) as a disease-causing candidate gene in the family. Five additional heterozygous missense variants in *KCNK3* were independently identified in 92 unrelated patients with familial pulmonary arterial hypertension and 230 patients with idiopathic pulmonary arterial hypertension. We used in silico bioinformatic tools to predict that all six novel variants would be damaging. Electrophysiological studies of the channel indicated that all these missense mutations resulted in loss of function, and the reduction in the potassium-channel current was remedied by the application of the phospholipase inhibitor ONO-RS-082.

Conclusions.—Our study identified the association of a novel gene, *KCNK3*, with familial and idiopathic pulmonary arterial hypertension. Mutations in this gene produced reduced potassium-channel current, which was successfully remedied by pharmacologic manipulation. (Funded by the National Institutes of Health.)

▶ In this impressive study by Ma et al published in *The New England Journal of Medicine,* genetic investigation of a family with an unidentified form of heritable pulmonary arterial hypertension (HPAH) results in identification of a causal mutation that sheds insight into a new mechanism of disease and a potential pharmacologic remedy.

The authors point out that 25% of familial PAH cases have unknown associated mutations. They investigated one such family using whole exome sequencing and identified a novel potassium channel mutation that conferred loss of function. The family did not carry mutations for *BMPR2, ALK1, ENG, SMAD9,* or *CAV1.*

The authors then investigated 10 additional probands with HPAH of unknown cause and identified 2 additional mutational variants of the same gene. The investigation was then expanded to include 82 unrelated cases of familial PAH and 230 cases of IPAH. Three more mutations were identified. All 5 additional mutations were found to be damaging. Extrapolation from their studied population would infer that as many as 1.3% of patients with PAH and 3.2% of patients with HPAH carry a mutation of this potassium channel gene.

The authors describe the affected protein, KCNK3, as a potassium channel that is sensitive to hypoxia and partially responsible for maintaining resting membrane potential in pulmonary artery smooth muscle impacting vascular tone. All identified mutations occurred in conserved regions (Fig 2 in the original article) resulting in loss of function at physiologic pH.

Next, the authors used ONO-RS-082, a compound known to be an activator of the KCNK3 protein and found recovery of function for some but not all of the mutations.

This study shows the power of modern scientific investigation and gives hope for a future of therapies tailored specifically to cause instead of focusing on disease modification.

C. D. Spradley, MD

Correction of Nonsense *BMPR2* and *SMAD9* Mutations by Ataluren in Pulmonary Arterial Hypertension
Drake KM, Dunmore BJ, McNelly LN, et al (Cleveland Clinic, OH; Univ of Cambridge School of Clinical Medicine, UK)
Am J Respir Cell Mol Biol 49:403-409, 2013

Heritable pulmonary arterial hypertension (HPAH) is a serious lung vascular disease caused by heterozygous mutations in the bone morphogenetic protein (BMP) pathway genes, *BMPR2* and *SMAD9*. One noncanonical function of BMP signaling regulates biogenesis of a subset of microRNAs. We have previously shown that this function is abrogated in patients with HPAH, making it a highly sensitive readout of BMP pathway integrity. Ataluren (PTC124) is an investigational drug that permits ribosomal readthrough of premature stop codons, resulting in a full-length protein. It exhibits oral bioavailability and limited toxicity in human trials. Here, we tested ataluren in lung- or blood-derived cells from patients with HPAH with nonsense mutations in *BMPR2* ($n = 6$) or *SMAD9* ($n = 1$). Ataluren significantly increased BMP-mediated microRNA processing in six of the seven cases. Moreover, rescue was achieved even for mutations exhibiting significant nonsense-mediated mRNA decay. Response to ataluren was dose dependent, and complete correction was achieved at therapeutic doses currently used in clinical trials for cystic fibrosis. BMP receptor (BMPR)-II protein levels were normalized and ligand-dependent phosphorylation of downstream target Smads was increased. Furthermore, the usually hyperproliferative phenotype of pulmonary artery endothelial and smooth muscle cells was reversed by ataluren. These results indicate that ataluren can effectively suppress a high proportion of *BMPR2* and *SMAD9* nonsense mutations and correct BMP signaling *in vitro*. Approximately 29%

of all HPAH mutations are nonsense point mutations. In light of this, we propose ataluren as a potential new personalized therapy for this significant subgroup of patients with PAH.

▶ Ataluren is a small molecule that promotes read through of premature stop codons generated by nonsense mutations. It is currently being clinically investigated in the treatment of cystic fibrosis and appears to be safe with potential efficacy.

Just more than 1/4 of all patients with idiopathic and familial pulmonary arterial hypertension (PAH) have a mutation in the bone morphogenic protein receptor II gene (*BMPR2*). Drake and colleagues investigated the efficacy of ataluren in inducing read through in a subset of 7 such mutations. Samples were derived from explanted lungs and the remainder from blood-derived cells.

Using upregulation of miRNA-27 (a downstream effect of the BMP pathway) as a signal, the authors were able to show the efficacy of ataluren across a variety of *BMPR2* point mutations (Fig 1 in the original article). This effect was not noted in an induced deletion mutation. Treatment with ataluren also resulted in a reduction in cell proliferation (believed to be pathologic in PAH) in the absence of cell death or senescence.

The authors point out that it is unclear whether changes seen at the bench level will translate to improvements in patients with advanced disease, but this finding provides hope for potential personalized therapy targeting the cause of disease in a subset of patients with PAH.

C. D. Spradley, MD

Pulmonary Artery Denervation to Treat Pulmonary Arterial Hypertension: The Single-Center, Prospective, First-in-Man PADN-1 Study (First-in-Man Pulmonary Artery Denervation for Treatment of Pulmonary Artery Hypertension)

Chen S-L, Zhang F-F, Xu J, et al (Nanjing Med Univ, China; et al)
J Am Coll Cardiol 62:1092-1100, 2013

Objectives.—This study was designed to test the safety and efficacy of pulmonary artery (PA) denervation (PADN) for patients with idiopathic PA hypertension (IPAH) not responding optimally to medical therapy.

Background.—Baroreceptors and sympathetic nerve fibers are localized in or near the bifurcation area of the main PA. We previously demonstrated that PADN completely abolished the experimentally elevated PA pressure responses to occlusion of the left interlobar PA.

Methods.—Of a total of 21 patients with IPAH, 13 patients received the PADN procedure, and the other 8 patients who refused the PADN procedure were assigned to the control group. PADN was performed at the bifurcation of the main PA, and at the ostial right and left PA. Serial echocardiography, right heart catheterization, and a 6-min walk test (6MWT) were performed. The primary endpoints were the change of PA pressure (PAP), tricuspid excursion (Tei) index, and 6MWT at 3 months follow-up.

Results.—Compared with the control group, at 3 months follow-up, the patients who underwent the PADN procedure showed significant reduction of mean PAP (from 55 ± 5 mm Hg to 36 ± 5 mm Hg, $p < 0.01$), and significant improvement of the 6MWT (from 324 ± 21 m to 491 ± 38 m, $p < 0.006$) and of the Tei index (from 0.7 ± 0.04 to 0.50 ± 0.04, $p < 0.001$).

Conclusions.—We report for the first time the effect of PADN on functional capacity and hemodynamics in patients with IPAH not responding optimally to medical therapy. Further randomized study is required to confirm the efficacy of PADN. (First-in-Man Pulmonary Artery Denervation for Treatment of Pulmonary Artery Hypertension [PADN-1] study; chiCTR-ONC-12002085).

▶ In this intriguing pilot study published in the *Journal of the American College of Cardiology* by Chen and colleagues, a novel interventional treatment for pulmonary arterial hypertension is explored. After informed consent, 13 of 21 patients with right heart catheterization—proven pulmonary artery hypertension (PAH) agreed to undergo the experimental procedure.

The procedure, pulmonary artery denervation, or PADN, was developed from the observation of a pulmo-pulmonary baroreceptor reflex that was described in the 1960s. The authors observed the same reflex in animal models of PAH and were able to improve hemodynamics in this model through radiofrequency ablation.

In the pilot study, the team selected 21 patients who had not responded to medical therapy, defined by only minor improvement in pulmonary artery pressure or insignificant improvement in exercise tolerance based on 6-minute walk distance. The 8 patients who declined the treatment were maintained on medical therapy. Interestingly, 12 of the 13 patients undergoing the procedure had all medications for treatment of PAH stopped after the procedure.

The reported results are astounding and include a 19—mm Hg decrease in mean PA and a 167-m improvement in 6-minute walk distance. This represents an unprecedented improvement in standard endpoints that eclipses all current medical therapy trials and, thus, invites careful scrutiny of this nonblinded, single-center pilot study. If these findings are replicated in larger well-designed studies, there will truly be reason for celebration.

C. D. Spradley, MD

Riociguat for the Treatment of Pulmonary Arterial Hypertension
Ghofrani H-A, for the PATENT-1 Study Group (Univ of Giessen and Marburg Lung Ctr, Germany; et al)
N Engl J Med 369:330-340, 2013

Background.—Riociguat, a soluble guanylate cyclase stimulator, has been shown in a phase 2 trial to be beneficial in the treatment of pulmonary arterial hypertension.

Methods.—In this phase 3, double-blind study, we randomly assigned 443 patients with symptomatic pulmonary arterial hypertension to receive placebo, riociguat in individually adjusted doses of up to 2.5 mg three times daily (2.5 mg-maximum group), or riociguat in individually adjusted doses that were capped at 1.5 mg three times daily (1.5 mg-maximum group). The 1.5 mg-maximum group was included for exploratory purposes, and the data from that group were analyzed descriptively. Patients who were receiving no other treatment for pulmonary arterial hypertension and patients who were receiving endothelin-receptor antagonists or (nonintravenous) prostanoids were eligible. The primary end point was the change from baseline to the end of week 12 in the distance walked in 6 minutes. Secondary end points included the change in pulmonary vascular resistance, N-terminal pro-brain natriuretic peptide (NT-proBNP) levels, World Health Organization (WHO) functional class, time to clinical worsening, score on the Borg dyspnea scale, quality-of-life variables, and safety.

Results.—By week 12, the 6-minute walk distance had increased by a mean of 30 m in the 2.5 mg-maximum group and had decreased by a mean of 6 m in the placebo group (least-squares mean difference, 36 m; 95% confidence interval, 20 to 52; $P < 0.001$). Prespecified subgroup analyses showed that riociguat improved the 6-minute walk distance both in patients who were receiving no other treatment for the disease and in those who were receiving endothelin-receptor antagonists or prostanoids. There were significant improvements in pulmonary vascular resistance ($P < 0.001$), NT-proBNP levels ($P < 0.001$), WHO functional class ($P = 0.003$), time to clinical worsening ($P = 0.005$), and Borg dyspnea score ($P = 0.002$). The most common serious adverse event in the placebo group and the 2.5 mg-maximum group was syncope (4% and 1%, respectively).

Conclusions.—Riociguat significantly improved exercise capacity and secondary efficacy end points in patients with pulmonary arterial hypertension. (Funded by Bayer HealthCare; PATENT-1 and PATENT-2 ClinicalTrials.gov numbers, NCT00810693 and NCT00863681, respectively).

▶ Chronic thromboembolic pulmonary hypertension (CTEPH) represents a unique disease state that is phenotypically similar to pulmonary arterial hypertension. There is a major difference, however. Sixty-three percent of patients with CTEPH can go to surgery (pulmonary endarterectomy) with the potential of being cured. These surgeries are performed at a handful of specialty centers and have improved the lives of thousands of patients. Unfortunately, some patients are not surgical candidates. Additionally, some eventually develop recurrent disease after surgery.

For these patients, clinicians frequently resort to therapies that have been studied and approved for the treatment of pulmonary arterial hypertension, not CTEPH. Only small case series guide this clinical decision. In this article published in the *New England Journal of Medicine* by Ghofrani and colleagues, the results of the CHEST 1 study are presented, and with that publication comes a new option for the management of CTEPH.

Riociguat, a soluble guanylate cyclase stimulator, was studied for efficacy and safety in this industry-sponsored, randomized, double-blind, placebo-controlled trial. Subjects receiving the agent garnered a placebo-adjusted increase of 46 m in the 6-minute walk at 16 weeks (Fig 2 in the original article). Statistically significant improvements in pulmonary vascular resistance, NT-Pro BNP, and functional class were also noted.

This study represents an important step forward in the management of a rare and debilitating disorder. Caution is advised, however, as the gold standard of treatment in CTEPH is surgical intervention with intent to cure. The availability of an oral therapy could potentially result in eligible patients missing that opportunity.

C. D. Spradley, MD

Riociguat for the Treatment of Chronic Thromboembolic Pulmonary Hypertension
Ghofrani H-A, for the CHEST-1 Study Group (Univ of Giessen and Marburg Lung Ctr, Germany)
N Engl J Med 369:319-329, 2013

Background.—Riociguat, a member of a new class of compounds (soluble guanylate cyclase stimulators), has been shown in previous clinical studies to be beneficial in the treatment of chronic thromboembolic pulmonary hypertension.

Methods.—In this phase 3, multicenter, randomized, double-blind, placebo-controlled study, we randomly assigned 261 patients with inoperable chronic thromboembolic pulmonary hypertension or persistent or recurrent pulmonary hypertension after pulmonary endarterectomy to receive placebo or riociguat. The primary end point was the change from baseline to the end of week 16 in the distance walked in 6 minutes. Secondary end points included changes from baseline in pulmonary vascular resistance, N-terminal pro—brain natriuretic peptide (NT-proBNP) level, World Health Organization (WHO) functional class, time to clinical worsening, Borg dyspnea score, quality-of-life variables, and safety.

Results.—By week 16, the 6-minute walk distance had increased by a mean of 39 m in the riociguat group, as compared with a mean decrease of 6 m in the placebo group (least-squares mean difference, 46 m; 95% confidence interval [CI], 25 to 67; P < 0.001). Pulmonary vascular resistance decreased by 226 dyn·sec·cm^{-5} in the riociguat group and increased by 23 dyn·sec·cm^{-5} in the placebo group (least-squares mean difference, −246 dyn·sec·cm^{-5}; 95% CI, −303 to −190; P < 0.001). Riociguat was also associated with significant improvements in the NT-proBNP level (P < 0.001) and WHO functional class (P = 0.003). The most common serious adverse events were right ventricular failure (in 3% of patients in each group) and syncope (in 2% of the riociguat group and in 3% of the placebo group).

Conclusions.—Riociguat significantly improved exercise capacity and pulmonary vascular resistance in patients with chronic thromboembolic pulmonary hypertension. (Funded by Bayer HealthCare; CHEST-1 and CHEST-2 ClinicalTrials.gov numbers, NCT00855465 and NCT00910429, respectively.)

▶ Published in the same issue of the *New England Journal of Medicine* as the CHEST 1 and CHEST 2 extension study, Ghofrani and colleagues present the results of the PATENT 1 trial and its extension study, PATENT 2. Here, riociguat is studied in group I pulmonary hypertension. The primary and secondary endpoints of the PATENT 1 trial are met in this industry-sponsored, randomized, double-blind, placebo-controlled trial of the first of a fourth class of directed therapy for pulmonary arterial hypertension.

Subjects receiving the full 2.5-mg dose of the soluble guanylate cyclase stimulator experienced a placebo-adjusted 36-m increase in 6-minute walk distance at 12 weeks (Fig 2 in the original article). The study included patients on endothelin receptor antagonists and inhaled prostacyclin analogs. Interestingly, treatment effect was noted in all groups, including those on no baseline therapy. The PATENT 2 extension study found additional improvement in walk distance with continued safety.

The dosing regimen was complex, but side effects were comparable to those of placebo. The drug was not studied in combination with intravenous or subcutaneous prostacyclin-based therapy and was also not studied in combination with PDE-5 inhibitors, which act along the same pathway.

Compared with SERAPHIN, the efficacy endpoints of PATENT 1 are less ambitious, but by the standards of prior studies, the results are strong.

C. D. Spradley, MD

Macitentan and Morbidity and Mortality in Pulmonary Arterial Hypertension
Pulido T, for the SERAPHIN Investigators (Ignacio Chávez Natl Heart Inst, Mexico City; et al)
N Engl J Med 369:809-818, 2013

Background.—Current therapies for pulmonary arterial hypertension have been adopted on the basis of short-term trials with exercise capacity as the primary end point. We assessed the efficacy of macitentan, a new dual endothelin-receptor antagonist, using a primary end point of morbidity and mortality in a long-term trial.

Methods.—We randomly assigned patients with symptomatic pulmonary arterial hypertension to receive placebo once daily, macitentan at a once-daily dose of 3 mg, or macitentan at a once-daily dose of 10 mg. Stable use of oral or inhaled therapy for pulmonary arterial hypertension, other than endothelin-receptor antagonists, was allowed at study entry. The primary end point was the time from the initiation of treatment to the first occurrence of a composite end point of death, atrial septostomy, lung transplantation, initiation of treatment with intravenous or subcutaneous prostanoids, or worsening of pulmonary arterial hypertension.

Results.—A total of 250 patients were randomly assigned to placebo, 250 to the 3-mg macitentan dose, and 242 to the 10-mg macitentan dose. The primary end point occurred in 46.4%, 38.0%, and 31.4% of the patients in these groups, respectively. The hazard ratio for the 3-mg macitentan dose as compared with placebo was 0.70 (97.5% confidence interval [CI], 0.52 to 0.96; $P = 0.01$), and the hazard ratio for the 10-mg macitentan dose as compared with placebo was 0.55 (97.5% CI, 0.39 to 0.76; $P < 0.001$). Worsening of pulmonary arterial hypertension was the most frequent primary end-point event. The effect of macitentan on this end point was observed regardless of whether the patient was receiving therapy for pulmonary arterial hypertension at baseline. Adverse events more frequently associated with macitentan than with placebo were headache, nasopharyngitis, and anemia.

Conclusions.—Macitentan significantly reduced morbidity and mortality among patients with pulmonary arterial hypertension in this event-driven study. (Funded by Actelion Pharmaceuticals; SERAPHIN ClinicalTrials.gov number, NCT00660179.)

▶ The year 2013 was a banner one for the treatment of pulmonary arterial hypertension (PAH). One of the biggest victories in the fight against this devastating disease was presented by Pulido et al in the *New England Journal of Medicine*. The industry-sponsored, double-blind, randomized, placebo-controlled SERAPHIN trial was a first in PAH therapeutics research. The study was an event-driven, long-term study evaluating morbidity and mortality in PAH patients receiving placebo or 1 of 2 doses of the dual endothelin receptor antagonist, macitentan.

The original study of epoprostenol published in 1986 was a 12-week study with a mortality endpoint. Subsequently, all therapeutic phase III trials in PAH have been short-term evaluations of clinical worsening, focusing primarily on improvement in 6-minute walk distance.[1]

This study evaluated long-term efficacy (3 years) with the primary composite endpoint of death, atrial septostomy, transplantation, initiation of treatment with intravenous or subcutaneous prostanoids, or worsening PAH. PAH worsening required all three of the following: 15% decrease in 6-minute walk distance, worsening of symptoms of pulmonary hypertension, and the need for additional treatment for PAH.

The primary endpoint was met in 46.4% of placebo patients, 38% of patients on 3 mg of macitentan, and 31.4% of patients on 10 mg of macitentan (Fig 1 in the original article). PAH worsening was the most commonly reached endpoint.

In addition to efficacy, macitentan was shown to be safe. Unlike its parent compound, bosentan, macitentan was not associated with significant liver function abnormalities, and unlike the selective endothelin agent, ambrisentan, it was not associated with more edema compared with placebo.

The report garnered criticism for the role played by the sponsor. Additionally, only a trend toward improved mortality was noted in the higher dose arm of the study over placebo. The authors point out, however, that death independent of clinical worsening is unlikely to occur as a first event.

This study introduces a powerful new tool in the fight against PAH and sets a high bar for future investigations.

C. D. Spradley, MD

Reference

1. Barst RJ, Rubin LJ, Long WA, et al. A comparison of continuous intravenous epoprostenol (prostacyclin) with conventional therapy for primary pulmonary hypertension. *N Engl J Med*. 1996;334:296-301.

5   Community-Acquired Pneumonia

Introduction

Pneumonia in the elderly was a common topic among studies published in 2013. Included in this section are three studies that provide additional insights in to the management of this population. Davydow et al, noting that hospitalizations in the elderly regardless of reason for admission frequently result in cognitive decline, performed a longitudinal study in pneumonia to determine the impact on mental function. On the prevention front, Juthani-Mehta et al reported on modifiable risk factors for development of pneumonia in community-dwelling elderly as an approach to reducing the incidence of the disease. A third area that has gained increasing attention, especially because of the reimbursement penalties associated with it, is readmission following an admission for pneumonia. The first step in reducing readmissions is to determine who is likely to require readmission. Shorr et al identified some of these risk factors in their report and also concluded that the organization and structure of the health care system may in part be at fault.

Risk factors for community-acquired pneumonia in all populations is a major research topic every year. In 2013 a number of risk factors were addressed. Van Vugt et al tried to identify whether pneumonia in patients with respiratory symptoms—specifically cough—could be ruled in or out with biomarkers such as C-reactive protein or procalcitonin. They reasoned that this would be valuable in settings in which chest x-ray was not readily available. Suissa et al took another look at the well-described increased risk of pneumonia in patients using inhaled corticosteroids. In a study of Quebec patients, the investigators were able to identify that the specific corticosteroid used may be an important component of the degree of risk. Vitamin D deficiency has been associated with reduced immunity and an increased incidence of respiratory infections. The obvious question is whether Vitamin D supplementation in deficient populations will reduce that risk. Multiple studies, including the one by Remmelts et al in a large Dutch population, have been unable to document a benefit of Vitamin D supplementation, however. To date, this remains an unresolved question. Identifying risks for drug-resistant disease or otherwise hard-to-treat patients is the topic of a study published by Shindo et al. This group looked at six specific known risk factors and tried to identify those that predicted drug resistance. The absolute number of risks, rather than weighting of specific risks, was a more useful tool in determining initial antibiotic treatment. Risks of contracting specific organisms are also a major concern. Methicillin-resistant staphylococcal aureus pneumonia is a particularly difficult pneumonia to treat and is increasingly identified in the community setting. Risk factors for this organism in the community setting are not well understood. Wooten et al studied a retrospective series of community-dwelling patients with this organism and found that the prior use of antibiotics was a major risk for the disease; however, prior hospitalization did not appear to be. With other specific organisms, the risk factors may be more obvious, and the main problem is to identify the degree of risk. Lanternier et al compared the impact of antitumor necrosis factor alpha (anti-TNFa) treatments, immunosuppressive drugs used in autoimmune illnesses, and their relationship to development of Legionnaire's pneumonia, which requires TNF alpha in the immune response.

Streptococcus pneumonia remains the most common bacterial infecting agent in community-acquired pneumonia. The patterns of disease have been of particular interest since the introduction of conjugate vaccine for children more than a decade ago. Griffin et al published a "decade later" study of pneumococcal disease that details the impact of the herd immunity that occurred after the introduction of conjugate vaccine in 2000 and the long-term outcome. A second study by Link-Gelles et al details the rise of serotypes not included in the original 7-valent vaccine in different geographic areas and the disturbing rate of antibiotic resistance in these serotypes.

Two additional studies address the difficulties in treating homeless patients contracting pneumonia (Jones et al) and the use of electronic medical record-embedded clinical decision support tools to assist physicians in prescribing appropriate and consistent antibiotic management (Litvin et al).

Janet R. Mauer, MD, MBA

Functional Disability, Cognitive Impairment, and Depression After Hospitalization for Pneumonia

Davydow DS, Hough CL, Levine DA, et al (Univ of Washington, Seattle; Univ of Michigan, Ann Arbor)
Am J Med 126:615-624, 2013

Objective.—The study objective was to examine whether hospitalization for pneumonia is associated with functional decline, cognitive impairment, and depression, and to compare this impairment with that seen after known disabling conditions, such as myocardial infarction or stroke.

Methods.—We used data from a prospective cohort of 1434 adults aged more than 50 years who survived 1711 hospitalizations for pneumonia, myocardial infarction, or stroke drawn from the Health and Retirement Study (1998-2010). Main outcome measures included the number of Activities and Instrumental Activities of Daily Living requiring assistance and the presence of cognitive impairment and substantial depressive symptoms.

Results.—Hospitalization for pneumonia was associated with 1.01 new impairments in Activities and Instrumental Activities of Daily Living (95% confidence interval [CI], 0.71-1.32) among patients without baseline functional impairment and 0.99 new impairments in Activities and Instrumental Activities of Daily Living (95% CI, 0.57-1.41) among those with mild-to-moderate baseline limitations, as well as moderate-to-severe cognitive impairment (odds ratio, 2.46; 95% CI, 1.60-3.79) and substantial depressive symptoms (odds ratio, 1.63; 95% CI, 1.06-2.51). Patients without baseline functional impairment who survived pneumonia hospitalization had more subsequent impairments in Activities and Instrumental Activities of Daily Living than those who survived myocardial infarction hospitalization. There were no significant differences in subsequent moderate-to-severe cognitive impairment or substantial depressive symptoms between patients who survived myocardial infarction or stroke and those who survived pneumonia.

Conclusions.—Hospitalization for pneumonia in older adults is associated with subsequent functional and cognitive impairment. Improved pneumonia prevention and interventions to ameliorate adverse sequelae during and after hospitalization may improve outcomes.

▶ Hospitalizations for chronic conditions in elderly patients are often associated with an overall worsening of their baseline state—a lower level of physical functionality after discharge as well as possible cognitive decline. Community-acquired pneumonia (CAP), however, is typically considered a discrete illness that is treatable and usually resolves completely. However, it is not known whether the insult of pneumonia transiently or permanently impacts the functional or mental baseline state of the elderly patient. This is an important question because pneumonia is extremely common in an aging population, and the health care system will need to plan for the impact of postpneumonia impairment if it is a common problem. The Davydow study is a longitudinal study that suggests that not only does such impairment occur, it may actually be worse than the declines observed after hospitalization for some chronic illnesses. In a second study published this year, Shah et al[1] showed that patients with even mild cognitive changes are more likely to develop pneumonia than patients without cognitive changes: patients with even mild cognitive changes often had accelerated changes after the pneumonia episode. With around 390 000 hospitalizations per year in older patients[2] and an anticipated near doubling of that number in around 25 years, it is very important to further study the postpneumonia status of elderly patients with an eye toward prevention and early intervention.

J. R. Maurer, MD

References

1. Shah FA, Pike F, Alvarez K, et al. Bidirectional relationship between cognitive function and pneumonia. *Am J Resp Crit Care Med.* 2013;188:586-592.
2. Thomas CP, Ryan M, Chapman JD, et al. Incidence and cost of pneumonia in medicare beneficiaries. *Chest.* 2012;142:973-981.

Modifiable Risk Factors for Pneumonia Requiring Hospitalization of Community-Dwelling Older Adults: The Health, Aging, and Body Composition Study

Juthani-Mehta M, for the Health ABC Study (Yale Univ, New Haven, CT; et al)
J Am Geriatr Soc 61:1111-1118, 2013

Objectives.—To identify novel modifiable risk factors, focusing on oral hygiene, for pneumonia requiring hospitalization of community-dwelling older adults.

Design.—Prospective observational cohort study.

Setting.—Memphis, Tennessee, and Pittsburgh, Pennsylvania.

Participants.—Of 3,075 well-functioning community-dwelling adults aged 70 to 79 enrolled in the Health, Aging, and Body Composition Study from 1997 to 1998, 1,441 had complete data in the data set of all variables used, a dental examination within 6 months of baseline, and were eligible for this study.

Measurements.—The primary outcome was pneumonia requiring hospitalization through 2008.

Results.—Of 1,441 participants, 193 were hospitalized for pneumonia. In a multivariable model, male sex (hazard ratio (HR) = 2.07, 95% confidence interval (CI) = 1.51–2.83), white race (HR = 1.44, 95% CI = 1.03–2.01), history of pneumonia (HR = 3.09, 95% CI = 1.86–5.14), pack-years of smoking (HR = 1.006, 95% CI = 1.001–1.011), and percentage of predicted forced expiratory volume in 1 minute (moderate vs mild lung disease or normal lung function, HR = 1.78, 95% CI = 1.28–2.48; severe lung disease vs mild lung disease or normal lung function, HR = 2.90, 95% CI = 1.51–5.57) were nonmodifiable risk factors for pneumonia. Incident mobility limitation (HR = 1.77, 95% CI = 1.32–2.38) and higher mean oral plaque score (HR = 1.29, 95% CI = 1.02–1.64) were modifiable risk factors for pneumonia. Average attributable fractions revealed that 11.5% of cases of pneumonia were attributed to incident mobility limitation and 10.3% to a mean oral plaque score of 1 or greater.

Conclusion.—Incident mobility limitation and higher mean oral plaque score were two modifiable risk factors that 22% of pneumonia requiring hospitalization could be attributed to. These data suggest innovative opportunities for pneumonia prevention among community-dwelling older adults.

▶ Because of the huge increase in community-acquired pneumonia—and the medical expense that that disease burden will generate—that is anticipated in the United States as the population ages over the next few decades, attention is beginning to focus on prevention. The first step is to determine what, if any, modifiable factors predispose the older population to developing pneumonia. Data in facility-confined patients, primarily nursing homes, have identified oral issues as important risk factors for pneumonia. These include oral care, swallowing difficulty, and plaque levels.[1,2] The current study assessed risk factors in community-dwelling adults and, interestingly, also found that oral plaque score was 1 of 2 modifiable risk factors in this population as well. Although this was an observational, registry database type of study that makes it difficult to establish direct relationships, these data are intriguing and should be further pursued in prospective, interventional trials, as improved oral care should be a low-cost, easy intervention.

J. R. Maurer, MD

References

1. Quagliarello V, Ginter S, Han L, Van Ness P, Allore H, Tinetti M. Modifiable risk factors for nursing home-acquired pneumonia. *Clin Infect Dis*. 2005;40:1-6.
2. El-Solh AA, Pietrantoni C, Bhat A, et al. Colonization of dental plaques: a reservoir of respiratory pathogens for hospital-acquired pneumonia in institutionalized elders. *Chest*. 2004;126:1575-1582.

Readmission Following Hospitalization for Pneumonia: The Impact of Pneumonia Type and Its Implication for Hospitals
Shorr AF, Zilberberg MD, Reichley R, et al (Washington Hosp Ctr, DC; EviMed Research Group, LLC, Goshen, MA; Barnes-Jewish Hosp, St Louis, MO)
Clin Infect Dis 57:362-367, 2013

Background.—Readmission rates following discharge after pneumonia are thought to represent the quality of care. Factors associated with readmission, however, remain poorly described. It is unclear if readmission rates vary based on pneumonia type.

Methods.—We retrospectively identified adults admitted to an index hospital with non-nosocomial pneumonia (January through December 2010) and who survived to discharge. We only included patients with bacterial evidence of infection. Readmission in the 30 days following discharge to any of 9 hospitals comprising the index hospital's healthcare system served as the primary end point. We recorded demographics, severity of illness, comorbidities, and infection-related factors. We noted whether the patient had healthcare-associated pneumonia (HCAP) versus community-acquired pneumonia. We utilized logistic regression analysis to determine factors independently associated with readmission.

Results.—The cohort included 977 subjects; 78.9% survived to discharge. The readmission rate equaled 20%. Neither disease severity nor the rate of initially inappropriate antibiotic therapy correlated with readmission. Subjects with HCAP were 7.5 (95% confidence interval [CI], 3.6–15.7) times more likely to be readmitted. Four HCAP criteria were independently associated with readmission: admission from long-term care (adjusted odds ratio [AOR], 2.2 [95% CI, 1.4–3.4]); immunosuppression (AOR, 1.9 [95% CI, 1.3–2.9]); prior antibiotics (AOR, 1.7 [95% CI, 1.2–2.6]); and prior hospitalization (AOR, 1.7 [95% CI, 1.1–2.5]).

Conclusions.—Readmission for pneumonia is common but varies based on pneumonia type. The variables associated with readmission do not reflect factors that hospitals directly control. Use of one rule to guide payment that fails to account for HCAP and the HCAP criteria on readmission seems inappropriate.

▶ High rates of readmission for certain diseases such as pneumonia have been targeted by the Centers for Medicare and Medicaid Services (CMS) as areas for improvement. To try to reduce these rates, CMS supports improved transitions in care and has implemented reduced payments for hospitals that have excessive readmission rates for acute myocardial infarctions, congestive heart failure, and pneumonia. COPD exacerbations and arthroplasties will be added to the CMS excess readmission program in fiscal year 2015. One of the challenges for physicians and hospitals is that there are few studies that identify the specific risk factors for readmission. A better understanding of the patients most likely to require readmission could be valuable on 2 fronts: it could help the providers better prepare a posthospitalization environment for the patient (eg, home care, multiple calls or visits) and help CMS better risk-adjust for hospitals that have high-risk discharges. This study tries to identify these risks with a retrospective analysis. The authors note that studies from outside the United States identify a lower readmission rate than that seen in US hospitals and suggest that "healthcare system organization and structure may be an important contributor to readmission rates." That is likely true. Other systems often have a better care transition structure. A valuable addition to this analysis would be a prospective study in which specific interventions designed for the high-risk readmission patients identified here were implemented at discharge to ensure adequate care in the early postdischarge timeframe.

J. R. Maurer, MD

Use of serum C reactive protein and procalcitonin concentrations in addition to symptoms and signs to predict pneumonia in patients presenting to primary care with acute cough: diagnostic study

van Vugt SF, on behalf of the GRACE consortium (Univ Med Ctr Utrecht, Netherlands; et al)
BMJ 346:f2450, 2013

Objectives.—To quantify the diagnostic accuracy of selected inflammatory markers in addition to symptoms and signs for predicting pneumonia and to derive a diagnostic tool.

Design.—Diagnostic study performed between 2007 and 2010. Participants had their history taken, underwent physical examination and measurement of C reactive protein (CRP) and procalcitonin in venous blood on the day they first consulted, and underwent chest radiography within seven days.

Setting.—Primary care centres in 12 European countries.

Participants.—Adults presenting with acute cough.

Main outcome measures.—Pneumonia as determined by radiologists, who were blind to all other information when they judged chest radiographs.

Results.—Of 3106 eligible patients, 286 were excluded because of missing or inadequate chest radiographs, leaving 2820 patients (mean age 50, 40% men) of whom 140 (5%) had pneumonia. Re-assessment of a subset of 1675 chest radiographs showed agreement in 94% (κ 0.45, 95% confidence interval 0.36 to 0.54). Six published "symptoms and signs models" varied in their discrimination (area under receiver operating characteristics curve (ROC) ranged from 0.55 (95% confidence interval 0.50 to 0.61) to 0.71 (0.66 to 0.76)). The optimal combination of clinical prediction items derived from our patients included absence of runny nose and presence of breathlessness, crackles and diminished breath sounds on auscultation, tachycardia, and fever, with an ROC area of 0.70 (0.65 to 0.75). Addition of CRP at the optimal cut off of >30 mg/L increased the ROC area to 0.77 (0.73 to 0.81) and improved the diagnostic classification (net reclassification improvement 28%). In the 1556 patients classified according to symptoms, signs, and CRP >30 mg/L as "low risk" (<2.5%) for pneumonia, the prevalence of pneumonia was 2%. In the 132 patients classified as "high risk" (>20%), the prevalence of pneumonia was 31%. The positive likelihood ratio of low, intermediate, and high risk for pneumonia was 0.4, 1.2, and 8.6 respectively. Measurement of procalcitonin added no relevant additional diagnostic information. A simplified diagnostic score based on symptoms, signs, and CRP >30 mg/L resulted in proportions of pneumonia of 0.7%, 3.8%, and 18.2% in the low, intermediate, and high risk group respectively.

Conclusions.—A clinical rule based on symptoms and signs to predict pneumonia in patients presenting to primary care with acute cough performed best in patients with mild or severe clinical presentation. Addition of CRP concentration at the optimal cut off of >30 mg/L improved diagnostic information, but measurement of procalcitonin concentration did not add clinically relevant information in this group.

▶ Biomarkers have been widely studied for their value in pneumonia to determine prognosis at the time of presentation and to follow up with patients under treatment for guidance in discharge planning and antibiotic management. This study looked at 2 of the most common biomarkers studied in pneumonia—procalcitonin and C-reactive protein (CRP)—to determine if these markers might actually be able to assist in distinguishing acute bronchitis from pneumonias in primary care settings in which the availability of chest x-rays may be limited. The authors selected patients with acute cough from a cross-sectional observational study, the GRACE-09 (Genomics to combat Resistance against Antibiotics in Community-acquired LRTI in Europe) study. In particular, the authors wondered if patients presenting with acute cough could have a more definitive diagnosis made of their lower respiratory tract infection if biomarkers were also measured. Disappointingly, only high levels of CRP added information to the classic findings of signs and symptoms suggestive of pneumonia, and the contribution of CRP was moderate at best. Procalcitonin was of little value. One of the most interesting aspects of this study is that it used data from the setting in which the issue of distinguishing between pneumonia and acute bronchitis is most often addressed—the primary care outpatient practice. Sixteen different primary care networks from across Europe participated. Traditionally, the use of biomarkers and other tools is done in secondary and tertiary settings; the use of primary care settings to conduct studies such as this that impact primary care is important.

J. R. Maurer, MD

Inhaled corticosteroids in COPD and the risk of serious pneumonia

Suissa S, Patenaude V, Lapi F, et al (McGill Univ, Montreal, Québec, Canada)
Thorax 68:1029-1036, 2013

Background.—Inhaled corticosteroids (ICS) are known to increase the risk of pneumonia in patients with chronic obstructive pulmonary disease (COPD). It is unclear whether the risk of pneumonia varies for different inhaled agents, particularly fluticasone and budesonide, and increases with the dose and long-term duration of use.

Methods.—We formed a new-user cohort of patients with COPD treated during 1990–2005. Subjects were identified using the Quebec health insurance databases and followed through 2007 or until a serious pneumonia event, defined as a first hospitalisation for or death from pneumonia. A nested case–control analysis was used to estimate the rate ratio (RR) of serious pneumonia associated with current ICS use, adjusted for age, sex, respiratory disease severity and comorbidity.

Results.—The cohort included 163 514 patients, of which 20 344 had a serious pneumonia event during the 5.4 years of follow-up (incidence rate 2.4/100/year). Current use of ICS was associated with a 69% increase in the rate of serious pneumonia (RR 1.69; 95% CI 1.63 to 1.75). The risk was sustained with long-term use and declined gradually after stopping ICS use, disappearing after 6 months (RR 1.08; 95% CI 0.99 to 1.17). The rate of serious pneumonia was higher with fluticasone (RR 2.01; 95% CI 1.93 to 2.10), increasing with the daily dose, but was much lower with budesonide (RR 1.17; 95% CI 1.09 to 1.26).

Conclusions.—ICS use by patients with COPD increases the risk of serious pneumonia. The risk is particularly elevated and dose related with fluticasone. While residual confounding cannot be ruled out, the results are consistent with those from recent randomised trials.

▶ Several studies have suggested that inhaled corticosteroids are associated with an increased risk of bacterial pneumonia in chronic obstructive pulmonary disorder (COPD) patients. Two large multicenter clinical treatment trials, the TORCH (Toward a Revolution in COPD Health) trial and the INSPIRE (Investigating New Standards for Prophylaxis in Reduction of Exacerbations) trial studied inhaled corticosteroids as part of 1 of 2 treatment arms for COPD. TORCH was a trial comparing inhaled fluticasone/salmeterol with placebo and the primary endpoint was mortality.[1] A secondary endpoint was morbidity related to exacerbations. INSPIRE was a trial comparing tiotropium and fluticasone/salmeterol in terms of efficacy with respect to exacerbations.[2] However, in both these studies, an adverse event finding in the analysis was an excess number of pneumonias in patients in the study arms in which inhaled corticosteroids were used—even though in both cases the absolute numbers of pneumonias were small. Subsequent meta-analysis on multiple studies evaluating inhaled corticosteroids in COPD have found mixed results of the impact of inhaled corticosteroids.[3,4] It has been speculated that part of this inconsistency may be caused by a differential effect of various inhaled corticosteroids. In this study, the authors assessed the Quebec population database of COPD patients and confirmed that the population using inhaled corticosteroids had a higher rate of pneumonia, but probably more importantly they found that fluticasone use created the highest risk and was dose-related, particularly compared with budesonide (the second most commonly used inhaled corticosteroid). This is consistent with both TORCH and INSPIRE in which the steroid used was fluticasone. Whether the difference between fluticasone and budesonide is real requires further evaluation. Of note, one of the meta-analyses found no increase in pneumonia with the use of inhaled corticosteroids evaluated budesonide, not fluticasone.[4] Fluticasone is generally considered a more potent drug and has a longer half-life, but its association with pneumonias may also be because it is used more often than budesonide in this population and possibly across a population of more severely ill patients.

J. R. Maurer, MD

References

1. Calverley PM, Anderson JA, Celli B, et al. Salmeterol and fluticasone propionate and survival in chronic obstructive pulmonary disease. *N Engl J Med.* 2007;356: 775-789.
2. Calverley PM, Stockley PA, Seemungal TA, et al. Reported pneumonia in patients with COPD: findings from the INSPIRE study. *Chest.* 2011;139:505-512.
3. Drummond MB, Dasenbrook EC, Pitz MW, Murphy DJ, Fan E. Inhaled corticosteroids in patients with stable chronic obstructive pulmonary disease: a systematic review and meta-analysis. *JAMA.* 2008;300:2407-2416.
4. Sin DD, Tashkin D, Zhang X, et al. Budesonide and the risk of pneumonia: a meta-analysis of individual patient data. *Lancet.* 2009;374:712-719.

The role of vitamin D supplementation in the risk of developing pneumonia: three independent case–control studies

Remmelts HHF, Spoorenberg SMC, Oosterheert JJ, et al (St Antonius Hosp, Nieuwegein, The Netherlands; Univ Med Ctr Utrecht, The Netherlands; et al)
Thorax 68:990-996, 2013

Background.—Vitamin D plays a role in host defence against infection. Vitamin D deficiency has been associated with an increased risk of respiratory tract infections in children and adults. This study aimed to examine whether vitamin D supplementation is associated with a lower pneumonia risk in adults.

Methods.—Three independent case–control studies were performed including a total of 33 726 cases with pneumonia in different settings with respect to hospitalisation status and a total of 105 243 controls. Cases and controls were matched by year of birth, gender and index date. The major outcome measure was exposure to vitamin D supplementation at the time of pneumonia diagnosis. Conditional logistic regression was used to compute ORs for the association between vitamin D supplementation and occurrence of pneumonia.

Results.—Vitamin D supplementation was not associated with a lower risk of pneumonia. In studies 1 and 2, adjustment for confounding resulted in non-significant ORs of 1.814 (95% CI 0.865 to 3.803) and 1.007 (95% CI 0.888 to 1.142), respectively. In study 3, after adjustment for confounding, the risk of pneumonia remained significantly higher among vitamin D users (OR 1.496, 95% CI 1.208 to 1.853). Additional analyses showed significant modification of the association through co-use of corticosteroids and drugs that affect bone mineralisation. For patients using these drugs, ORs below one were found combined with higher ORs for patients not using these drugs.

Conclusions.—This study showed no preventive association between vitamin D supplementation and the risk of pneumonia in adults.

▶ Vitamin D deficiency has been documented in various populations around the world, particularly in the elderly and in those who have limited sun exposure.[1,2] Even within highly developed countries such as the United States, different segments of the population may have very different vitamin D intake and levels,[3] and deficiency is common. Among the health concerns associated with vitamin D deficiency are a potential, although controversial, increased risk for respiratory tract infections.[4,5] It has been postulated that immunomodulary effects of vitamin D may be important in preventing these infections.[6] However, studies about the impact of vitamin D levels as risk factors for infection are far from conclusive. In this large set of 3 case-control studies of almost 140 000 Dutch people, almost one-quarter of whom had pneumonia, there was no protective effect for those taking vitamin D. In a second multicenter, placebo-controlled trial in which patients were given vitamin D to assess its potential role in preventing colorectal adenoma, upper respiratory tract symptom diaries were kept. This trial showed no impact of vitamin D supplementation in reducing the rate of upper respiratory tract infections.[7] The role of vitamin D in infection prevention remains unclear and requires further study in large populations.

J. R. Maurer, MD

References

1. Lips P. Vitamin D deficiency and secondary hyperparathyroidism in the elderly: consequences for bone loss and fractures and therapeutic implications. *Endocr Rev.* 2001;22:477-501.
2. Pearce SH, Cheetham TD. Diagnosis and management of vitamin D deficiency. *BMJ.* 2010;340:b5664.
3. Yetley EA. Assessing the vitamin D status of the US population. *Am J Clin Nutr.* 2008;88:558S-564S.
4. Berry DJ, Hesketh K, Power C, Hyppönen E. Vitamin D status has a linear association with seasonal infections and lung function in British adults. *Br J Nutr.* 2011;106:1433-1440.
5. Ginde AA, Mansbach JM, Camargo CA Jr. Association between serus 25-hydroxy vitamin D level and upper respiratory tract infection in the Third National Health and Nutrition Examination Survey. *Arch Intern Med.* 2009;169:384-390.
6. Aranow C. Vitamin D and the immune system. *J Investig Med.* 2011;59:881-886.
7. Rees JR, Hendricks K, Barry EL, et al. Vitamin D3 supplementation and upper respiratory tract infections in a randomized, controlled trial. *Clin Infect Dis.* 2013; 57:1384-1392.

Risk Factors for Drug-Resistant Pathogens in Community-acquired and Healthcare-associated Pneumonia

Shindo Y, on behalf of the Central Japan Lung Study Group (Nagoya Univ, Japan; et al)
Am J Respir Crit Care Med 188:985-995, 2013

Rationale.—Identification of patients with drug-resistant pathogens at initial diagnosis is essential for treatment of pneumonia.

Objectives.—To elucidate clinical features of community-acquired pneumonia (CAP) and healthcare-associated pneumonia (HCAP), and to clarify risk factors for drug-resistant pathogens in patients with CAP and HCAP.

Methods.—A prospective observational study was conducted in hospitalized patients with pneumonia at 10 institutions in Japan. Pathogens identified as not susceptible to ceftriaxone, ampicillin-sulbactam, macrolides, and respiratory fluoroquinolones were defined as CAP drug-resistant pathogens (CAP-DRPs).

Measurements and Main Results.—In total, 1,413 patients (887 CAP and 526 HCAP) were analyzed. CAP-DRPs were more frequently found in patients with HCAP (26.6%) than in patients with CAP (8.6%). Independent risk factors for CAP-DRPs were almost identical in patients with CAP and HCAP. These included prior hospitalization (adjusted odds ratio [AOR], 2.06; 95% confidence interval [CI], 1.23−3.43), immunosuppression (AOR, 2.31; 95% CI, 1.05−5.11), previous antibiotic use (AOR, 2.45; 95% CI, 1.51−3.98), use of gastric acid−suppressive agents (AOR, 2.22; 95% CI, 1.39−3.57), tube feeding (AOR, 2.43; 95% CI,

1.18–5.00), and nonambulatory status (AOR, 2.45; 95% CI, 1.40–4.30) in the combined patients with CAP and HCAP. The area under the receiver operating characteristic curve for counting the number of risk factors was 0.79 (95% CI, 0.74–0.84).

Conclusions.—The clinical profile of HCAP was different from that of CAP. However, physicians can predict drug resistance in patients with either CAP or HCAP by taking account of the cumulative number of the risk factors.

Clinical trial registered with https://upload.umin.ac.jp/cgi-open-bin/ctr/ctr.cgi?function=brows&action=brows&type=summary&recptno=R000 004001&language=E; number UMIN000003306.

▶ In the 2005 Guidelines of the American Thoracic Society and the Infectious Diseases Society of America, the groups identified a new category of pneumonia called *health care–associated pneumonia* (HCAP).[1] It differed from hospital-acquired pneumonia in that it did not occur within the context of a hospitalization but did occur in the setting of recent or ongoing interface with health care institutions, such as nursing homes, dialysis centers, and homecare wound care. This category of pneumonia was separated out because of the concern that this type of patient would have more complicated causal organisms or resistance to antibiotics. The concept of HCAP has been the focus of many studies and is a controversial concept. That stems in part from the fact that HCAP seems to be different in different geographic regions. For example, HCAP in the United States has been reported to present with more resistant organisms than routine community-acquired pneumonia[2]; however, in Europe and Japan, the types of organisms in HCAP patients more closely resemble those of community-acquired pneumonia.[3,4] This article addresses the issue of determining an appropriate approach to initial antibiotic therapy and identified 6 specific risk factors for antibiotic resistance in CAP or HCAP patients. Interestingly, although HCAP patients had a higher rate of resistance, the risk factors predicting resistance were almost identical in the 2 groups. The study found that, unlike previous studies identifying risk factors,[5] weighting of the risks was not particularly helpful. Simply counting the number and assigning an increased risk (with the implication for broader antibiotic treatment) for those with 2 or more factors was adequate. This study requires validation in other geographic areas, but if the findings are confirmed, it would simplify the approach to HCAP and could be universally applicable.

J. R. Maurer, MD

References

1. American Thoracic Society, Infectious Diseases Society of America. Guidelines for the management of adults with hospital-acquired, ventilator-associated, and healthcare-associated pneumonia. *Am J Respir Crit Care Med.* 2005;171:388-416.
2. Kollef MH, Shorr A, Tabak YP, Gupta V, Liu LZ, Johannes RS. Epidemiology and outcomes of health-care-associated pneumonia: results from a large US database of culture-positive pneumonia. *Chest.* 2005;128:3854-3862.
3. Chalmers JD, Taylor JK, Singanayagam A, et al. Epidemiology, antibiotic therapy, and clinical outcomes in health care-associated pneumonia: a UK cohort study. *Clin Infect Dis.* 2011;53:107-113.

4. Maruyama T, Gabazza EC, Morser J, et al. Community-acquired pneumonia and nursing home-acquired pneumonia in the very elderly patients. *Respir Med.* 2010; 104:584-592.

5. Aliberti S, Di Pasquale M, Zanaboni AM, et al. Stratifying risk factors for multidrug-resistant pathogens in hospitalized patients coming from the community with pneumonia. *Clin Infect Dis.* 2012;54:470-478.

Risk factors for methicillin-resistant *Staphylococcus aureus* in patients with community-onset and hospital-onset pneumonia
Wooten DA, Winston LG (Univ of California, San Francisco)
Respir Med 107:1266-1270, 2013

Objectives.—The risk factors for methicillin-resistant *Staphylococcus aureus* (MRSA) pneumonia have not been fully characterized and are likely to be different depending on whether infection is acquired in the community or the hospital.

Methods.—We conducted a case-control study of 619 adults hospitalized between 2005 and 2010 with either MRSA or methicillin-sensitive *S. aureus* (MSSA) pneumonia. Patients with a respiratory culture within 48 h of hospitalization had community-onset pneumonia whereas patients with a culture collected after this time point had hospital-onset pneumonia.

Results.—Among patients with community-onset disease, the risk for MRSA was increased by tobacco use (OR 2.31, CI 1.23—4.31), chronic obstructive pulmonary disease (OR 3.76, CI 1.74—8.08), and recent antibiotic exposure (OR 4.87, CI 2.35—10.1) in multivariate analysis while patients with hospital-onset disease had an increased MRSA risk with tobacco use (OR 2.66, CI 1.38—5.14), illicit drug use (OR 3.52, CI 2.21—5.59), and recent antibiotic exposure (OR 2.04, CI 3.54—13.01). Hospitalization within the prior three months was associated with decreased risk (OR 0.64, CI 0.46—0.89) in multivariate analysis.

Conclusions.—This study suggests there are common and distinct risk factors for MRSA pneumonia based on location of onset. The decreased risk for MRSA pneumonia associated with recent hospitalization is unexpected and warrants further investigation.

Summary.—This case-control study showed that there are common and distinct risk factors associated with MRSA pneumonia depending on whether the infection onset is in the hospital or in the community. Recent hospitalization was unexpectedly shown to be associated with decreased risk for MRSA pneumonia and warrants further investigation.

▶ Methicillin-resistant *Staphylococcus aureus* (MRSA) is an increasingly common and feared cause of both community-acquired and hospital-acquired pneumonias. It is often severe, difficult to treat, and highly morbid for its victims. When patients present with skin infections, the possibility of MRSA is always considered; however, it is less clear what the community risk factors for MRSA pneumonia are, and it is rarely an initial consideration in patients unless they have recently been in a health care setting. In the author's group of 619 patients with *S aureus* pneumonia, 44% had MRSA. Of those with *S aureus* pneumonia, 37% had community-acquired disease. Prior antibiotic exposure was a major risk factor in both community-acquired disease and hospital-onset disease; however, interestingly, hospitalization within the previous 3 months was not (Table 2 in the original article). Another interesting finding was that MRSA-infected and methicillin-sensitive *S aureus*–infected patients had similar risks for intensive care unit admission and mortality at 30 days. This is consistent with other studies that show similar outcomes from resistant or sensitive organisms as long as the appropriate therapy is started when the patient presents.[1] The information in this study is informative but should be tempered by the methodology used to capture it, which is a retrospective chart review. In addition, the disease onset was dated from a positive culture not from onset of symptomology, which could have misclassified some community-acquired disease as hospital-onset disease. Nevertheless, the results suggest that we should better define risk factors for *S aureus* pneumonias to ensure early appropriate treatment and improved outcomes.

J. R. Maurer, MD

Reference

1. Athanassa Z, Siempos II, Falagas ME. Impact of methicillin resistance on mortality in Staphylococcus aureus VAP: a systematic review. *Eur Respir J*. 2008;31: 625-632.

Incidence and Risk Factors of *Legionella pneumophila* Pneumonia During Anti-Tumor Necrosis Factor Therapy: A Prospective French Study

Lanternier F, for the Research Axed on Tolerance of Biotherapies Group (Université Paris Descartes, France; et al)
Chest 144:990-998, 2013

Objective.—Our objective was to describe the incidence and risk factors of legionellosis associated with tumor necrosis factor (TNF)-α antagonist use.

Methods.—From February 1, 2004, to January 31, 2007, we prospectively collected all cases of legionellosis among French patients receiving TNF-α antagonists in the Research Axed on Tolerance of Biotherapies (RATIO) national registry. We conducted an incidence study with the French population as a reference and a case-control analysis with four control subjects receiving TNF-α antagonists per case of legionellosis.

Results.—Twenty-seven cases of legionellosis were reported. The overall annual incidence rate of legionellosis for patients receiving TNF-α antagonists, adjusted for age and sex, was 46.7 (95% CI, 0.0-125.7) per 100,000 patient-years. The overall standardized incidence ratio (SIR) was 13.1 (95% CI, 9.0-19.1; $P < .0001$) and was higher for patients receiving infliximab (SIR, 15.3 [95% CI, 8.5-27.6; $P < .0001$]) or adalimumab (SIR, 37.7 [95% CI, 21.9-64.9; $P < .0001$]) than etanercept (SIR, 3.0

[95% CI, 1.00-9.2; *P* =.06]). In the case-control analysis, exposure to adalimumab (OR, 8.7 [95% CI, 2.1-35.1]) or infliximab (OR, 9.2 [95% CI, 1.9-45.4]) vs etanercept was an independent risk factor for legionellosis.

Conclusions.—The incidence rate of legionellosis for patients receiving TNF-α antagonists is high, and the risk is higher for patients receiving anti-TNF-α monoclonal antibodies than soluble TNF-receptor therapy. In case of pneumonia occurring during TNF-α antagonist therapy, specific urine antigen detection should be performed and antibiotic therapy should cover legionellosis.

Trial Registry.—ClinicalTrials.gov; No.: NCT00224562; URL: www.clinicaltrials.gov.

▶ Anti–tumor necrosis factor alpha (TNF-α) antibodies and soluble receptor are widely used in treatment of various autoinflammatory diseases such as rheumatoid arthritis, ankylosing spondylitis, psoriatic arthritis, and Crohn disease. Anti–TNF-α preparations and other monoclonal antibodies or modulators of necessity interfere with the normal function of the immune system and predispose those requiring these treatments to multiple, often opportunistic, infections from common and uncommon organisms. Fungal infections and tuberculosis have been the most commonly reported. The immune response to these types of infections requires granuloma formation and maintenance, which is interfered with by the intracellular infection control disruption of TNF antagonists. *Legionella pneumophila* is also an intracellular organism, and TNF-α is required as part of the immune response to this organism. The authors of this study previously reported a case series of *L pneumophila* in patients using TNF-α.[1] They then embarked on a 3-year prospective, multicenter study hoping to identify both the incidence and risk factors for opportunistic and severe bacterial infections in this population. *Legionella* infections tended to be severe with acute respiratory distress syndrome in 7 cases. Extrapulmonary manifestations including abnormal mental status, abdominal pain, diarrhea, and a smattering of other symptoms occurred in 14 of the patients. Only 1 patient was known to have died from the *Legionella*, although 2 others were lost to follow-up. The authors suggest that patients being treated with anti–TNF-α that develop pneumonia have sporadic urine antigen testing for *Legionella* and that any such patient presenting with pneumonia initially be given antibiotic treatment that covers *Legionella*. Most of the pneumonias occur with anti–TNF-α monoclonal antibodies; in someone who develops *Legionella* pneumonia, but requires restarting of anti–TNF-α therapy, it may be wise to use a product such as etanercept, which blocks TNF-α activity by a different mechanism.

J. R. Maurer, MD

Reference

1. Tubach F, Ravaud P, Salmon-Céron D, et al. Recherce Axée sur la Tolerance des Biotherapies Group. Emergence of Legionella pneumophila pneumonia in patients receiving tumor necrosis factor-alpha antagonists. *Clin Infect Dis.* 2006;43:e95-e100.

U.S. Hospitalizations for Pneumonia after a Decade of Pneumococcal Vaccination

Griffin MR, Zhu Y, Moore MR, et al (Vanderbilt Univ School of Medicine, Nashville, TN; Ctrs for Disease Control and Prevention, Atlanta, GA)
N Engl J Med 369:155-163, 2013

Background.—The introduction of 7-valent pneumococcal conjugate vaccine (PCV7) into the U.S. childhood immunization schedule in 2000 has substantially reduced the incidence of vaccine-serotype invasive pneumococcal disease in young children and in unvaccinated older children and adults. By 2004, hospitalizations associated with pneumonia from any cause had also declined markedly among young children. Because of concerns about increases in disease caused by nonvaccine serotypes, we wanted to determine whether the reduction in pneumonia-related hospitalizations among young children had been sustained through 2009 and whether such hospitalizations in older age groups had also declined.

Methods.—We estimated annual rates of hospitalization for pneumonia from any cause using the Nationwide Inpatient Sample database. The reason for hospitalization was classified as pneumonia if pneumonia was the first listed diagnosis or if it was listed after a first diagnosis of sepsis, meningitis, or empyema. Average annual rates of pneumonia-related hospitalizations from 1997 through 1999 (before the introduction of PCV7) and from 2007 through 2009 (well after its introduction) were used to estimate annual declines in hospitalizations due to pneumonia.

Results.—The annual rate of hospitalization for pneumonia among children younger than 2 years of age declined by 551.1 per 100,000 children (95% confidence interval [CI], 445.1 to 657.1), which translates to 47,000 fewer hospitalizations annually than expected on the basis of the rates before PCV7 was introduced. The rate for adults 85 years of age or older declined by 1300.8 per 100,000 (95% CI, 984.0 to 1617.6), which translates to 73,000 fewer hospitalizations annually. For the three age groups of 18 to 39 years, 65 to 74 years, and 75 to 84 years, the annual rate of hospitalization for pneumonia declined by 8.4 per 100,000 (95% CI, 0.6 to 16.2), 85.3 per 100,000 (95% CI, 7.0 to 163.6), and 359.8 per 100,000 (95% CI, 199.6 to 520.0), respectively. Overall, we estimated an age-adjusted annual reduction of 54.8 per 100,000 (95% CI, 41.0 to 68.5), or 168,000 fewer hospitalizations for pneumonia annually.

Conclusions.—Declines in hospitalizations for childhood pneumonia were sustained during the decade after the introduction of PCV7. Substantial reductions in hospitalizations for pneumonia among adults were also observed.

▶ The introduction of pneumococcal conjugate vaccine (PCV7) in 2000 for use in infants had a dramatic impact on pneumococcal disease in the United States. Not only did the incidence of pneumococcal disease decrease dramatically in the vaccinated children, it also decreased significantly in unvaccinated patients, particularly the elderly. The elimination of nasopharyngeal carriage of the serotypes included in the PCV7 vaccine by the children who were immunized removed a critical step in the pathogenesis of pneumococcal disease by reducing the transmission from person to person. This herd immunity was dramatic, but was it sustained? This report is an update of a study documenting the decline in pneumonia admissions in the United States in the first few years after the introduction of the vaccine.[1] There has been concern that these early gains from the vaccine may not have been sustained because within a few years of the vaccine introduction, nonvaccine serotypes began to emerge and increase in prevalence. They now account for a substantial portion of pneumococcal disease. This study used data collected by the Agency for Healthcare Research and Quality (AHRQ), which collects discharge diagnoses on a sample of 20% of US hospitalizations. The findings were that the decreased hospitalizations for pneumonia were sustained throughout the decade after PCV7 introduction in both children and adults (Figs 2A and 3A in the original article) despite the observed serotype replacement by nonvaccine serotypes. This is good news, but how long this sustained impact might have lasted will never be known, as PCV7 was replaced with PCV13 containing 13 serotypes in 2010, and the vaccine use has been broadened to other populations. We look forward to an analysis of the further impact of this new immunization approach.

J. R. Maurer, MD

Reference

1. Grijalva CG, Nuorti JP, Arbogast PG, Martin SW, Edwards KM, Griffin MR. Decline in pneumonia admissions after routine childhood immunisation with pneumococcal conjugate vaccine in the USA: a time-series analysis. *Lancet.* 2007;369:1179-1186.

Geographic and Temporal Trends in Antimicrobial Nonsusceptibility in Streptococcus pneumoniae in the Post-vaccine era in the United States
Link-Gelles R, Thomas A, Lynfield R, et al (Ctrs for Disease Control and Prevention, Atlanta, GA; Oregon Public Health Division, Portland; Minnesota Dept of Health, Minneapolis; et al)
J Infect Dis 208:1266-1273, 2013

Background.—We examined whether observed increases in antibiotic nonsusceptible nonvaccine serotypes after introduction of pneumococcal conjugate vaccine in the United States in 2000 were driven primarily by vaccine or antibiotic use.

Methods.—Using active surveillance data, we evaluated geographic and temporal differences in serotype distribution and within-serotype differences during 2000–2009. We compared nonsusceptibility to penicillin and erythromycin by geography after standardizing differences across time, place, and serotype by regressing standardized versus crude proportions. A regression slope (RS) approaching zero indicates greater importance of the standardizing factor.

Results.—Through 2000—2006, geographic differences in nonsusceptibility were better explained by within-serotype prevalence of nonsusceptibility (RS 0.32, 95% confidence interval [CI], .08—.55 for penicillin) than
by geographic differences in serotype distribution (RS 0.71, 95% CI,
.44—.97). From 2007—2009, serotype distribution differences became
more important for penicillin (within-serotype RS 0.52, 95% CI,
.11—.93; serotype distribution RS 0.57, 95% CI, .14—1.0).

Conclusions.—Differential nonsusceptibility, within individual serotypes, accounts for most geographic variation in nonsusceptibility, suggesting selective pressure from antibiotic use, rather than differences in
serotype distribution, mainly determines nonsusceptibility patterns.
Recent trends suggest geographic differences in serotype distribution
may be affecting the prevalence of nonsusceptibility, possibly due to
decreases in the number of nonsusceptible serotypes.

▶ Pneumococcal conjugate vaccine (PCV7) was introduced in 2000 and cov-
ered 7 serotypes of *Streptococcus pneumoniae* that accounted for 78% of
strains that had developed resistance to penicillin. In the wake of the widespread use of PCV7 in young children, disease from those strains has decreased
by 99% in the United States.[1] However, in a phenomenon known as *serotype
replacement*, several other strains of *S pneumoniae* have increased rapidly
and have replaced the PCV7 strains as a cause of pneumococcal disease.
Unfortunately, several of these replacement strains have shown significant
resistance to antibiotics. This study "assessed geographical, serotype and temporal variation in the frequency of drug nonsusceptibility." The authors hoped
to determine if vaccine use that allowed nonsusceptible serotypes to emerge
was more responsible for the new antibiotic resistance than the use of antibiotics. In the pre-PCV7 era, the authors state, antibiotic use appeared to "select for
non-susceptible strains within each serotype rather than to alter the distribution
of serotypes." The authors note that in the post-PCV7 era, the same pattern of
selectivity within the newly emerged serotypes seems to be developing, again
supporting selective antibiotic pressure as an important factor in nonsusceptibility. The impact of the new PCV13 conjugate strain with 13 serotypes (including the notoriously resistant strain 19A) is unknown. However, we can likely
expect emergence of more antibiotic-resistant strains that will have significance
for public health prevention and intervention strategies.

J. R. Maurer, MD

Reference

1. Centers for Disease Control and Prevention. Invasive pneumococcal disease in
children 5 years after conjugate vaccine introduction—eight states, 1998—2005.
MMWR Morb Mortal Wkly Rep. 2008;57:144-148.

Admission Decisions and Outcomes of Community-Acquired Pneumonia in the Homeless Population: A Review of 172 Patients in an Urban Setting
Jones B, Gundlapalli AV, Jones JP, et al (Univ of Utah, Salt Lake City; Kaiser Permanente, Pasadena, CA; et al)
Am J Public Health 103:S289-S293, 2013

Objectives.—We compared admission rates, outcomes, and performance of the CURB-65 mortality prediction score of homeless patients and nonhomeless patients with community-acquired pneumonia (CAP).

Methods.—We compared homeless (n = 172) and nonhomeless (n = 1897) patients presenting to a Salt Lake City, Utah, emergency department with CAP from 1996 to 2006. In the homeless cohort, we measured referral from and follow-up with the local homeless health care clinic and arrangement of medical housing.

Results.—Homeless patients were younger (44 vs 59 years; P < .001) and had lower CURB-65 scores and higher hospitalization risk (severity-adjusted odds ratio = 1.89; 95% confidence interval = 1.33, 2.69) than did nonhomeless patients, with a similar length of stay, median inpatient cost, and median outpatient cost, even after severity adjustment. Of homeless patients, 22% were referred from the homeless health care clinic to the emergency department; 54% of outpatients and 51% of hospital patients were referred back to the clinic, and medical housing was arranged for 23%.

Conclusions.—A large cohort of homeless patients with CAP demonstrated higher hospitalization risk than but similar length of stay and costs as nonhomeless patients. The strong relationship between the hospital and homeless health care clinic may have contributed to this finding.

▶ In 2012, the US Department of Housing and Urban Development reported more than 630 000 homeless people in the United States.[1] Health care for the homeless population in this country is little studied and predominantly urgent or emergent. It is probably the most shattered part of a broken health care system because of the many requirements for coordination to ensure that this socially isolated population accesses and adheres to appropriated preventive and treatment strategies. The study cited here assesses various components of the management of community-acquired pneumonia (CAP), a common medical issue, in this population. Not surprisingly, the usual tools used to predict severity and need for hospitalization were not often followed because of the psychosocial issues that the patients had. Thus, the hospitalization rate was much higher than that of the nonhomeless CAP patients, even though severity of disease was lower. This particular group of homeless patients was fortunate in that they had access to a clinic that serves that population and, therefore, many were referred there after hospitalization. In the absence of such an arrangement, transitions in care can be nonexistent. As the authors note, "we need more programs that effectively establish a strong relationship between primary care providers, community housing, and acute care facilities for homeless patients."

J. R. Maurer, MD

Reference

1. *The 2012 Point-in-Time Estimates of Homelessness. 2012 Annual Homelessness Assessment Report.* 2012. Washington, DC: The U.S. Department of Housing and Urban Development; 2012.

Use of an Electronic Health Record Clinical Decision Support Tool to Improve Antibiotic Prescribing for Acute Respiratory Infections: The ABX-TRIP Study

Litvin CB, Ornstein SM, Wessell AM, et al (Med Univ of South Carolina, Charleston)
J Gen Intern Med 28:810-816, 2013

Background.—Antibiotics are often inappropriately prescribed for acute respiratory infections (ARIs).

Objective.—To assess the impact of a clinical decision support system (CDSS) on antibiotic prescribing for ARIs.

Design.—A two-phase, 27-month demonstration project.

Setting.—Nine primary care practices in PPRNet, a practice-based research network whose members use a common electronic health record (EHR).

Participants.—Thirty-nine providers were included in the project.

Intervention.—A CDSS was designed as an EHR progress note template. To facilitate CDSS implementation, each practice participated in two to three site visits, sent representatives to two project meetings, and received quarterly performance reports on antibiotic prescribing for ARIs.

Main Outcome Measures.—1) Use of antibiotics for inappropriate indications. 2) Use of broad spectrum antibiotics when inappropriate. 3) Use of antibiotics for sinusitis and bronchitis.

Key Results.—The CDSS was used 38,592 times during the 27-month intervention; its use was sustained for the study duration. Use of antibiotics for encounters at which diagnoses for which antibiotics are rarely appropriate did not significantly change through the course of the study (estimated 27-month change, 1.57% [95% CI, −5.35%, 8.49%] in adults and −1.89% [95% CI, −9.03%, 5.26%] in children). However, use of broad spectrum antibiotics for ARI encounters improved significantly (estimated 27 month change, −16.30%, [95% CI, −24.81%, −7.79%] in adults and −16.30 [95% CI, −23.29%, −9.31%] in children). Prescribing for bronchitis did not change significantly, but use of broad spectrum antibiotics for sinusitis declined.

Conclusions.—This multi-method intervention appears to have had a sustained impact on reducing the use of broad spectrum antibiotics for

ARIs. This intervention shows promise for promoting judicious antibiotic use in primary care.

▶ Antibiotics remain an area of overuse or misuse, particularly in primary care practices in which sinusitis, bronchitis, otitis, and other common infections are frequently seen but only occasionally require antibiotic therapy. Physicians and other prescribers are well aware of the overuse of antibiotics through multiple educational campaigns and medical society statements, such as the Choosing Wisely Initiative.[1] Yet, still more than half of acute respiratory visits result in an antibiotic prescription.[2] So, why does this practice continue? Multiple pressures on the health care professionals, including limited time to educate patients, patient expectations, and uncertainty about diagnosis in the moment seem to outweigh the more global concerns about increased antibiotic resistance and potential complications. This article describes an effort to improve antibiotic prescribing practices by using an electronic health record—embedded decision support tool that provides guidance for evidence-supported prescribing. Similar to previous efforts to change prescribing patterns, this intervention was only moderately successful. While it did seem to reduce the use of broad-spectrum antibiotics where not appropriate, it was less successful in reducing the use of any antibiotic in an inappropriate setting. Practice behaviors are very hard to change, even when support information is right there for the prescriber to use. Even point-of-care decision support is unlikely to be very effective unless combined with financial disincentives to discourage inappropriate prescribing.

J. R. Maurer, MD

References

1. www.choosingwisely.org. Accessed December 29, 2013.
2. Grijalva CG, Nuorti JP, Griffin MR. Antibiotic prescription rates for acute respiratory tract infections in US ambulatory settings. *JAMA.* 2009;302:758-766.

6 Lung Transplantation

Introduction

The section on lung transplantation for 2014 begins with four articles that focus on different aspects of the immunology of transplantation. All potential lung transplant recipients are screened for the presence of common preformed antibodies and, if the levels of such antibodies are high enough, steps are taken to ensure that these patients receive donor organs to which they are not likely to react immunologically. Brugiere et al present some of the first longer-term outcome data on recipients with pre-existing antibodies. Anti-HLA antibodies can also develop after transplant in a subgroup of recipients and produce a fulminant and problematic type of rejection, unlike classic T-lymphocyte-mediated acute rejection. Since this can occur months to years after transplant and in a minority of patients, few reports have detailed this type of process. Witt et al report on the presentation and outcomes of a relatively large cohort of patients with this type of rejection and document the poor prognosis. Tiriveedhi et al add a new dimension to the topic of preformed antibodies in potential recipients by noting that other types of antibodies than the commonly measured antihuman leukocyte—directed antibodies (HLA)—in this case tissue-restricted self-antigens—may be important in outcomes and may be important to measure and address prior to transplant. On a different but related note, Cantu et al report on the potential of utilizing the genetic makeup of a recipient (and potential donors) to identify innate immune pathways, personalize immunosuppressive approaches, and address potential immunologic problems proactively.

Two studies focus on changes in the recipient population that the lung allocation score, a standard national ranking system for potential transplant recipients, has created since its introduction in 2005. In part, this system was intended to reduce disparities in access to transplant for minorities and women. The study by Wille et al reports interesting results, especially with respect to the impact on women. A second report by Thabut et al addresses the impact of the lung allocation score on the cystic fibrosis transplant population.

Expanded criteria for donors and potential transplant recipients, as well as the outcomes achieved by patients in the expanded criteria sets, are the topics of three studies. Two reviews based on the United Network for Organ Sharing database reported outcomes for recipients receiving donor organs greater than 55 years old. One of the reviews, by Bittle et al, is included here. Shigemura et al studied the outcomes of lung transplant recipients in the setting of a previous lung volume reduction surgery. The report notes a significant rate of surgical complications that has not previously been emphasized in this population. Retransplantation is another area of expansion. The more patients who are transplanted, the more who are likely to eventually develop graft failure and seek redo surgery. Kilic et al analyzed 390 cases of retransplant and identified the characteristics of those most likely to benefit.

Several important studies of infection, a remaining significant morbidity for transplant recipients, were published in 2013. Three are included here. Clostridium difficile, which is a nosocomial epidemic in the United States, has also been identified as an important infection in transplant recipients. The study by Lee et al is the first large series of these infections reported and emphasizes both the impact on morbidity and mortality. Of note is the high incidence of infections and that at least half the infections are in the early posttransplant period when immunosuppression is maximum. Cytomegalovirus (CMV) remains a primary infection as well. Ghassemieh et al report an interesting post-hoc finding from a prospective, randomized immunosuppression trial that the TOR-inhibitor, rapamycin, resulted in fewer CMV infections than more conventional immunosuppression. Not only are CMV and other viruses in the herpes virus family the cause of potentially lethal infection, members of the group have also been implicated in development of posttransplant lymphoproliferative disease (PTLD), also potentially lethal. Jaksch et al report on a single-center (but large population) reduction in the rate of PTLD following prophylactic administration of CMV immune globulin to high-risk patients.

The biggest threat to lung transplant recipients continues to be loss of lung function, classically identified as bronchiolitis obliterans or a picture of bronchiolitis on pulmonary functions termed bronchiolitis obliterans syndrome. In recent years, two major developments have 1) broadened our understanding of the development of posttransplant bronchiolitis, and 2) expanded the concepts of graft dysfunction beyond the pathology of bronchiolitis obliterans. In the studies included here, Griffin et al expand in an important prospective study upon the popular hypothesis of aspiration via gastric reflux as a mechanism of graft injury early posttransplant period. Parasheva et al describe one form of restrictive allograft dysfunction (RAD), an acute fibrinoid organizing pneumonia resulting is significant restrictive graft dysfunction quite different from bronchiolitis obliterans.

The last report in this section is about pulmonary rehabilitation pretransplantation. While it is widely prescribed for patients, the impact on posttransplant outcomes has rarely been reported. Li et al have published the first study that supports the benefit of pretransplant rehabilitation in outcomes.

Janet R. Mauer, MD, MBA

Lung Transplantation in Patients with Pretransplantation Donor-Specific Antibodies Detected by Luminex Assay

Brugière O, Suberbielle C, Thabut G, et al (Hôpital Bichat, Paris, France; et al)
Transplantation 95:761-765, 2013

Background.—New methods of solid-phase assays, such as Luminex assay, with high sensitivity in detecting anti—human leukocyte antigen (HLA) antibodies (Abs), have increased the proportion of sensitized candidates waiting for lung transplantation (LTx). However, how to apply these results clinically during graft allocation is debated: strict exclusion of candidates with Luminex-positive results can lead to lost opportunities for Tx. We retrospectively analyzed the clinical impact of pre-LTx Luminex-detected Abs on post-LTx outcomes for patients who underwent LTx before the availability of Luminex assay.

Methods.—We analyzed data for 56 successive patients who underwent LTx before 2008 and were considered to not have anti-HLA Abs by then-available methods of detection at the date of their LTx. Pre-LTx sera from these patients were retested by Luminex assay. Using log-rank test, freedom from bronchiolitis obliterans syndrome (BOS) and graft survival were compared between patients with and without pre-LTx Luminex-detected anti-HLA Abs classes I and II and donor-specific Abs (DSA) classes I and II.

Results.—Freedom from bronchiolitis obliterans syndrome was lower, and mortality was higher for patients with than those without pre-LTx Luminex-detected DSA class II ($P = 0.004$ and $P = 0.007$, respectively) but did not differ for patients with and without DSA class I or anti-HLA Abs class I or II.

Conclusions.—It suggests to avoid attributing graft with forbidden antigens to sensitized candidates with Luminex-detected DSA class II and to evaluate the role of specific posttransplantation protocols for LTx candidates who require emergency LTx.

▶ Preformed anti—human leukocyte (anti-HLA) antibodies in potential transplant recipients are a known risk for rejection and early mortality, particularly in renal transplantation. Patients with certain levels of antibodies are typically prematched against potential suitable donors to ensure compatibility or may be pretreated to remove antibodies. In recent years, the widespread availability of a much more sensitive assay for preformed antibodies, the Luminex assay, has shown that many—possibly as many as half of potential recipients—have some level of preformed anti-HLA antibodies. This has left many transplant centers with a perplexing question: How important are these antibodies in the outcomes of patients? Could they be responsible for some of the early graft dysfunction? What role, if any, do they contribute to long-term graft survival? And, if they do impact the graft, how important is that impact? This study starts to evaluate the potential impact of these antibodies, particularly on intermediate and later outcomes. These preliminary data suggest the antibodies impact outcomes; however, this retrospective study needs to be confirmed by a large,

carefully designed prospective evaluation, as the outcome could have significant implications for donor and recipient matching.

J. R. Maurer, MD

Acute antibody-mediated rejection after lung transplantation
Witt CA, Gaut JP, Yusen RD, et al (Washington Univ School of Medicine, St
Louis, MO)
J Heart Lung Transplant 32:1034-1040, 2013

Background.—Antibody-mediated rejection (AMR) after lung transplantation remains enigmatic, and there is no consensus on the characteristic clinical, immunologic and histologic features.

Methods.—We performed a retrospective, single-center cohort study
and identified cases of acute AMR based on the presence of circulating
donor-specific human leukocyte antigen (HLA) antibodies (DSA), histologic evidence of acute lung injury, C4d deposition and clinical allograft
dysfunction.

Results.—We identified 21 recipients with acute AMR based on the
aforementioned criteria. AMR occurred a median 258 days after transplantation; 7 recipients developed AMR within 45 days of transplantation. All patients had clinical allograft dysfunction, DSA, histology of
acute lung injury and capillary endothelial C4d deposition. Fifteen recipients improved clinically and survived to hospital discharge, but 6 died of
refractory AMR. One survivor had bronchiolitis obliterans syndrome at
the time of AMR diagnosis; 13 of the 14 remaining survivors developed
chronic lung allograft dysfunction (CLAD) during follow-up. Overall,
15 recipients died during the study period, and the median survival after
the diagnosis of AMR was 593 days.

Conclusions.—Acute AMR can be a fulminant form of lung rejection,
and survivors are at increased risk of developing CLAD. The constellation
of acute lung injury, DSA and capillary endothelial C4d deposition is compelling for acute AMR in recipients with allograft dysfunction. This clin-
icopathologic definition requires validation in a multicenter cohort, but
may serve as a foundation for future studies to further characterize AMR.

▶ Classic acute rejection in lung transplant recipients is primarily T-cell mediated and directed against foreign human leukocyte antigens (HLA) expressed in
the graft. However, there are also antibody-mediated types of graft rejection.
A hyperacute type of rejection, although uncommon, does occur rapidly within
hours or days of the transplant and is mostly likely caused by preformed antibodies in the recipient that were undetected before the surgery. Another type
of antibody-mediated acute rejection can be observed months or years from
the transplant. This type of acute rejection occurs in a relatively small number
of patients, so most transplant centers do not have a large experience with it.
In fact, in this report, only 21 cases occurred in a population of 501 transplants
(484 patients). Another important study this year looking at 441 recipients

identified 59 that developed antibodies specific to donor HLA. That report found that the development of antibodies predicts a significantly worse outcome in terms of morbidity and mortality for the patient.[1] The purpose of this study was to define more precisely in a relatively large cohort of these cases the clinical, pathologic, and immunologic, features of this entity so that precisely directed therapies can be developed and used. Early intervention in such cases is important not only because the diffuse lung damage that typically occurs results in many deaths but also because those who survive almost all develop subsequent chronic lung allograft dysfunction and impaired quality of life.

J. R. Maurer, MD

Reference

1. Snyder LD, Wang Z, Chen DF, et al. Implications for human leukocyte antigen antibodies after lung transplantation: a 10-year experience in 441 patients. *Chest.* 2013;144:226-233.

Pre-transplant antibodies to Kα1 tubulin and collagen-V in lung transplantation: Clinical correlations
Tiriveedhi V, Gautam B, Sarma NJ, et al (Washington Univ School of Medicine, St Louis, MO; et al)
J Heart Lung Transplant 32:807-814, 2013

Background.—Immune responses to lung-associated self-antigens (SAgs) have been implicated in chronic lung allograft rejection. The goals of this study were to determine the prevalence of pre-existing antibodies (Abs) to the SAgs in pulmonary diseases and the association between pre-existing Abs to SAgs and the development of primary graft dysfunction (PGD), donor-specific antibodies (DSA), and chronic rejection.

Methods.—Pre- and post-transplant sera were analyzed from 317 lung transplant (LTx) recipients between 2000 and 2011 with diagnosis of chronic obstructive disease ($n = 161$), idiopathic pulmonary fibrosis (IPF; $n = 50$), cystic fibrosis (CF; $n = 55$), and others ($n = 51$). Samples were analyzed for Abs to SAgs by enzyme-linked immunosorbent assay, and DSA and cytokines by Luminex. The clinical diagnosis of PGD and bronchiolitis obliterans syndrome (BOS) was based on International Society for Heart and Lung Transplantation guidelines.

Results.—The overall prevalence of Abs to SAgs was 22.71%, including 18% in chronic obstructive pulmonary disease ($p = 0.033$), 34% in IPF ($p = 0.0006$), 29% in CF ($p = 0.0023$), and 19.6% in other diagnoses ($p = 0.044$). The incidence of PGD (88% vs 54%, $p < 0.05$), DSA (70% vs 45%, $p < 0.01$), and BOS (90% vs 38% ($p < 0.001$) after LTx was significantly higher in patients with pre-LTx Abs to SAgs than without. Pro-inflammatory cytokines (interleukin-1β, interleukin-17, and interferon-γ) were elevated in patients who had pre-LTx Abs to SAgs, along with a reduction in anti-inflammatory interleukin-10.

Conclusions.—Patients with IPF and CF have the highest prevalence of Abs to SAgs. Patients with pre-existing Abs to SAgs are at increased risk for development of PGD, DSA, and BOS. Strategies to remove pre-existing Abs to SAgs should be considered to improve lung allograft outcome.

▶ In addition to the antihuman leukocyte antigen antibodies that have been shown to form in lung and other solid organ transplants and to participate in antibody-mediated rejection episodes, tissue-restricted self-antigens (SAgs) may also be an important stimulator of antibody production. In the lung, SAgs that have been identified as important to inciting antibody production are collagen-V and Kα1 tubulin. Donor-specific antibodies to these tissue antigens have been linked to the development of chronic lung allograft dysfunction, specifically bronchiolitis obliterans.[1] Further evidence that these antibodies may be linked to graft dysfunction has been demonstrated by the use of preemptive treatment with immunoglobulin. Patients treated with immunoglobulin or other approaches who had successful removal of the antibodies have been reported to have better survival and lower graft-related morbidity.[2] This study further defines the epidemiology of these antigens in the various diseases that present for transplant. Not surprisingly, patients with idiopathic pulmonary fibrosis, which may be an immune-related disease, and patients with cystic fibrosis, who have significant ongoing chronic inflammation in their lungs, are most likely to have these antibodies pretransplant. A prospective study is indicated (and probably underway) to determine if routine removal of the antibodies before transplant or in the perioperative period improves outcomes.

J. R. Maurer, MD

References

1. Hachem RR, Tiriveedhi V, Patterson GA, Aloush A, Trulock EP, Mohanakumar T. Antibodies to K-alpha 1 tubulin and collagen V are associated with chronic rejection after lung transplantation. *Am J Transplant.* 2012;12:2164-2171.
2. Hachem RR, Yusen RD, Meyers BF, et al. Anti-human leukocyte antigen antibodies and preemptive antibody-directed therapy after lung transplantation. *J Heart Lung Transplant.* 2010;29:973-980.

Gene Set Enrichment Analysis Identifies Key Innate Immune Pathways in Primary Graft Dysfunction After Lung Transplantation
Cantu E, for the CTOT Investigators (Univ of Pennsylvania, Philadelphia; et al)
Am J Transplant 13:1898-1904, 2013

We hypothesized alterations in gene expression could identify important pathways involved in transplant lung injury. Broncho alveolar lavage fluid (BALF) was sampled from donors prior to procurement and in recipients within an hour of reperfusion as part of the NIAID Clinical Trials in Organ Transplantation Study. Twenty-three patients with Grade 3 primary graft dysfunction (PGD) were frequency matched with controls based on donor age and recipient diagnosis. RNA was analyzed using the Human

Gene 1.0 ST array. Normalized mRNA expression was transformed and differences between donor and postreperfusion values were ranked then tested using Gene Set Enrichment Analysis. Three-hundred sixty-two gene sets were upregulated, with eight meeting significance (familywise-error rate, FWER p-value < 0.05), including the NOD-like receptor inflammasome (NLR; $p < 0.001$), toll-like receptors (TLR; $p < 0.001$), IL-1 receptor ($p = 0.001$), myeloid differentiation primary response gene 88 ($p = 0.001$), NFkB activation by nontypeable *Haemophilus influenzae* ($p = 0.001$), TLR4 ($p = 0.008$) and TLR 9 ($p = 0.018$). The top five ranked individual transcripts from these pathways based on rank metric score are predominantly present in the NLR and TLR pathways, including IL1β (1.162), NLRP3 (1.135), IL1α (0.952), IL6 (0.931) and CCL4 (0.842). Gene set enrichment analyses implicate inflammasome—mediated and innate immune signaling pathways as key mediators of the development of PGD in lung transplant patients.

▶ Ultimately, the most likely pathway through which lung transplantation will move to achieve a significantly improved rate of long-term survival and diminished morbidity will be through individualized management. That will require understanding the genetic makeup of each individual and using that information not only to match with an appropriate donor but also to use the most appropriate immunosuppressive therapy in the appropriate dose based on the recipient's unique genome. Genetic information should also help direct anti-infective prophylaxis and other treatment strategies. We are not, of course, quite there yet. This study by Cantu et al is focused on identifying the genes that are expressed in severe primary graft dysfunction. The data point to specific gene expression that is involved in primary graft dysfunction, and that data may help us not only predict severe primary graft dysfunction but also suggest therapies to prevent or ameliorate it. This is just the beginning of research into an area that promises a very bright future for transplant recipients and sufferers of many other conditions.

J. R. Maurer, MD

Disparities in lung transplantation before and after introduction of the lung allocation score
Wille KM, Harrington KF, deAndrade JA, et al (Univ of Alabama at Birmingham)
J Heart Lung Transplant 32:684-692, 2013

Background.—In May 2005, the Lung Allocation Score (LAS) became the primary method for determining allocation of lungs for organ transplantation for those at least 12 years of age in the United States. During the pre-LAS period, black patients were more likely than white patients to become too sick or die while awaiting transplant. The association between gender and lung transplant outcomes has not been widely studied.
Methods.—Black and white patients aged ≥18 years registered on the United Network for Organ Sharing (UNOS) lung transplantation waiting

list from January 1, 2000, to May 3, 2005 (pre-LAS, $n = 8,765$), and from May 4, 2005, to September 4, 2010 (LAS, $n = 8,806$), were included. Logistic regression analyses were based on smaller cohorts derived from patients listed in the first 2 years of each era (2,350 pre-LAS, and 2,446 LAS) to allow for follow-up time. Lung transplantation was the primary outcome measure. Multivariable analyses were performed within each interval to determine the odds that a patient would die or receive a lung transplant within 3 years of listing.

Results.—In the pre-LAS era, black patients were more likely than white patients to become too sick for transplantation or die within 3 years of waiting list registration (43.8% vs 30.8%; odds ratio [OR], 1.84; $p < 0.001$). Race was not associated with death or becoming too sick while listed for transplantation in the LAS era (14.0% vs 13.3%; OR, 0.93; $p = 0.74$). Black patients were less likely to undergo transplantation in the pre-LAS era (56.3% vs 69.2%; OR, 0.54; $p < 0.001$) but not in the LAS era (86.0% vs 86.7%; OR, 1.07; $p = 0.74$). Women were more likely than men to die or become too sick for transplantation within 3 years of listing in the LAS era (16.1% vs 11.3%; OR, 1.58; $p < 0.001$) compared with the pre-LAS era (33.4% vs 30.7%; OR, 1.19; $p = 0.08$).

Conclusion.—Racial disparities in lung transplantation have decreased with the implementation of LAS as the method of organ allocation; however, gender disparities may have actually increased in the LAS era.

▶ The Lung Allocation Score (LAS) that was implemented in 2005 for the allocation of donor organs to lung transplant recipients essentially created organ distribution on the basis of sickest first compared with the less-standardized system existing at the time that allocated organs primarily to recipients basically by how long they had been on the wait list. This approach created inflated wait lists so that potential recipients could accrue wait time. In the era of the LAS, the lists became much smaller and, as designed, the listed potential recipients became much sicker. The hope was that the new system would be fairer and eliminate some of the disparities that seemed to exist in the old system. The authors' finding that the LAS system may actually create a greater disadvantage for women is intriguing, especially because the scoring in this system uses objective data. There are several possibilities why this may be true, but the most intriguing is that a given set of objective measurements of disease severity may not mean the same in a man and a woman. This is suggested by studies of chronic obstructive pulmonary disease survival in men and women.[1] And that means that a separate scoring system or weighting of scores should be considered for women who are awaiting transplant.

J. R. Maurer, MD

Reference

1. Machado MC, Krishnan JA, Buist SA, et al. Sex differences in survival of oxygen-dependent patients with chronic obstructive pulmonary disease. *Am J Respir Crit Care Med.* 2006;174:524-529.

Survival Benefit of Lung Transplant for Cystic Fibrosis since Lung Allocation Score Implementation

Thabut G, Christie JD, Mal H, et al (Hôpital Bichat, Paris, France; Univ of Pennsylvania, Philadelphia; et al)
Am J Respir Crit Care Med 187:1335-1340, 2013

Rationale.—The survival benefit of lung transplantation (LT) in adult patients with cystic fibrosis (CF) is debated.

Objectives.—We sought to assess the survival benefit of LT in adult patients with CF.

Methods.—We used data from the United Network for Organ Sharing Registry to identify adult patients with CF on a wait list for LT in the United States between 2005 and 2009. Survival times while on the wait list and after LT were modeled by use of a Cox model that incorporated transplantation status as a time-dependent covariate. Evolution in lung allocation score (LAS) while on the wait list was used as a surrogate for disease severity. We fitted a model for the joint distribution of survival and longitudinal disease process (LAS over time).

Measurements and Main Results.—A total of 704 adult patients with CF were registered on a wait list during the study period. The cumulative incidence of LT was 39.3% (95% confidence interval, 35.6—42.9%) at 3 months and 64.7% (61.0—68.4%) at 12 months, whereas the incidence of death while on the wait list at the same times was 8.5% (6.4—10.6%) and 12.9% (10.3—15.5%), respectively. Survival after LT was 96.5% (94.7—98.2%) at 3 months; 88.4% (85.1—91.8%) at 12 months; and 67.8% (59.9—76.8%) at 3 years. LT conferred a 69% reduction in the instantaneous risk of death (51—80%). The interaction between LAS and LT was significant: the higher the LAS, the greater the survival benefit of LT ($P < 0.001$).

Conclusions.—LT confers a survival benefit for adult patients with CF.

▶ Before the implementation of the Lung Allocation Score (LAS) system for allocating donor organs to potential transplant recipients, organs were allocated on a wait-time basis. That is, those who had been on the wait list the longest received the organs as they became available (with a few exceptions designed to ensure a compatible donor/recipient match). It was often argued before the use of LAS that patients with chronic obstructive pulmonary disease (COPD) and those with cystic fibrosis (CF) could receive organs and suffer postoperative complications that actually shortened their lives relative to what their survival might have been had they not received their transplant. That could happen because the survival of patients with those diagnoses is hard to predict precisely once they reach end stage; thus, many patients might have been listed earlier than necessary. It was argued that not only might it be unethical for these patients to undergo transplant and, by so doing, shorten their survival, but that this also cheated others who were waiting and who would almost certainly have a survival advantage with a transplant. With the LAS in place, only the sickest patients (across all diseases) receive the organs. The net effect of this realignment in allocation has been that the percentage of the total transplants per year has decreased for both COPD and CF patients; the percentage of patients with idiopathic pulmonary fibrosis has nearly doubled. The study reported here confirms that those CF patients undergoing transplant are truly the sickest of the CF population and should put to rest the argument that the CF patients may not benefit from the transplant.

J. R. Maurer, MD

The use of lung donors older than 55 years: A review of the United Network of Organ Sharing database
Bittle GJ, Sanchez PG, Kon ZN, et al (Univ of Maryland School of Medicine, Baltimore)
J Heart Lung Transplant 32:760-768, 2013

Background.—Current lung transplantation guidelines stipulate that the ideal donor is aged younger than 55 years, but several institutions have reported that outcomes using donors aged 55 years and older are comparable with those of younger donors.

Methods.—We retrospectively reviewed the United Network for Organ Sharing (UNOS) database to identify all adult lung transplants between 2000 and 2010 in the United States. Patients were stratified by donor age 18 to 34 (reference), 35 to 54, 55 to 64, and ≥65 years. Primary outcomes included survival at 30 days and at 1, 3, and 5 years and rates of bronchiolitis obliterans syndrome (BOS). Survival was assessed using the Kaplan-Meier method. Risk factors for mortality were identified by multivariable Cox and logistic regression.

Results.—We identified 10,666 recipients with median follow-up of 3 years (range, 0–10 years). Older donors were more likely to have died of cardiovascular or cerebrovascular causes, but there were no differences in recipient diagnosis, lung allocation score, or incidence of BOS as a function of donor age. The use of donors aged 55 to 64 years was not a risk factor for mortality at 1 year (odds ratio, 1.1; $p = 0.304$) or 3 years (odds ratio, 0.923; $p = 0.571$) compared with the reference group; however, use of donors aged >65 years was associated with increased mortality at both time points (odds ratio, 2.8 and 2.4, $p < 0.02$).

Conclusions.—Outcomes after lung transplantation using donors aged 55 to 64 years were similar to those observed with donors meeting conventional age criteria. Donors aged ≥65 years, however, were associated with decreased intermediate-term survival, although there was no increased risk of BOS for this group.

▶ Only a few years ago, there were very strict, but usually unwritten, restrictions around potential lung donors. For example, any infiltrates, impaired oxygenation, smoking history, and even age greater than 45 years were exclusions. However, those constraints left a small universe of donors for an ever-growing number of people with end-stage lung disease in need of organs. This led progressively to the loosening of criteria and an increased use of so-called *marginal* donors. Probably the extension of the age criteria has been the easiest to justify, as there is little good evidence that older lungs, although they have some increase in compliance and minimal functional loss, have higher risk of graft morbidity or loss than younger lungs. In the decade 2000 to 2010, the United Network for Organ Sharing (UNOS) database recorded 1008 donors age 55 years or older with 104 of those age greater than 64. The only group that had a reduced survival were those who received organs older than 64 years. The authors note that this is consistent with most of the published literature (small studies) about donor age. Another study reported this year using the same database came to a similar conclusion.[1] A close look at the deaths in this group shows that almost all of the excess deaths occurred early after the transplants. This suggests that the older organs may have been given to sicker patients or older patients, particularly in the last 5 years of the decade when the lung allocation system focused on distribution to sickest first. With the small number of grafts from donors aged 65 or more, the early mortality may reflect a bias in distribution of the organs as much as the age of the organ.

J. R. Maurer, MD

Reference

1. Baldwin MR, Peterson ER, Easthausen I, et al. Donor age and early graft failure after lung transplantation: a Cohort Study. *Am J Transplant.* 2013;13:2685-2695.

Lung Transplantation After Lung Volume Reduction Surgery

Shigemura N, Gilbert S, Bhama JK, et al (Univ of Pittsburgh Med Ctr, PA)
Transplantation 96:421-425, 2013

Background.—Lung volume reduction surgery (LVRS) as a bridge to lung transplantation was first advocated in 1995 and published studies have supported the concept but with limited data. The risk-benefit tradeoffs of the combined procedure have not been thoroughly examined, although substantial information regarding LVRS has emerged.

Methods.—Of 177 patients who underwent lung transplantation for end-stage emphysema between 2002 and 2009 at our center, 25 had prior LVRS (22 bilateral and 3 unilateral). Lung transplantation was performed 22.9 ± 15.9 months after LVRS. We compared in-hospital morbidity, functional capacity, and long-term outcomes of patients who underwent LVRS before lung transplantation with a matched cohort of patients without prior LVRS to assess the influence of LVRS on posttransplantation morbidity and mortality.

Results.—The incidence of postoperative bleeding requiring reexploration and the incidence of renal dysfunction requiring dialysis were higher in patients with LVRS before lung transplantation. Posttransplantation peak forced expiratory volume in 1 s was worse in patients with LVRS before lung transplantation (56.7% vs. 78.8%; $P<0.05$). Five-year survival

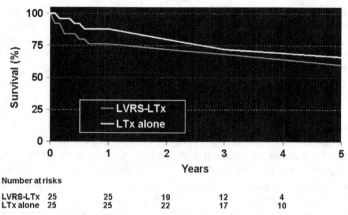

FIGURE 1.—Comparison of patient survival after lung transplantation between double lung transplant after LVRS (LVRS-Lung Transplant Group) and double lung transplant without prior LVRS (Lung Transplant Alone Group). (Reprinted from Shigemura N, Gilbert S, Bhama JK, et al. Lung transplantation after lung volume reduction surgery. *Transplantation.* 2013;96:421-425, with permission from Lippincott Williams & Wilkins.)

was not significantly different (59.7% in patients with LVRS before lung transplantation vs. 66.2% in patients with lung transplantation alone). In multivariate analysis, age more than 65 years, prolonged cardiopulmonary bypass time, and severe pulmonary hypertension were significant predictors for mortality ($P<0.05$).

Conclusions.—Although LVRS remains a viable option as a bridge to lung transplantation in appropriately selected patients, LVRS before lung transplantation can impart substantial morbidity and compromised functional capacity after lung transplantation. LVRS should not be easily considered as a bridge to transplantation for all lung transplant candidates (Fig 1).

▶ Lung volume reduction surgery (LVRS) is sometimes used as a bridge to lung transplantation in selected patients who have a particular set of characteristics: apical predominant disease and poor exercise tolerance. Several series of patients underwent LVRS followed by transplant, and in most of those studies there has been little negative impact on outcome of transplant with the staged procedures. This study is a bit different in that it presents a relatively large series from a single center, and nearly all of the transplants performed were double lung transplants. Although overall 5-year survival with the staged procedure was not significantly different from that of the transplant-only group, the morbidity in the staged group was much greater. The study reports a sobering rate of significant surgical complications, especially in the double lung transplants. Also notable is that the patients who underwent the staged procedure enjoyed only about a 2-year reprieve from transplant with their LVRS. Certainly, this information should be part of the shared decision-making process when a patient is trying to decide the best course of action.

J. R. Maurer, MD

Functional Status Is Highly Predictive of Outcomes After Redo Lung Transplantation: An Analysis of 390 Cases in the Modern Era

Kilic A, Beaty CA, Merlo CA, et al (Johns Hopkins Hosp, Baltimore, MD)
Ann Thorac Surg 96:1804-1811, 2013

Background.—The aim of this study was to evaluate whether functional status is a predictor of outcomes after redo lung transplantation (LTx).

Methods.—Adults undergoing redo LTx after implementation of the Lung Allocation Score (May 2005 to December 2010) were identified in the United Network for Organ Sharing database. Patients were stratified into three groups based on functional status as measured before redo LTx by the Karnofsky scale: (1) no assistance required, (2) some assistance required, and (3) total assistance required. Outcomes after redo LTx were compared based on these preoperative functional cohorts.

Results.—A total of 390 redo LTx were identified: 44 (11%) required no functional assistance, 176 (45%) required some assistance, and 170 (44%) required total assistance preoperatively. Overall survival at 1 year after redo LTx was significantly reduced in the total assistance group (56% versus 82% no assistance, versus 82% some assistance; $p < 0.001$). After risk adjustment, recipients requiring total assistance preoperatively were at significant risk for 1-year mortality (odds ratio 3.72, $p = 0.02$). Overall, the preoperative functional assessment outperformed the Lung Allocation Score in predicting 1-year survival after redo LTx (c-index: 0.68 versus 0.58). Transplant survivors who required total assistance before redo LTx were also at increased risk of requiring total assistance after redo LTx (26% versus 0% no assistance, versus 3% some assistance; $p < 0.001$).

Conclusions.—These data suggest that performing redo LTx in patients requiring total functional assistance is associated with significant risk of early mortality and continued functional limitation, findings that may have important implications in organ allocation.

▶ The role of retransplantation in lung transplantation, where the numbers of potential recipients always exceeds the number of available donors, remains a controversial issue. At 3%[1] of the overall transplants per year, the number remains fairly small. However, the number of previous transplant recipients seeking retransplant is likely to increase substantially over the next decade. It is well documented that the rate of chronic lung allograft dysfunction increases and worsens the longer the transplant recipient survives. Increasing numbers of transplants per year and longer-surviving transplants as well as the use of a less-selective group of donor organs (in the past sometimes called *marginal* organs) will increase the number of patients seeking retransplant. These patients will necessarily be competing with first-time recipients for the available grafts, so it is very important to start to define—as the authors have started to do in this report—the characteristics of patients seeking retransplant that lead to good and less good outcomes.

J. R. Maurer, MD

Reference

1. Adult Lung Transplantation Statistics. http://www.ishlt.org/registries/slides. Accessed 12/7/2013.

Clostridium difficile infection increases mortality risk in lung transplant recipients
Lee JT, Kelly RF, Hertz MI, et al (Univ of Minnesota, Minneapolis)
J Heart Lung Transplant 32:1020-1026, 2013

Background.—*Clostridium difficile* infection (CDI) and associated mortality in solid organ transplant recipients is rising, but data are scarce in lung transplant recipients. We aimed to characterize CDI and its effect on mortality in a large cohort of lung transplant recipients.

Methods.—Lung transplant recipients were identified from our transplant database from 2000 to 2011. Cox proportional hazard models were used to calculate hazard ratios for CDI and death after adjusting for potential confounders identified from bivariate analysis.

Results.—We identified 388 patients (196 female, 192 male), with a median age of 56 years (range, 8–75 years), during the study period. CDI developed after transplant in 89 (22.9%), with 27 (7.0%) developing CDI during the initial hospitalization at a mean diagnosis of 12.7 ± 11.4 days. Incidence varied widely each year (median, 24%; range, 5%–32%), with the highest rates in 2007 to 2008. Post-operative length of stay was identified as a significant predictor of CDI (hazard ratio [HR], 1.02; 95% confidence interval [CI], 1.01–1.03). Early CDI was an independent significant predictor of death (HR, 1.96; 95% CI, 1.14–3.36) as well as CDI anytime after transplant (HR, 1.61; 95% CI, 1.02–2.52).

Conclusions.—CDI rates varied widely from 2000 through 2011, with the highest rates in 2007 to 2008. Lung transplant recipients who developed CDI had a higher risk of death, especially when CDI occurred in the first 6 months after transplant.

▶ *Clostridium difficile* is rapidly becoming the most common nosocomial infection in the United States. In some areas in the country, it has actually surpassed methicillin-resistant *Staphylococcus aureus* in incidence and become the most important hospital-acquired infection.[1] Not only is this infection increasing in incidence and morbidity in hospitalized patients, it is beginning to be seen in the community as well. The changing epidemiology to larger populations with less comorbidity has been associated with the emergence of a very virulent strain of *C difficile*, NAP1/BI/027. Not only is this strain very virulent, it is typically resistant to fluoroquinolones, has higher toxin production, and is resistant to typical treatment strategies. A few years ago, the incidence and importance of *C difficile* began to be reported in solid organ transplant patients.[2-4] These early reports, when they included lung transplant recipients, had only small numbers, and little could be concluded about the morbidity and mortality of the infection in that population. This is the first large series of lung transplant recipients, and it confirms that this infection confers a significant risk for increased morbidity and mortality. Perhaps more significant is the large number of lung transplant recipients in this series, nearly one-quarter, who developed the infection. Infections were concentrated in the first 6 months after transplant, but almost half occurred beyond that time frame. There is clearly an urgent need to control these infections, especially because they do not respond well to antibiotic therapy. The authors correctly stress approaches to prevention of infection in the institutional setting and the ongoing pursuit of a vaccine. They don't mention a newer approach to treatment that has been shown in several studies recently to be successful, the use of fecal transplant[5] to restore normal colonic flora. That may be a reasonable approach in this population, as it avoids the use of additional antibiotics.

J. R. Maurer, MD

References

1. Miller BA, Chen LF, Sexton DJ, Anderson DJ. Comparison of the burdens of hospital-onset, healthcare facility-associated Clostridium difficile infection and of healthcare-associated infection due to methicillin-resistant Staphylococcus aureus in community hospitals. *Infect Control Hosp Epidemiol.* 2011;32:387-390.
2. Theunissen C, Knoop C, Nonhoff C, et al. Clostridium difficile colitis in cystic fibrosis patients with and without lung transplantation. *Transpl Infect Dis.* 2008;10: 240-244.
3. Boutros M, Al-Shaibi M, Chan G, et al. Clostridium difficile colitis: increasing incidence, risk factors, and outcomes in solid organ transplant recipients. *Transplantation.* 2012;93:1051-1057.
4. Gunderson CC, Gupta MR, Lopz F, et al. Clostridium difficile colitis in lung transplantation. *Transpl Infect Dis.* 2008;10:245-251.
5. Lo Vecchio A, Cohen MB. Fecal microbiota transplantation for Clostridium difficile infection: benefits and barriers. *Curr Opin Gastroenterol.* 2014;30:47-53.

Decreased incidence of cytomegalovirus infection with sirolimus in a post hoc randomized, multicenter study in lung transplantation
Ghassemieh B, Ahya VN, Baz MA, et al (Univ of Chicago Med Ctr, IL; Hosp of the Univ of Pennsylvania, Philadelphia; Univ of Florida School of Medicine, Gainesville; et al)
J Heart Lung Transplant 32:701-706, 2013

Background.—Cytomegalovirus (CMV) is the most common opportunistic infection in lung transplantation. A recent multicenter, randomized trial (the AIRSAC study) comparing sirolimus to azathioprine in lung transplant recipients showed a decreased incidence of CMV events in the sirolimus cohort. To better characterize this relationship of decreased incidence of CMV events with sirolimus, we examined known risk factors and characteristics of CMV events from the AIRSAC database.

Methods.—The AIRSAC database included 181 lung transplant patients from 8 U.S.-based lung transplant centers that were randomized to sirolimus or azathioprine at 3 months post-transplantation. CMV incidence, prophylaxis, diagnosis and treatment data were all prospectively collected. Prophylaxis and treatment of CMV were at the discretion of each institution.

Results.—The overall incidence of any CMV event was decreased in the sirolimus arm when compared with the azathioprine arm at 1 year after lung transplantation (relative risk [RR] = 0.67, confidence interval [CI] 0.55 to 0.82, $p < 0.01$). This decreased incidence of CMV events with sirolimus remained significant after adjusting for confounding factors of CMV serostatus and CMV prophylaxis.

Conclusions.—These data support results from other solid-organ transplantation studies and suggest further investigation of this agent in the treatment of lung transplant recipients at high risk for CMV events.

▶ The data in this report are a fortunate side benefit of a multicenter prospective study[1] that was designed to look at an entirely different question—whether azathioprine or sirolimus is a better long-term immunosuppressant in lung transplant recipients in terms of graft dysfunction and mortality. Thus, the participating centers did not use a standard regimen for prophylaxis against cytomegalovirus (CMV), still a significant infectious threat to lung transplants particularly if a previously uninfected recipient received a donor with evidence of previous infection (D$^+$/R$^-$). The finding that CMV disease was less common in the sirolimus-treated patients—even in the face of different prophylaxis regimens—is consistent with findings in other types of solid organ transplants. But that finding probably has more importance in lung transplants because CMV, especially in higher-risk lung transplant recipients, tends to be a more severe disease with more mortality and morbidity than in other types of transplants. The differential impact of sirolimus and azathioprine on CMV disease may be a more important finding of this study than the original primary outcomes. A prospective study comparing sirolimus with azathioprine or mycophenolate and using a common strategy around CMV would be very helpful in better understanding the importance of the impact on CMV. This may also better guide immunosuppressive strategies in higher-risk patients.

J. R. Maurer, MD

Reference

1. Bhorade S, Ahya VN, Baz MA, et al. Comparison of sirolimus with azathioprine in a tacrolimus-based immunosuppressive regimen in lung transplantation. *Am J Respir Crit Care Med.* 2011;183:379-387.

Effect of Cytomegalovirus Immunoglobulin on the Incidence of Lymphoproliferative Disease After Lung Transplantation: Single-Center Experience With 1157 Patients

Jaksch P, Wiedemann D, Kocher A, et al (Med Univ of Vienna, Austria)
Transplantation 95:766-772, 2013

Background.—Posttransplantation lymphoproliferative disorder (PTLD), a complication of lung transplantation with an incidence ranging from as much as 20%, is mainly associated with Epstein-Barr virus (EBV) infection. In renal transplantation, the use of immunoglobulin (Ig) cytomegalovirus (CMV) prophylaxis, which contains anti-EBV antibodies, resulted in a significant lower incidence of PTLD. In this study, we report our experience with PTLD in lung transplantation with CMV Ig prophylaxis.

Methods.—One-thousand one-hundred fifty-seven consecutive patients who underwent lung transplantation at the Medical University of Vienna between November 1989 and December 2011 were included in this retrospective analysis on PTLD. CMV prophylaxis consisted in all patients of antiviral drugs (ganciclovir/valganciclovir) combined with anti-CMV Ig for 4 weeks.

Results.—A total of 18 patients (1.5%) developed PTLD of B cell origin. Fifteen patients were diagnosed in the first posttransplantation year, and three patients, beyond 1 year. One- and three-year survival after diagnosis of PTLD was 50% and 38%, respectively.

Conclusion.—The incidence of PTLD in our center is extremely low when compared with the scientific literature. We hypothesize that CMV Ig prophylaxis also protects from EBV-associated PTLD.

▶ Posttransplant lymphoproliferative disease (PTLD) is a risk in transplant patients and is more common in lung transplants than in other solid organ transplants, probably because of the more intensive immunosuppression required in those patients. Most cases of PTLD are B-cell proliferative disorders, and Epstein-Barr virus (EBV) can be detected in the cells. The greatest risk of PTLD development is in patients who are EBV negative at the time of transplant and either receive EBV-positive grafts or develop de novo EBV infection. The rates of PTLD in lung transplant recipients vary from less than 5% to more than 20% and tend to be related to the intensity of the immunosuppression used. Unfortunately, treatments—usually consisting of pulling back immunosuppression or using antitumor regimens—are only partially successful, and the disease has a high mortality rate. This article describes another approach, more of a preventive approach that may be useful in reducing the incidence of PTLD in high-risk patients. This particular program reports using cytomegalovirus immunoglobulin for one month after transplant in all patients. Although that is a very expensive strategy and likely not practical for most programs, the data from this large population does suggest that the approach might be beneficial in EBV-naïve recipients, as only 5 of the cases of PTLD that occurred in this large cohort were in that high-risk group.

J. R. Maurer, MD

Aspiration and Allograft Injury Secondary to Gastroesophageal Reflux Occur in the Immediate Post-Lung Transplantation Period (Prospective Clinical Trial)

Griffin SM, Robertson AGN, Bredenoord AJ, et al (Royal Victoria Infirmary, Newcastle upon Tyne, UK; Sint Antonius Hosp, Nieuwegein, The Netherlands; et al)

Ann Surg 258:705-712, 2013

Objectives.—To provide novel pilot data to quantify reflux, aspiration, and allograft injury immediately post–lung transplantation.

Background.—Asymptomatic reflux/aspiration, associated with allograft dysfunction, occurs in lung transplant recipients. Early fundoplication has been advocated. Indications for surgery include elevated biomarkers of aspiration (bile salts) in bronchoalveolar lavage fluid (BALF). Measurements have been mostly documented after the immediate posttransplant period. We report the first prospective study of reflux/aspiration immediately posttransplantation to date.

Methods.—Lung transplant recipients were recruited over 12 months. At 1 month posttransplantation, patients completed a Reflux Symptom Index questionnaire and underwent objective assessment for reflux (manometry and pH/impedance). Testing was performed on maintenance proton pump inhibitor. BALF was assessed for pepsin, bile salts, interleukin-8 and neutrophils.

Results.—Eighteen lung transplant recipients, median age of 46 years (range: 22–59 years), were recruited. Eight of 18 patients had abnormal esophageal peristalsis. Five of 17 patients were positive on Reflux Symptom Index questionnaire. Twelve of 17 patients had reflux. Three patients exclusively had weakly acid reflux. Median acid exposure was 4.8% (range: 1%–79.9%) and median esophageal volume exposure was 1.6% (range: 0.7–5.5). There was a median of 72 reflux events (range: 27–147) per 24 hours. A correlation existed between Reflux Symptom Index score and proximal reflux ($r = 0.533$, $P = 0.006$). Pepsin was detected in 11 of 15 BALF samples signifying aspiration (median: 18 ng/mL; range: 0–43). Bile salts were undetectable, using spectrophotometry and rarely detectable using dual mass spectrometry (2/15) (levels 0.2 and 1.2 μmol/L). Lavage interleukin-8 and neutrophil levels were elevated. A correlation existed between proximal reflux events and neutrophilia ($r = 0.52$, $P = 0.03$).

Conclusions.—Lung transplant recipients should be routinely assessed for reflux/aspiration within the first month posttransplant. Reflux/aspiration can be present early postoperatively. Pepsin was detected suggesting aspiration. Bile salts were rarely detected. Proximal reflux events correlated with neutrophilia, linked to allograft dysfunction and mortality. These results support the need for early assessment of reflux/aspiration, which may inform fundoplication.

▶ For the last 10 years or so, multiple studies have identified a high incidence of gastric reflux and aspiration in both pre-lung transplant and post-lung transplant patients. This finding has led, in most lung transplant programs, to routine assessment for presence of gastric reflux in transplant candidates and, when found, various types of treatments of gastric reflux in an attempt to prevent the aspiration. This varies from the use of medication, primarily proton pump inhibitors, to the widespread use of fundal plication to reduce the likelihood of aspiration. The concern about gastric aspiration is that it predisposes to chronic lung allograft dysfunction, primarily bronchiolitis.[1,2] The exact mechanism of the injury that results in a risk to lung function is still being investigated. It has been postulated that injury to the bronchial epithelium may result in increased expression of alloantigens. Animal studies have found that gastric aspiration can recruit CD8[+] T-cells and result in bronchiolitis obliterans.[3] The purpose of the current, prospective study is to better define the characteristics of reflux in the early period after transplant and to better quantify and understand the importance of these events. This is only a pilot study, and we need much more prospective data around the importance of these aspiration events and the best way to manage them. Hopefully, more long-term prospective studies are on the way.

J. R. Maurer, MD

References

1. Robertson AG, Griffin SM, Murphy D, et al. Targeting allograft injury and inflammation in the management of post-lung transplant bronchiolitis obliterans syndrome. *Am J Transplant.* 2009;9:1272-1278.
2. D'Ovidio F, Mura M, Ridsdale R, et al. The effect of reflux and bile acid aspiration on the lung allograft and its surfactant and innate immunity molecules SP-A and SP-D. *Am J Transplant.* 2006;6:1930-1938.
3. Hartwig MG, Appel JZ, Li B, et al. Chronic aspiration of gastric fluid accelerates pulmonary allograft dysfunction in a rat model of lung transplantation. *J Thorac Cardiovasc Surg.* 2006;131:209-217.

Acute Fibrinoid Organizing Pneumonia after Lung Transplantation

Paraskeva M, McLean C, Ellis S, et al (Alfred Hosp, Melbourne, Australia; et al)
Am J Respir Crit Care Med 187:1360-1368, 2013

Rationale.—The barrier to long-term success after lung transplantation is the development of chronic lung allograft dysfunction. As the experience with lung transplantation accrues, it has become increasingly apparent that not all chronic allograft dysfunction is consistent with the traditionally recognized small-airway histological process of obliterative bronchiolitis (OB).

Objectives.—To identify and describe chronic allograft dysfunction that is not consistent with the well-described bronchiolitis obliterans syndrome and to further characterize a novel histopathological process, acute fibrinoid organizing pneumonia (AFOP), that has led invariably to respiratory decline and death after lung transplantation.

Methods.—We evaluated 194 bilateral lung transplant recipients, identifying 87 individuals who developed chronic allograft dysfunction. They were then classified according to features on spirometry, chest imaging, and histopathological specimens.

Measurements and Main Results.—Two main phenotypes of chronic allograft dysfunction were identified; 39 (45%) recipients were categorized as having developed OB and 22 (25%) as having AFOP. Survival in those who developed AFOP was significantly worse than in those who developed OB (median time to death 101 vs. 294 d; $P = 0.02$), with all exhibiting a rapid decline in respiratory function leading to death.

Conclusions.—AFOP is a novel form of chronic allograft dysfunction exhibiting spirometric, radiological, and histopathological characteristics that differentiate it from OB. The further characterization of chronic allograft dysfunction and its heterogeneous manifestations will allow the targeting of clinical and experimental efforts to prevent and treat chronic allograft dysfunction.

▶ Concepts of lung function loss after lung transplantation have expanded to include a variety of changes besides the classical description of obliterative bronchiolitis or bronchiolitis obliterans syndrome (BOS). In fact, a more general term, *chronic lung allograft dysfunction* (CLAD), is now applied to the constellation of changes that can occur in transplanted lungs as a result of rejection sequelae or other insults. One of the most common nonbronchiolitic findings is a restrictive functional loss that has been termed *restrictive allograft syndrome* (RAS). Paraskeva et al describe one form of this, acute fibrinoid organizing pneumonia, in 25% of those patients with loss of lung function. This group of patients had a more rapid downhill course than patients with classical BOS. In a second study reported in 2013, Mihalek et al[1] noted that the finding of interstitial pneumonitis on transbronchial biopsy done during surveillance or for a clinical indication was associated with a greater risk of BOS development. This suggests a correlation with parenchymal and bronchiolar disease. This more precise delineation of the changes in posttransplant lungs is important in helping to define the underlying pathogenesis and in accurately determining prognosis and management.

J. R. Maurer, MD

Reference

1. Mihalek AD, Rosas IO, Padera RF Jr, et al. Interstitial pneumonitis and the risk of chronic allograft rejection in lung transplant recipients. *Chest*. 2013;143:1430-1435.

Pulmonary rehabilitation in lung transplant candidates

Li M, Mathur S, Chowdhury NA, et al (Univ Health Network, Toronto, Ontario, Canada)

J Heart Lung Transplant 32:626-632, 2013

Background.—While awaiting lung transplantation, candidates may participate in pulmonary rehabilitation to improve their fitness for surgery. However, pulmonary rehabilitation outcomes have not been systematically evaluated in lung transplant candidates.

Methods.—This investigation was a retrospective cohort study of 345 pre-transplant pulmonary rehabilitation participants who received a lung transplant between January 2004 and June 2009 and had available pre-transplant exercise data. Data extracted included: 6-minute walk tests at standard intervals; exercise training details; health-related quality-of-life (HRQL) measures; and early post-transplant outcomes. Paired t-tests were used to examine changes in the 6MW distance (6MWD), exercise training volume and HRQL during the pre-transplant period. We evaluated the association between pre-transplant 6MWD and transplant hospitalization outcomes.

Results.—The final 6MWD prior to transplantation was only 15 m less than the listing 6MWD ($n = 200$; $p = 0.002$). Exercise training volumes increased slightly from the start of the pulmonary rehabilitation program until transplant: treadmill, increase 0.69 ml/kg/min ($n = 238$; $p < 0.0001$); biceps resistance training, 18 lbs. × reps ($n = 286$; $p < 0.0001$); and quadriceps resistance training, 15 lbs. × reps ($n = 278$; $p < 0.0001$). HRQL measures declined. A greater final 6MWD prior to transplant correlated with a shorter length of stay in the hospital ($n = 207$; $p = 0.003$).

Conclusions.—Exercise capacity and training volumes are well preserved among lung transplant candidates participating in pulmonary rehabilitation, even in the setting of severe, progressive lung disease. Participants with greater exercise capacity prior to transplantation have more favorable early post-transplant outcomes.

▶ Virtually all patients awaiting lung transplant (with the possible exception of patients with severe pulmonary hypertension) are required to participate in pulmonary rehabilitation. This has been a consistent requirement since the first successful transplants were performed in the 1980s. Interestingly, the role of this approach—that is, whether it is really helpful in preparing patients for transplant and whether it makes a difference in the outcomes—has been little studied. An evaluation of the role of pulmonary rehabilitation is important because it can be difficult for very sick preoperative patients to get to pulmonary rehabilitation programs, and these programs add an additional cost. This study helps justify this approach to preoperative management. Although another study has found that transplant candidates who are more functional pretransplant have lower mortality posttransplant, that study did not address the role of pulmonary rehabilitation in influencing the functional capacity.[1] This study documents that functional capacity is preserved in those who participate in rehabilitation and that those with higher functional capacity have better outcomes—supporting the role of preoperative pulmonary rehabilitation.

J. R. Maurer, MD

Reference

1. Kawut SM, O'Shea MK, Bartels MN, Wilt JS, Sonett JR, Arcasoy SM. Exercise testing determines survival in patients with diffuse parenchymal lung disease evaluated for lung transplantation. *Respir Med.* 2005;99:1431-1439.

7   Sleep Disorders

Introduction

In this YEAR BOOK's sleep medicine selections, I have chosen articles that further enforce (or refute) some of our current practices. An example is the article entitled "Impact of Treatment with Continuous Positive Airway Pressure (CPAP) on Weight in Obstructive Sleep Apnea." I think many of our patients expect to lose weight once they start CPAP. I think many of us have probably told our patients that they would lose weight. This article challenges those ideas. Then let's examine the evidence of adeno-tonsillectomy on pediatric obstructive sleep apnea. Does adenotonsillec-tomy affect behavioral outcomes? I encourage you to read these articles. In addition, while many of us know that oral appliances are recommended as treatment in those with mild to moderate sleep apnea, the data on out-comes in those with severe obstructive sleep apnea has not been studied as well. In this YEAR BOOK, I've included two articles examining outcomes in studies that included this population. These articles examine longer-term endpoints and health-related outcomes. I feel both of these articles are clinically relevant to our practice today, particularly as there is a growing acceptance of its usefulness and its increasing availability. Besides oral appliances and CPAP, newer devices are coming down the pipeline. Read "Novel and Emerging Nonpositive Airway Pressure Therapies for Sleep Apnea" to find out more.

Additional selections include articles on sleep health. Please read the articles entitled "Effects of Experimental Sleep Restriction on Caloric Intake and Activity Energy Expenditure," "The Face of Sleepiness: Improvement in Appearance after Treatment of Sleep Apnea," and "Self-reported Sleep and β-Amyloid Deposition in Community-Dwelling Older Adults." All may lend supportive arguments for our patients to get more sleep and better sleep.

Phenotypes are a hot topic, and obstructive sleep apnea is no exception. I really enjoyed the article entitled "Defining phenotypic causes of obstruc-tive sleep apnea." The creation of the PALM scale is a new way to think about the causes and potential treatments that exist for our patients. I expect that we will hear more of this in the future.

These and others wrap up another year of important movements in the field of sleep medicine. I hope that you will find the selections clinically applicable to your practice and a joy to read.

Shirley F. Jones, MD, FCCP, DABSAM

Central Sleep Apnea and Heart Failure

Randomized Controlled trial of Noninvasive Positive Pressure Ventilation (NPPV) Versus Servoventilation in Patients with CPAP-Induced Central Sleep Apnea (Complex Sleep Apnea)

Dellweg D, Kerl J, Hoehn E, et al (Kloster Grafschaft, Schmallenberg, Germany)
Sleep 36:1163-1171, 2013

Study Objectives.—To compare the treatment effect of noninvasive positive pressure ventilation (NPPV) and anticyclic servoventilation in patients with continuous positive airway pressure (CPAP)-induced central sleep apnea (complex sleep apnea).

Design.—Randomized controlled trial.

Setting.—Sleep center.

Patients.—Thirty patients who developed complex sleep apnea syndrome (CompSAS) during CPAP treatment.

Interventions.—NPPV or servoventilation.

Measurements and Results.—Patients were randomized to NPPV or servo-ventilation. Full polysomnography (PSG) was performed after 6 weeks. On CPAP prior to randomization, patients in the NPPV and servoventilator arm had comparable apnea-hypopnea indices (AHI, 28.6 ± 6.5 versus 27.7 ± 9.7 events/h (mean ± standard deviation [SD])), apnea indices (AI, 19 ± 5.6 versus 21.1 ± 8.6 events/h), central apnea indices (CAI, 16.7 ± 5.4 versus 18.2 ± 7.1 events/h), oxygen desaturation indices (ODI, 17.5 ± 13.1 versus 24.3 ± 11.9 events/h). During initial titration NPPV and servoventilation significantly improved the AHI (9.1 ± 4.3 versus 9 ± 6.4 events/h), AI (2 ± 3.1 versus 3.5 ± 4.5 events/h) CAI (2 ± 3.1 versus 2.5 ± 3.9 events/h) and ODI (10.1 ± 4.5 versus 8.9 ± 8.4 events/h) when compared to CPAP treatment (all $P < 0.05$). After 6 weeks we observed the following differences: AHI (16.5 ± 8 versus 7.4 ± 4.2 events/h, $P = 0.027$), AI (10.4 ± 5.9 versus 1.7 ± 1.9 events/h, $P = 0.001$), CAI (10.2 ± 5.1 versus 1.5 ± 1.7 events/h, $P < 0.0001$)) and ODI (21.1 ± 9.2 versus 4.8 ± 3.4 events/h, $P < 0.0001$) for NPPV and servoventilation, respectively. Other sleep parameters were unaffected by any form of treatment.

Conclusions.—After 6 weeks, servoventilation treated respiratory events more effectively than NPPV in patients with complex sleep apnea syndrome.

▶ The prevalence of complex sleep apnea is 15% of patients undergoing polysomnography at a large referral center. Clinical characteristics of patients with complex sleep apnea are similar to those with obstructive sleep apnea syndrome.[1] No reliable clinical markers are predictive of the appearance of complex sleep apnea.[2] Furthermore, there are no published guidelines on how to treat or who to treat. Complex sleep apnea is best thought of as a dynamic process with some individuals' apnea resolving and others in whom the complex apnea continues. Furthermore, Cassel et al reported the development of complex sleep apnea at 3-month follow-up in patients who had no evidence of it initially.[3] This finding only adds to the difficulty of treating this entity.

In this article, at 6 week follow-up those randomly assigned to noninvasive positive pressure ventilation (NPPV) had significantly higher apnea-hypopnea indices (AHI) than those receiving servoventilation. Central events represent the greatest number of respiratory events at follow-up, despite the fact that both groups had similar AHI on the titration night. It is unclear from this study why NPPV failed to control the complex sleep apnea at follow-up, but what I think we can glean from this study plus the existing literature is that this group of patients needs close follow-up because there are no clear predictors of the course for complex sleep apnea and that servoventilation appears to treat complex apnea more effectively over time compared with NPPV.

S. F. Jones, MD, FCCP, DABSM

References

1. Morgenthaler TI, Kagramanov V, Hanak V, Decker PA. Complex sleep apnea syndrome: is it a unique clinical syndrome? *Sleep.* 2006;36:1203-1209.
2. Kuźniar TJ, Morgenthaler TI. Treatment of complex sleep apnea syndrome. *Chest.* 2012;142:1049-1057.
3. Cassel W, Canisius S, Becker HF, et al. A prospective polysomnographic study on the evolution of complex sleep apnoea. *Eur Respir J.* 2011;38:329-337.

Consequences of Sleep-Disordered Breathing

An Official American Thoracic Society Clinical Practice Guideline: Sleep Apnea, Sleepiness, and Driving Risk in Noncommercial Drivers: An Update of a 1994 Statement
Strohl KP, on behalf of the ATS Ad Hoc Committee on Sleep Apnea, Sleepiness, and Driving Risk in Noncommercial Drivers
Am J Respir Crit Care Med 187:1259-1266, 2013

Background.—Sleepiness may account for up to 20% of crashes on monotonous roads, especially highways. Obstructive sleep apnea (OSA) is the most common medical disorder that causes excessive daytime sleepiness, increasing the risk for drowsy driving two to three times. The purpose of these guidelines is to update the 1994 American Thoracic Society Statement that described the relationships among sleepiness, sleep apnea, and driving risk.

Methods.—A multidisciplinary panel was convened to develop evidence-based clinical practice guidelines for the management of sleepy driving due to OSA. Pragmatic systematic reviews were performed, and the Grading of Recommendations, Assessment, Development, and Evaluation approach was used to formulate and grade the recommendations. Critical outcomes included crash-related mortality and real crashes, whereas important outcomes included near-miss crashes and driving performance.

Results.—A strong recommendation was made for treatment of confirmed OSA with continuous positive airway pressure to reduce driving risk, rather than no treatment, which was supported by moderate-quality evidence. Weak recommendations were made for expeditious diagnostic evaluation and initiation of treatment and against the use of stimulant medications or empiric continuous positive airway pressure to reduce driving risk. The weak recommendations were supported by very low–quality evidence. Additional suggestions included routinely determining the driving risk, inquiring about additional causes of sleepiness, educating patients about the risks of excessive sleepiness, and encouraging clinicians to become familiar with relevant laws.

Discussion.—The recommendations presented in this guideline are based on the current evidence, and will require an update as new evidence and/or technologies becomes available.

▶ This is an update of the previous statement (which was last published in 1994!). A lot has happened since that time: litigations, drowsy driving laws passed in some states, and overall an increase in public awareness. So an update on this statement is timely (and overdue). The authors of the report are well-recognized experts in the field of sleep medicine and driving safety who have reviewed the available literature. Obstructive sleep apnea is associated with an increased risk of motor vehicle accidents. Furthermore, considering the possible number of near misses on the roadways today, it is important that our patients are aware of the public risk of drowsy driving and the importance of treatment and education. It is important that a timely evaluation and diagnostic testing is performed on high-risk individuals. There is emphasis on use of home sleep testing in the appropriate candidate. This, of course, would expedite diagnosis and management.

S. F. Jones, MD, FCCP, DABSM

Does autotitrating positive airway pressure therapy improve postoperative outcome in patients at risk for obstructive sleep apnea syndrome? A randomized controlled clinical trial
O'Gorman SM, Gay PC, Morgenthaler TI (Mayo Clinic, Rochester, MN)
Chest 144:72-78, 2013

Background.—Obstructive sleep apnea has been associated with postoperative complications. We hypothesized that postoperative autotitrating positive airway pressure (APAP) applied to patients at high risk for obstructive sleep apnea would shorten hospital stay and reduce postoperative complications.

Methods.—Included were patients aged 18 to 100 years scheduled for elective total knee or hip arthroplasty who were able to give informed consent. Patients without contraindication to positive airway pressure therapy were divided into a high- or low-risk group on the basis of the Flemons sleep apnea clinical score. Low-risk patients received standard care. High-risk patients were randomized to receive standard care or standard care plus postoperative APAP. All patients were administered a predismissal cardiorespiratory sleep study. The primary end point was length of stay, and secondary end points were a range of postoperative complications.

Results.—One hundred thirty-eight patients were enrolled in the study (52 in the low-risk group, 86 in the high-risk group). Within the high-risk group, 43 were randomized to standard care and 43 to standard care plus postoperative APAP. There were no significant differences in the length of stay ($P = .65$) or any of the secondary end points between the randomized groups. On subgroup analysis of patients with an apnea-hypopnea index of ≥ 15, patients randomized to APAP had a longer postoperative stay (median, 5 vs 4 days; $P = .02$).

Conclusions.—The role for empirical postoperative APAP requires further study, but the findings did not show benefit for APAP applied postoperatively to positive airway pressure-naive patients at high risk for sleep apnea.

▶ More than a decade ago, a case-control study reported that obstructive sleep apnea was associated with an increased risk in postoperative complications including unplanned transfers to the intensive care unit and longer length of stay. Patients not using their continuous positive airway pressure (CPAP) machine before hospitalization had higher rates of serious complications compared with home CPAP users.[1] This article is important in that it aimed to investigate the effect of postoperative CPAP on length of stay and complication rate.

The study has interesting findings. The investigators screened more than 2000 patients for this study and still fell short of the targeted enrollment (not from lack of trying, obviously). No significant differences in length of stay or complications were noted between those receiving standard therapy or standard therapy plus autotitrating PAP (APAP). The authors actually observed a longer length of stay and longer times spent with hypoxia in patients with AHI greater than 15 who received APAP than in those patients randomly selected to usual care plus APAP. They also reported a residual AHI of 13.5 while on APAP! What could explain the seemingly opposite results of the initial hypothesis? It is these details, which, in my opinion, draw the greatest interest (and inquiry). The authors' discussion is lively and draws many possibilities to explain these results, but I think the one that deserves real consideration is that central apneas may have a greater presence in the postoperative period, which would explain why the APAP was not effective. Also, the population studied included only those who were CPAP naïve. Less than 4 hours of APAP use was achieved on most of the nights (excluding the first): definitely noncompliance. The postoperative period is not the best time to introduce nightly wear of CPAP in naïve patients.

I believe additional studies should be performed in this area. I think the preoperative period is the best time (if time is permitting) to introduce PAP and that perhaps Bilevel ventilation with backup rate is needed.

S. F. Jones, MD, FCCP, DABSM

Reference

1. Gupta RM, Parvizi J, Hanssen AD, Gay PC. Postoperative complications in patients with obstructive sleep apnea syndrome undergoing hip or knee replacement: a case-control study. *Mayo Clin Proc.* 2001;76:897-905.

CPAP Treatment and Benefits

Impact of Group Education on Continuous Positive Airway Pressure Adherence

Lettieri CJ, Walter RJ (Walter Reed Natl Military Med Ctr, Bethesda, MD)
J Clin Sleep Med 9:537-541, 2013

Study Objectives.—To compare the impact of a group educational program versus individual education on continuous positive airway pressure (CPAP) adherence.

Methods.—Post hoc assessment of a performance improvement initiative designed to improve clinic efficiency, access to care, and time to initiate therapy. Consecutive patients newly diagnosed with obstructive sleep apnea (OSA) initiating CPAP therapy participated in either an individual or group educational program. The content and information was similar in both strategies.

Results.—Of 2,116 included patients, 1,032 received education regarding OSA and CPAP through a group clinic, and 1,084 received individual education. Among the cohort, 76.6% were men, mean age 48.3 ± 9.2 years, mean body mass index 29.6 ± 4.6 kg/m^2, and mean apnea-hypopnea index was 33.3 ± 24.4 events/hour. Baseline characteristics were similar between groups. CPAP adherence was significantly greater in those participating in a group program than those receiving individual education. Specifically, CPAP was used for more nights (67.2% vs. 62.1%, $p = 0.02$) and more hours per night during nights used (4.3 ± 2.1 vs. 3.7 ± 2.8, $p = 0.03$). Further, fewer individuals discontinued therapy (10.6% vs. 14.5%, $p < 0.001$), more achieved regular use of CPAP (45.2%. vs. 40.6%, $p = 0.08$), and time to initiate therapy was shorter (13.2 ± 3.1 versus 24.6 ± 7.4 days, $p < 0.001$). Group education resulted in a 3- to 4-fold increase in the number of patients seen per unit time.

Conclusions.—A group educational program facilitated improved CPAP adherence. If confirmed by prospective randomized studies, group CPAP education may be an appropriate alternative to individual counseling, may improve acceptance of and adherence to therapy, and decrease time to treatment.

▶ I read this article with enthusiasm because I find the topic of continuous positive airway pressure (CPAP) adherence interesting and because I see the applicability in a busy clinical practice. In a practice with many referrals, we must find ways to be efficient and deliver outstanding service and, most importantly, provide excellent care for our patients. Of course, this all needs to be done early in the course of CPAP initiation, a time in which patterns of adherence (or not) emerge.

In this article, the authors evaluated adherence in patients who received education in an individual or group construct. By using group therapy, more patients could be seen in one time period compared, hence, improved efficiency. Subjects who received group education used their CPAP for more hours per night and a greater portion of nights than those who received individual attention. But alas! Although there is a statistically significant improvement in the adherence numbers, the mean hours of use and portion of nights used as a group are still less than ideal and fall below the CMS definition of compliance. Nevertheless, a positive note is that group therapy is feasible to use in the clinical setting with adherence rates that are better than those of individual education.

In my practice setting, we attempted a group education initiative for a short time. I think there were certain patients who found a group setting enjoyable, and for others it was not. By gaining a better understanding of the patient and medical-related factors, along with the technical challenges of CPAP adherence, we can adjust our methods of CPAP education and hopefully improve the current rates of treatment acceptance. I encourage you to read the article by Wickwire et al (also a selection in the YEAR BOOK).[1]

S. F. Jones, MD, FCCP, DABSM

Reference

1. Wickwire EM, Lettieri CJ, Cairns AA, Collop NA. Maximizing positive airway pressure adherence in adults. *Chest*. 2013;144:680-693.

Maximizing Positive Airway Pressure Adherence in Adults: A Common-Sense Approach
Wickwire EM, Lettieri CJ, Cairns AA, et al (Pulmonary Disease and Critical Care Associates, Columbia, MD; Uniformed Services Univ and Walter Reed Natl Military Med Ctr, Bethesda, MD; et al)
Chest 144:680-693, 2013

Positive airway pressure (PAP) therapy is considered the most efficacious treatment of obstructive sleep apnea (OSA), especially moderate to severe OSA, and remains the most commonly prescribed. Yet suboptimal adherence presents a challenge to sleep-medicine clinicians. The purpose of the current review is to highlight the efficacy of published interventions to improve PAP adherence and to suggest a patient-centered clinical approach to enhancing PAP usage.

▶ Nonadherence to continuous positive airway pressure (CPAP) is a common and daily problem clinicians see in practice. Although technologies continue to advance the field to make the prescribed pressure more acceptable, patient-related factors are important. We need to understand the multiple variables that make treatment so difficult for our patients, or otherwise we will continue to see rates of CPAP abandonment at 25%,[1] and long-term treatment adherence in less than 50% of patients.[2] This article nicely outlines patient, medical, and psychiatric disease-related factors and equipment-related issues associated with adherence. The available data on interventions that have been tried are reviewed. I think many of us focus on education, making it the center of our methods to promote adherence, but that alone is not enough. It is likely that we need to understand what inhibits our patients from CPAP use just as much as what is the best intervention. Individualization and interdisciplinary teams are important. There is a need for behavioral specialists on the team, and I think (and hope) that more sleep centers will incorporate such experts.

S. F. Jones, MD, FCCP, DABSM

References

1. van Zeller M, Severo M, Santos AC, Drummond M. 5-year APAP adherence in OSA patients—do first impressions matter? *Respir Med.* 2013;107:2046-2052.
2. Weaver TE, Grunstein RR. Adherence to continuous positive airway pressure therapy: the challenge to effective treatment. *Proc Am Thorac Soc.* 2008;5:173-178.

The Face of Sleepiness: Improvement in Appearance after Treatment of Sleep Apnea

Chervin RD, Ruzicka DL, Vahabzadeh A, et al (Univ of Michigan, Ann Arbor; et al)

J Clin Sleep Med 9:845-852, 2013

Study Objectives.—Anecdote but no formal evidence suggests that facial appearance improves after hypersomnolent patients with obstructive sleep apnea are treated. We investigated whether masked volunteer raters can identify post- rather than pre-treatment images as looking more alert, and whether impressions are predicted by any objective changes on highly precise 3-dimensional digital photogrammetry.

Methods.—Participants included 20 adults with obstructive sleep apnea on polysomnography and excessive sleepiness on Epworth Sleepiness Scales. Photogrammetry was performed before and after $\geq$ 2 months of adherent use of positive airway pressure. Twenty-two raters then assessed pre- and post-treatment facial images, paired side-by-side in random order.

Results.—Subjects included 14 men and 6 women, with mean age 45 ± 11 (SD) years and mean baseline apnea/hypopnea index of 26 ± 21. The 22 raters twice as often identified post-treatment rather than pre-treatment images to look more alert ($p = 0.0053$), more youthful ($p = 0.026$), more attractive ($p = 0.0068$), and more likely to reflect the treated state ($p = 0.015$). Photogrammetry documented post-treatment decreases in forehead surface volume and decreased infraorbital and cheek redness, but no narrowing of the interpalpebral fissure. Decreased deep NREM sleep at baseline, and pre- to post-treatment decrements in facial redness showed promise as predictors of improved subjective ratings for alertness.

Conclusions.—Patients with obstructive sleep apnea are perceived to appear more alert, more youthful, and more attractive after adherent use of positive airway pressure. Objective changes in facial surface volume and color were identified. Post-treatment decrements in redness may inform subjective impressions of improved alertness.

▶ We commonly associate bags or circles under the eyes as indicators of poor sleep. In patients with obstructive sleep apnea, can use of continuous positive airway pressure (CPAP) correct/improve facial appearance, and is this detectable subjectively and objectively? This article by Chervin et al focuses on these questions. Objective changes in appearance were measured using photogrammetry, which has been used in plastic surgery. Interestingly, changes in infraorbital surface volume (what we know as bags under the eyes) were not significantly changed. Post-CPAP images were consistently selected as more youthful, alert, and attractive by reviewers. It is interesting that nonmedical reviewers were correct more often than medical reviewers at identifying the post-CPAP images as improved in appearance. Objectively, a decrease in facial color redness in the infraorbital and cheek redness was detected in post-CPAP images by photogrammetry. This is the first study of its kind to my knowledge. Because lay people are able to discern that a post-CPAP image appears more youthful, alert, and attractive, this may provide motivation for patients to adhere to therapy.

S. F. Jones, MD, FCCP, DABSM

5-Years APAP adherence in OSA patients — Do first impressions matter?
van Zeller M, Severo M, Santos AC, et al (Centro Hospitalar de São João, Porto, Portugal; Univ of Porto Med School, Portugal)
Respir Med 107:2046-2052, 2013

Background.—Although continuous positive airway pressure (CPAP) is effective in treating obstructive sleep apnoea (OSA), inadequate adherence remains a major cause of treatment failure. This study aimed to determine long term adherence to auto adjusting-CPAP (APAP) and its influencing factors including the role of initial compliance.

Methods.—Eighty-eight male patients with newly diagnosed moderate/severe OSA were included. After initiation of APAP treatment, patients had periodic follow-up appointments at 2 weeks, 6 months and then annually for at least 5 years. Patient's compliance to therapy was assessed in each appointment and predictors to treatment abandonment and poor compliance were evaluated.

Results.—The studied population had a mean age of 53.8 years and mean apnoea—hypopnoea index of 52.71/h.

The mean time of follow-up was 5.2 (± 1.6) years, during that time 22 (25%) patients abandoned APAP, those who maintained treatment had good compliance to it since 94% of them used it more than 4 h/day for at least 70% of days.

A significant negative association was found between age, % of days and mean time of APAP use on 12th day and 6th month and the risk of abandoning. APAP use lower than 33% and 57% of days at 12th day and 6th month, respectively had high specificity (~100%) to detect treatment abandonment.

Conclusions.—The majority of patients adheres to long term APAP treatment and has good compliance after 5-years of follow-up. Age and initial compliance (% days of use and mean hour/day) have the ability to predict future adherence, as soon as 12 days and 6 months after initiation.

▶ Although continuous positive airway pressure (CPAP) is first-line therapy for obstructive sleep apnea (OSA), adherence to therapy is difficult for many patients. It is estimated that up to 83% of patients use their CPAP machines less than 4 hours per night for less than 70% of nights.[1] While recognizing the association between OSA and cardiovascular morbidity and mortality, clinicians need to be able to identify early who is going to be nonadherent to therapy and consider alternative treatments for OSA or methods to improve adherence. Recognition should ideally occur before the patient abandons therapy with CPAP and is lost to follow-up.

The authors in this study performed 5-year longitudinal follow-up of 88 men with moderate to severe OSA. Subjects received an autotitrating PAP (APAP) machine and were followed up at regular intervals. Overall, 25% of the study subjects abandoned treatment. The first visit was at 12 days on average, and APAP use lower than 33% at the 12th day had a 100% specificity to detect treatment abandonment. There was also a negative relationship between age and risk of abandonment. Patients who report problems during the first night of APAP use the treatment less than those who do not.[2] If signs of abandonment are seen as early as 12th day, for how long should we continue to ask our patients to keep using PAP before we switch therapies or initiate an intervention strategy to promote adherence? What is the ideal strategy to improve adherence? That answer is not clear.

On a positive note, the treatment adherence in this study was high. Seventy percent of subjects still used PAP at 5 years, with 94% of patients using it for at least 4 hours per night on 70% of nights. Although this study did not find an association between apnea–hypopnea index and abandonment, the study included only patients with moderate to severe OSA. Disease severity has been found to be a weak but consistent factor to CPAP use.[3] For those who abandon therapy, the authors summarize that first impressions seem to last. I would agree with that.

S. F. Jones, MD, FCCP, DABSM

References

1. Weaver TE, Grunstein RR. Adherence to continuous positive airway pressure therapy: the challenge to effective treatment. *Proc Am Thorac Soc.* 2008;5:173-178.
2. Lewis KE, Seale L, Bartle IE, Watkins AJ, Ebden P. Early predictors of CPAP use for the treatment of obstructive sleep apnea. *Sleep.* 2004;27:134-138.
3. Sawyer AM, Gooneratne NS, Marcus CL, Ofer D, Richards KC, Weaver TE. A systematic review of CPAP adherence across age groups: clinical and empiric insights for developing CPAP adherence interventions. *Sleep Med Rev.* 2011;15: 343-356.

Impact of Treatment with Continuous Positive Airway Pressure (CPAP) on Weight in Obstructive Sleep Apnea

Quan SF, Budhiraja R, Clarke DP, et al (Brigham and Women's Hosp and Harvard Med School, Boston, MA; Univ of Arizona, Tucson; et al)

J Clin Sleep Med 9:989-993, 2013

Study Objective.—To determine the impact of continuous positive airway pressure (CPAP) on weight change in persons with obstructive sleep apnea (OSA).

Design, Setting, and Participants.—The Apnea Positive Pressure Long-term Efficacy Study (APPLES) was a 6-month, randomized, double-blinded sham-controlled multicenter clinical trial conducted at 5 sites in the United States. Of 1,105 participants with an apnea hypopnea index ≥ 10 events/hour initially randomized, 812 had body weight measured at baseline and after 6 months of study.

Intervention.—CPAP or Sham CPAP.

Measurements.—Body weight, height, hours of CPAP or Sham CPAP use, Epworth Sleepiness Scale score.

Results.—Participants randomized to CPAP gained 0.35 ± 5.01 kg, whereas those on Sham CPAP lost 0.70 ± 4.03 kg (mean ± SD, $p = 0.001$). Amount of weight gain with CPAP was related to hours of device adherence, with each hour per night of use predicting a 0.42 kg increase in weight. This association was not noted in the Sham CPAP group. CPAP participants who used their device ≥ 4 h per night on ≥ 70% of nights gained the most weight over 6 months in comparison to non-adherent CPAP participants (1.0 ± 5.3 vs. −0.3 ± 5.0 kg, $p = 0.014$).

Conclusions.—OSA patients using CPAP may gain a modest amount of weight with the greatest weight gain found in those most compliant with CPAP (Table 2).

▶ Obesity is one of the most important risk factors for obstructive sleep apnea (OSA). A one—standard deviation increase in the body mass index (BMI) and

TABLE 2.—Change in Weight Over 6 Months Stratified by CPAP Adherence and Treatment Group

Treatment (N)	Timepoint	> 4 Hours and 70% Nights	Hours Adherent	Weight (kg)	Weight Change (kg)
Sham (251)	Baseline	No	2.5 ± 1.7	96.3 ± 21.7[a]	−0.7 ± 4.1
	6 months			95.6 ± 21.7	
CPAP (202)	Baseline	No	3.3 ± 1.7	94.9 ± 20.6[b]	−0.2 ± 5.0
	6 months			94.7 ± 20.5	
Sham (84)	Baseline	Yes	6.3 ± 1.0	94.7 ± 19.9[b]	−0.3 ± 3.1
	6 months			94.5 ± 20.1	
CPAP (170)	Baseline	Yes	6.5 ± 1.1	97.0 ± 25.1[c]	1.0 ± 5.3
	6 months			98.0 ± 25.6	

[a]$p = 0.008$, Baseline vs. 6 months.
[b]$p > 0.05$, Baseline vs. 6 months.
[c]$p = 0.014$, Baseline vs. 6 months.

neck circumference is associated with 4-fold and 5-fold increase in risk of sleep-disordered breathing, respectively.[1] But there is also evidence to support the bidirectionality between obesity and OSA. Furthermore, OSA is associated with symptoms of fatigue and hypersomnia, which can impact the degree to which patients may feel empowered to begin healthy weight loss behaviors. So, theoretically, it would seem that treatment of OSA (and its symptoms) with continuous positive airway pressure (CPAP) would improve or facilitate weight loss. If it were only so easy...

In a retrospective study by Redenius,[2] CPAP use of 4 or more hours for at least 70% of the time was not associated with weight loss. One of the criticisms of the Redenius study is that sleep duration was not monitored. Quan and colleagues draw upon this work in this article. This article is drawn from the research being conducted in the APPLES trial, a well-designed 6-month, randomized, double-blind, sham-controlled, multicenter trial examining neuro-cognitive outcomes in patients with OSA.[3] The authors report a slight weight gain in patients receiving CPAP vs sham (Fig 2 in the original article) with closer review of the data supporting that compliant CPAP users (mean hours of use was 6.5 h/night) experienced greater weight gain than compliant sham users (Table 2). There was no effect modification of the Epworth Sleepiness Score.

How does CPAP adherence promote weight gain? Although it still remains unclear, the answer is likely multifactorial. Perhaps there is greater energy expenditure in patients with untreated OSA owing to the work of breathing, and with CPAP treatment, the energy expenditure lessens. This study specifically does not address the caloric intake between groups. But perhaps consistent calorie intake and decreased energy expenditure in CPAP patients may have led to the observed findings. The authors have a nice discussion in the article. In practice, some patients hope that use of CPAP will facilitate weight loss. Again, it is not that easy. Certainly, CPAP should still be offered as therapy for OSA. We should not deter our patients from its use with this study's findings; however, patients should look to other means of achieving weight loss and not rely on CPAP alone.

S. F. Jones, MD, FCCP, DABSM

References

1. Young T, Palta M, Dempsey J, Skatrud J, Weber S, Badr S. The occurence of sleep disordered breathing among middle aged adults. *N Engl J Med.* 1993;328: 1230-1235.
2. Redenius R, Murphy C, O'Neill E, et al. Does CPAP lead to change in BMI? *J Clin Sleep Med.* 2008 Jun 15;4(3):205-209.
3. Kushida CA, Nichols DA, Quan SF, et al. The Apnea Positive Pressure Long-term Efficacy Study (APPLES): rationale, design, methods, and procedures. *J Clin Sleep Med.* 2006;2:288-300.

Effect of CPAP on Blood Pressure in Patients With Obstructive Sleep Apnea and Resistant Hypertension: The HIPARCO Randomized Clinical Trial
Martínez-García M-A, for the Spanish Sleep Network (Hospital Universitario y Politécnico La Fe, Valencia, Spain)
JAMA 310:2407-2415, 2013

Importance.—More than 70% of patients with resistant hypertension have obstructive sleep apnea (OSA). However, there is little evidence about the effect of continuous positive airway pressure (CPAP) treatment on blood pressure in patients with resistant hypertension.

Objective.—To assess the effect of CPAP treatment on blood pressure values and nocturnal blood pressure patterns in patients with resistant hypertension and OSA.

Design, Setting, and Participants.—Open-label, randomized, multicenter clinical trial of parallel groups with blinded end point design conducted in 24 teaching hospitals in Spain involving 194 patients with resistant hypertension and an apnea-hypopnea index (AHI) of 15 or higher. Data were collected from June 2009 to October 2011.

Interventions.—CPAP or no therapy while maintaining usual blood pressure control medication.

Main Outcomes and Measures.—The primary end point was the change in 24-hour mean blood pressure after 12 weeks. Secondary end points included changes in other blood pressure values and changes in nocturnal blood pressure patterns. Both intention-to-treat (ITT) and per-protocol analyses were performed.

Results.—A total of 194 patients were randomly assigned to receive CPAP (n = 98) or no CPAP (control; n = 96). The mean AHI was 40.4 (SD, 18.9) and an average of 3.8 antihypertensive drugs were taken per patient. Baseline 24-hour mean blood pressure was 103.4 mm Hg; systolic blood pressure (SBP), 144.2 mm Hg; and diastolic blood pressure (DBP), 83 mm Hg. At baseline, 25.8% of patients displayed a dipper pattern (a decrease of at least 10% in the average nighttime blood pressure compared with the average daytime blood pressure). The percentage of patients using CPAP for 4 or more hours per day was 72.4%. When the changes in blood pressure over the study period were compared between groups by ITT, the CPAP group achieved a greater decrease in 24-hour mean blood pressure (3.1 mm Hg [95% CI, 0.6 to 5.6]; $P = .02$) and 24-hour DBP (3.2 mm Hg [95% CI, 1.0 to 5.4]; $P = .005$), but not in 24-hour SBP (3.1 mm Hg [95% CI, −0.6 to 6.7]; $P = .10$) compared with the control group. Moreover, the percentage of patients displaying a nocturnal blood pressure dipper pattern at the 12-week follow-up was greater in the CPAP group than in the control group (35.9% vs 21.6%; adjusted odds ratio [OR], 2.4 [95% CI, 1.2 to 5.1]; $P = .02$). There was a significant positive correlation between hours of CPAP use and the decrease in 24-hour mean blood pressure ($r = 0.29$, $P = .006$), SBP ($r = 0.25$; $P = .02$), and DBP ($r = 0.30$, $P = .005$).

Conclusions and Relevance.—Among patients with OSA and resistant hypertension, CPAP treatment for 12 weeks compared with control resulted in a decrease in 24-hour mean and diastolic blood pressure and an improvement in the nocturnal blood pressure pattern. Further research is warranted to assess longer-term health outcomes.

Trial Registration.—clinicaltrials.gov Identifier: NCT00616265.

▶ Studies indicate modest decreases in blood pressure with continuous positive airway pressure (CPAP) in patients with obstructive sleep apnea. This study is unique in that the population studied had resistant hypertension. The mean number of antihypertensive medications in subjects in this study was 3.8. The study was performed at multiple institutions in Spain, which is an important strength. The authors reported greater reductions in mean 24-hour blood pressure and 24-hour diastolic blood in those receiving CPAP (Fig 2 in the original article). The overall compliance with CPAP in this study was 71% and data supported a correlation between CPAP use and effect on blood pressure. The recovery of the dipper nocturnal blood pressure pattern in the CPAP group plus the decrease in the number of nocturnal risers is important because the phenotypes have increased cardiovascular risk and even modest degrees in reducing blood pressure can improve cardiovascular mortality.

S. F. Jones, MD, FCCP, DABSM

Diagnosis of Sleep-Disordered Breathing

Defining Phenotypic Causes of Obstructive Sleep Apnea: Identification of Novel Therapeutic Targets

Eckert DJ, White DP, Jordan AS, et al (Brigham and Women's Hosp and Harvard Med School, Boston, MA)

Am J Respir Crit Care Med 188:996-1004, 2013

Rationale.—The pathophysiologic causes of obstructive sleep apnea (OSA) likely vary among patients but have not been well characterized.

Objectives.—To define carefully the proportion of key anatomic and nonanatomic contributions in a relatively large cohort of patients with OSA and control subjects to identify pathophysiologic targets for future novel therapies for OSA.

Methods.—Seventy-five men and women with and without OSA aged 20–65 years were studied on three separate nights. Initially, the apnea-hypopnea index was determined by polysomnography followed by determination of anatomic (passive critical closing pressure of the upper airway [Pcrit]) and nonanatomic (genioglossus muscle responsiveness, arousal threshold, and respiratory control stability; loop gain) contributions to OSA.

Measurements and Main Results.—Pathophysiologic traits varied substantially among participants. A total of 36% of patients with OSA had minimal genioglossus muscle responsiveness during sleep, 37% had a low arousal threshold, and 36% had high loop gain. A total of 28% had

TABLE 3.—Pcrit, Arousal Threshold, Loop Gain, and Muscle Responsiveness Scale (the PALM Scale)

PALM Category	Proportion of Patients	Category Cut-Offs	Patient Features	Possible Treatment Targets
1	23%	Pcrit greater than +2 cm H_2O	Highly collapsible upper airway 62% have one or more nonanatomic traits in the vulnerable* range 23% have poor muscle responsiveness 38% have a low arousal threshold 29% have high loop gain 23% have two or more potentially contributing factors All have severe OSA: AHI = 76 (53 −100); range, 31–122 events per hour; REM/non-REM = 0.8[†] BMI = 37 ± 6; range, 28–45 kg/m²; age = 46 ± 11; range, 24–60 y; 8%♀	Major anatomic or mechanical intervention likely required (e.g., CPAP)
2	58%	Pcrit −2 to +2 cm H_2O	Moderately collapsible upper airway Overall severe OSA: AHI = 32 (19 −55); wide range, 10–112 events per hour; REM/non-NREM = 1.2[†] BMI = 35 ± 6; range, 23–46 kg/m²; age = 47 ± 11; range, 20–65 y; 33%♀	Candidate for one or a combination of targeted therapies
2a	36%	Pcrit −2 to +2 cm H_2O without nonanatomic vulnerability	Moderately collapsible upper airway; primarily anatomically driven None have nonanatomic traits in the vulnerable* range	Anatomic intervention (e.g., CPAP, mandibular advancement splint, upper airway surgery, positional therapy, or weight loss)
2b	64%	Pcrit −2 to +2 cm H_2O with nonanatomic vulnerability	Moderately collapsible upper airway and 100% have one or more nonanatomic traits in the vulnerable* range 52% have poor muscle responsiveness 48% have a low arousal threshold 50% have high loop gain 33% have two or more potentially contributing factors	A combination of anatomic and nonanatomic interventions is likely required (e.g., mandibular advancement splint or weight loss plus oxygen or a sleep consolidation aid)

(Continued)

TABLE 3.—(*Continued*)

PALM Category	Proportion of Patients	Category Cut-Offs	Patient Features	Possible Treatment Targets
3	19%	Pcrit less than -2 cm H_2O	Some vulnerability to upper airway collapse 100% have one or more nonanatomic traits in the vulnerable* range 55% have poor muscle responsiveness 45% have a low arousal threshold 70% have high loop gain 55% have two or more potentially contributing factors Overall mild-moderate OSA: AHI = 19 (13–37); range, 11–59 events per hour; REM/non-REM = = 3.3[†] BMI = 34 ± 5; range, 26–42 kg/m²; age = 47 ± 12; range, 26–64 y; 27%♀	Candidate for one or a combination of targeted therapies with an increased likelihood that nonanatomic interventions (e.g., oxygen or a sleep consolidation aid) would be beneficial in these patients

Definition of abbreviations: AHI = apnea-hypopnea index; BMI = body mass index; CPAP = continuous positive airway pressure; OSA = obstructive sleep apnea; Pcrit = pharyngeal critical closing pressure.

*Definitions of "vulnerable" for nonanatomic traits: poor muscle responsiveness; greater than -0.1% maximum genioglossus electromyographic activity/–cm H_2O epiglottic pressure, low arousal threshold; greater than -15 cm H_2O, and high loop gain; less than -5 dimensionless. Refer to the text for further detail.

[†]REM/non-REM AHI ratio was only calculated in patients who had greater than 30 minutes of REM sleep during their diagnostic study (64% of PALM category 1, 58% of PALM category 2, and 46% of PALM category 3 patients).

multiple nonanatomic features. Although overall the upper airway was more collapsible in patients with OSA (Pcrit, 0.3 [−1.5 to 1.9] vs.−6.2 [−12.4 to −3.6] cm H_2O; $P < 0.01$), 19% had a relatively noncollapsible upper airway similar to many of the control subjects (Pcrit, −2 to −5 cm H_2O). In these patients, loop gain was almost twice as high as patients with a Pcrit greater than −2 cm H_2O (−5.9 [−8.8 to −4.5] vs. −3.2 [−4.8 to −2.4] dimensionless; $P = 0.01$). A three-point scale for weighting the relative contribution of the traits is proposed. It suggests that nonanatomic features play an important role in 56% of patients with OSA.

Conclusions.—This study confirms that OSA is a heterogeneous disorder. Although Pcrit-anatomy is an important determinant, abnormalities in nonanatomic traits are also present in most patients with OSA (Table 3).

▶ I think this is a great article! This article has brought together the multiple pathophysiologic factors in obstructive sleep apnea (OSA). For a while we have known about the importance of the critical closing pressure of the upper airway, the ventilatory responsiveness or loop gain, the respiratory arousal threshold, and the responsiveness of the pharyngeal dilators. However, Eckert and colleagues have collectively measured those variables in patients with and without OSA. With that comes the idea of discrete phenotypic causes of OSA. I feel that many of us have been searching for understanding of reasons for sleep-disordered breathing and feel that the treatments target predominantly anatomic factors (eg, continuous positive airway pressure, oral appliances). How we integrate other factors such as loop gain, arousal threshold, and muscle responsiveness into the management of the individual instead of the disease is a real step in the right direction. The authors introduce the Pcrit, Arousal Threshold, Loop Gain, and Muscle Responsiveness (PALM) scale (Table 3) and describe important differences between those with and without OSA and how therapeutic targets might differ among categories. This is such a new and refreshing way of thinking about OSA, its pathophysiology, and its management. Although certainly additional testing and research are needed, the idea of the PALM scale could facilitate research of treatment targeting such phenotypes.

S. F. Jones, MD, FCCP, DABSM

Non-CPAP Treatment of Sleep-Disordered Breathing

Novel and Emerging Nonpositive Airway Pressure Therapies for Sleep Apnea

Park JG, Morgenthaler TM, Gay PC (Mayo Clinic College of Medicine, Rochester, MN)
Chest 144:1946-1952, 2013

CPAP therapy has remained the standard of care for the treatment of sleep apnea for nearly 4 decades. Its overall effectiveness, however, has been limited by incomplete adherence despite many efforts to improve comfort. Conventional alternative therapies include oral appliances and upper airway surgeries. Recently, several innovative alternatives to CPAP have been developed. These novel approaches include means to increase arousal thresholds, electrical nerve stimulation, oral vacuum devices, and nasal expiratory resistive devices. We will review the physiologic mechanisms and the current evidence for these novel treatments.

▶ Sleep-disordered breathing is characterized by repetitive narrowing of the upper airway during sleep.[1] The illness is associated with increased all-cause mortality and cardiovascular-related mortality compared with those without sleep-disordered breathing.[2] Although continuous positive airway pressure (CPAP) is a first-line treatment for sleep-disordered breathing, compliance is less than optimal with nearly half of patients intolerant to CPAP.[3] New treatments, particularly those that do not involve positive airway pressure, are needed. In this review article, the authors nicely summarize the literature on nasal expiratory positive airway pressure (Provent; Ventus Medical inc). The available literature supports modest improvements in apnea–hypopnea index (AHI), but the method probably should be reserved for those with mild obstructive sleep apnea or those intolerant of CPAP.[4] The device's ability to reduce AHI by at least 50% in less than half of study subjects combined with its intolerance in another study[5] restricts its overall use. It is currently available on the market.

Another therapy currently still under testing and not yet approved for clinical use is the hypoglossal nerve stimulator. The literature on this device shows greater degrees of improvement in the AHI. Expect to hear more about this device in the near future. Because it is an implantable device, data on cost and maintenance follow-up are needed. Furthermore, health-related outcome data such as effect on cardiovascular endpoints are not available on any of the devices mentioned.

S. F. Jones, MD, FCCP, DABSM

References

1. Young T, Palta M, Dempsey J, Skatrud J, Weber S, Badr S. The occurrence of sleep-disordered breathing among middle-aged adults. *N Engl J Med.* 1993;328:1230-1235.
2. Young T, Finn L, Peppard PE, et al. Sleep disordered breathing and mortality: eighteen-year follow-up of the Wisconsin sleep cohort. *Sleep.* 2008;31:1071-1078.
3. Kribbs NB, Pack AI, Kline LR, et al. Objective measurement of patterns of nasal CPAP use by patients with obstructive sleep apnea. *Am Rev Respir Dis.* 1993;147:887-895.
4. Colrain IM, Brooks S, Black J. A pilot evaluation of a nasal expiratory resistance device for the treatment of obstructive sleep apnea. *J Clin Sleep Med.* 2008;4:426-433.
5. Kryger MH, Berry RB, Massie CA. Long-term use of a nasal expiratory positive airway pressure (EPAP) device as a treatment for obstructive sleep apnea (OSA). *J Clin Sleep Med.* 2011;7:449-453.

Health Outcomes of Continuous Positive Airway Pressure versus Oral Appliance Treatment for Obstructive Sleep Apnea: A Randomized Controlled Trial

Phillips CL, Grunstein RR, Darendeliler MA, et al (Royal North Shore Hosp, St. Leonards, Australia; Woolcock Inst of Med Res, New South Wales, Australia; Univ of Sydney, Australia)
Am J Respir Crit Care Med 187:879-887, 2013

Rationale.—Continuous positive airway pressure (CPAP) and mandibular advancement device (MAD) therapy are commonly used to treat obstructive sleep apnea (OSA). Differences in efficacy and compliance of these treatments are likely to influence improvements in health outcomes.

Objectives.—To compare health effects after 1 month of optimal CPAP and MAD therapy in OSA.

Methods.—In this randomized crossover trial, we compared the effects of 1 month each of CPAP and MAD treatment on cardiovascular and neurobehavioral outcomes.

Measurements and Main Results.—Cardiovascular (24-h blood pressure, arterial stiffness), neurobehavioral (subjective sleepiness, driving simulator performance), and quality of life (Functional Outcomes of Sleep Questionnaire, Short Form-36) were compared between treatments. Our primary outcome was 24-hour mean arterial pressure. A total of 126 patients with moderate-severe OSA (apnea hypopnea index [AHI], 25.6 [SD 12.3]) were randomly assigned to a treatment order and 108 completed the trial with both devices. CPAP was more efficacious than MAD in reducing AHI (CPAP AHI, 4.5 ± 6.6/h; MAD AHI, 11.1 ± 12.1/h; $P < 0.01$) but reported compliance was higher on MAD (MAD, 6.50 ± 1.3 h per night vs. CPAP, 5.20 ± 2 h per night; $P < 0.00001$). The 24-hour mean arterial pressure was not inferior on treatment with MAD compared with CPAP (CPAP-MAD difference, 0.2 mm Hg [95% confidence interval, -0.7 to 1.1]); however, overall, neither treatment improved blood pressure. In contrast, sleepiness, driving simulator performance, and disease-specific quality of life improved on both treatments by similar amounts, although MAD was superior to CPAP for improving four general quality-of-life domains.

Conclusions.—Important health outcomes were similar after 1 month of optimal MAD and CPAP treatment in patients with moderate-severe OSA. The results may be explained by greater efficacy of CPAP being offset by inferior compliance relative to MAD, resulting in similar effectiveness. Clinical trial registered with https://www.anzctr.org.au (ACTRN 12607000289415).

▶ Treatment of obstructive sleep apnea (OSA) with continuous positive airway pressure (CPAP) has been shown to produce a number of clinical benefits. However, despite the obvious benefits, adherence to CPAP is less than optimal in practice. This leaves a great number of patients either with no treatment or partial treatment. Oral appliances have been used primarily in patients with mild to moderate OSA, and, when compared with CPAP, patients prefer oral appliance. But does oral appliance produce the same clinical benefits to blood pressure, quality of life, and sleepiness as CPAP? This report is important in that it is the largest study of its kind and was well designed. The authors included patients with severe OSA (34% of the population in this study), a group that is often excluded in studies involving oral appliances. The authors report similar health outcomes after 1 month of treatment with oral appliance and CPAP. This was a noninferiority trial. Further interesting aspects lie in the details of the study. Although the primary outcome of the difference in the 24-hour mean arterial pressure showed no difference between groups, the presence of comorbid hypertension was not an inclusion criteria in this trial, so the effect on blood pressure overall in the study was not significant between groups. As other studies have shown, oral appliance does not reduce the apnea hypopnea index (AHI) as well as CPAP. Despite this difference, this appears to have no effect on the subjective measures of sleepiness, quality of life, and driving simulation. Just how much residual AHI remains in patients treated with oral appliance? Fig 2 in the original article indicates that in almost 40% of patients, oral appliance was deemed a treatment failure defined as AHI not lowered by at least 50% of baseline AHI. The graph of the overall treatment in Fig 2 of the original article supports that many of the subjects had AHI between 20 and 60 on oral appliance. I think that is too much residual apnea, and, in practice, I would prefer that my patient use CPAP if that is the case.

Although the authors argue that because of the results in this study, we should offer oral appliance to patients with severe OSA, I am not sure that I agree with that entirely. There are no reliable indicators of who responds to oral appliance. Furthermore, compliance cannot be monitored reliably, and we have to rely mainly on subjective compliance (as in this study). While I am sure that the technology will advance in the near future to measure compliance with oral appliance, it is not here yet. Until these conditions are met, I think more research is needed before we can offer oral appliance as standard therapy for severe OSA in my opinion, but this article definitely encompasses the spirit of comparative effectiveness research.

S. F. Jones, MD, FCCP, DABSM

Oral Appliance Versus Continuous Positive Airway Pressure in Obstructive Sleep Apnea Syndrome: A 2-Year Follow-up
Doff MHJ, Hoekema A, Wijkstra PJ, et al (Univ of Groningen, The Netherlands)
Sleep 36:1289-1296, 2013

Study Objectives.—Oral appliance therapy has emerged as an important alternative to continuous positive airway pressure (CPAP) in treating patients with obstructive sleep apnea syndrome (OSAS). In this study we report about the subjective and objective treatment outcome of oral appliance therapy and CPAP in patients with OSAS.

Design.—Cohort study of a previously conducted randomized clinical trial.

Setting.—University Medical Center, Groningen, The Netherlands.

Patients or Participants.—One hundred three patients with OSAS.

Interventions.—CPAP and oral appliance therapy (Thornton Adjustable Positioner type-1, Airway Management, Inc., Dallas, TX, USA).

Measurements and Results.—Objective (polysomnography) and subjective (Epworth Sleepiness Scale, Functional Outcomes of Sleep Questionnaire, Medical Outcomes Study 36-item Short Form Health Survey [SF-36]) parameters were assessed after 1 and 2 years of treatment. Treatment was considered successful when the apnea-hypopnea index (AHI) was < 5 or showed substantial reduction, defined as reduction in the index of at least 50% from the baseline value to a value of < 20 in a patient without OSAS symptoms while undergoing therapy. Regarding the proportions of successful treatments, no significant difference was found between oral appliance therapy and CPAP in treating mild to severe OSAS in a 2-year follow-up. More patients (not significant) dropped out under oral appliance therapy (47%) compared with CPAP (33%). Both therapies showed substantial improvements in polysomnographic and neurobehavioral outcomes. However, CPAP was more effective in lowering the AHI and showed higher oxyhemoglobin saturation levels compared to oral appliance therapy ($P < 0.05$).

Conclusions.—Oral appliance therapy should be considered as a viable treatment alternative to continuous positive airway pressure (CPAP) in patients with mild to moderate obstructive sleep apnea syndrome (OSAS). In patients with severe OSAS, CPAP remains the treatment of first choice.

Clinical Trial Information.—The original randomized clinical trial, of which this study is a 2-year follow-up, is registered at ISRCTN.org; identifier: ISRCTN18174167; trial name: Management of the obstructive sleep apnea-hypopnea syndrome: oral appliance versus continuous positive airway pressure therapy; URL: http://www.controlled-trials.com/ISRCTN18174167.

▶ According to the practice parameters published by the American Academy of Sleep Medicine, oral appliances (OAs) are indicated for use in patients with mild to moderate obstructive sleep apnea (OSA) who prefer OAs to continuous positive airway pressure (CPAP) or who do not respond to CPAP, are not appropriate candidates for CPAP, or who fail treatment attempts with CPAP.[1] The findings in this study support those recommendations. There are, however, findings in the Doff study that are worth mentioning. In this study, Doff et al included patients with severe OSA (approximately 50% of subjects). Recall that the guideline issued by the American Academy of Sleep Medicine did not include patients with severe OSA. Treatment was considered successful if the apnea-hypopnea index (AHI) improved to less than 5 events per hour or reduced by at least 50% from the baseline to a value of less than 20 in patients with OSA but without symptoms. As a whole, OAs were just as successful as CPAP in achieving the primary and secondary outcomes of proportion of successful treatments at different time points and neurobehavioral outcomes, respectively. Success was achieved in 52.9% of subjects receiving OAs and in 67.3% of subjects receiving CPAP as a whole. These rates were not significant.

When examining the subgroup of severe OSA, success was achieved in half of those receiving OAs, but in nearly 75% of those receiving CPAP. Although CPAP may be a better option compared with OA for those with severe OSA, it is notable that OA is still a viable option with success half of the time. Furthermore, other studies support that OAs are a preferred option compared with CPAP.[2] It is interesting to note that in the Doff study, there were more dropouts in the group initially randomly selected to receive OAs, perhaps reflective of the deteriorating success rates in the OA group or that the AHI was significantly lower in the CPAP group compared with OA after 1 and 2 years (Fig 2 in the original article). I think what we can glean from this study is that OA is a viable option for our patients, but careful attention should be paid with follow-up polysomnography with the OA in place to ensure that the AHI has improved and to follow-up with dental and sleep medicine specialists. Research into monitoring compliance with OAs should become mainstream in the future as is the current practice with CPAP.

S. F. Jones, MD, FCCP, DABSM

References

1. Kushida CA, Morgenthaler TI, Littner MR, et al. Practice parameters for the treatment of snoring and obstructive sleep apnea with oral appliances: an update for 2005. *Sleep.* 2006;29:240-243.
2. Barnes M, McEvoy RD, Banks S, et al. Efficacy of positive airway pressure and oral appliance in mild to moderate obstructive sleep apnea. *Am J Respir Crit Care Med.* 2004;170:656-664.

Effectiveness of Lifestyle Interventions on Obstructive Sleep Apnea (OSA): Systematic Review and Meta-Analysis

Araghi MH, Chen Y-F, Jagielski A, et al (Univ of Birmingham, UK; et al)
Sleep 36:1553-1562, 2013

Background.—Obstructive sleep apnea (OSA) is a common sleep disorder associated with several adverse health outcomes. Given the close association between OSA and obesity, lifestyle and dietary interventions are commonly recommended to patients, but the evidence for their impact on OSA has not been systematically examined.

Objectives.—To conduct a systematic review and meta-analysis to assess the impact of weight loss through diet and physical activity on measures of OSA: apnea-hypopnea index (AHI) and oxygen desaturation index of 4% (ODI4).

Methods.—A systematic search was performed to identify publications using Medline (1948-2011 week 40), EMBASE (from 1988-2011 week 40), and CINAHL (from 1982-2011 week 40). The inverse variance method was used to weight studies and the random effects model was used to analyze data.

Results.—Seven randomized controlled trials (519 participants) showed that weight reduction programs were associated with a decrease in AHI

(−6.04 events/h [95% confidence interval −11.18, −0.90]) with substantial heterogeneity between studies ($I^2 = 86\%$). Nine uncontrolled before-after studies (250 participants) showed a significant decrease in AHI (−12.26 events/h [95% confidence interval −18.51, −6.02]). Four uncontrolled before-after studies (97 participants) with ODI4 as outcome also showed a significant decrease in ODI4 (−18.91 episodes/h [95% confidence interval −23.40, −14.43]).

Conclusions.—Published evidence suggests that weight loss through lifestyle and dietary interventions results in improvements in obstructive sleep apnea parameters, but is insufficient to normalize them. The changes in obstructive sleep apnea parameters could, however, be clinically relevant in some patients by reducing obstructive sleep apnea severity. These promising preliminary results need confirmation through larger randomized studies including more intensive weight loss approaches.

▶ Weight loss is routinely recommended in addition to continuous positive airway pressure (CPAP) in obese patients with obstructive sleep apnea (OSA). This article aimed to evaluate the effectiveness of lifestyle interventions (further classified into diet, exercise, or diet and exercise subcategories) on apnea hypopnea index (AHI) and oxygen desaturation index (ODI). It is important to recognize that there was substantial heterogeneity between studies, but a modest reduction in AHI can be achieved with weight loss. Of the studies that measured ODI, weight loss had greater impact on ODI. Exercise alone seemed to have the least impact on OSA. The analysis included a total of 21 articles and 893 patients, a small number overall with durations of study periods from as little as 4 weeks to as long as 24 weeks. The authors performed a metaregression analysis showing that the greatest weight loss is associated with the greatest improvements in AHI (Fig 8 in the original article). This is also supported by the surgical weight loss literature with the great reductions in body mass index associated with the greatest reductions in the AHI.[1] It is important to note the lack of neurobehavioral endpoints in the studies examined. Very few studies included measures of sleepiness or symptoms. These should be included in future studies.

This article supports that lifestyle intervention alone cannot be expected to normalize or cure OSA. Furthermore, because we know that many of our patients regain weight that is lost, follow-up is emphasized. Despite the arduous task of reviewing the literature and its analysis, we still do not know which specific lifestyle intervention we should recommend to our patients, how to implement them, or the best method of delivery. It is likely that an individualized approach is needed with close attention to follow-up.

S. F. Jones, MD, FCCP, DABSM

Reference

1. Greenburg DL, Lettieri CJ, Eliasson AH. Effects of surgical weight loss on measures of obstructive sleep apnea: a meta-analysis. *Am J Med.* 2009;122:535-542.

Non-Pulmonary Sleep

Effects of Experimental Sleep Restriction on Caloric Intake and Activity Energy Expenditure

Calvin AD, Carter RE, Adachi T, et al (Mayo Clinic, Rochester, MN; Showa Univ, Tokyo, Japan; et al)

Chest 144:79-86, 2013

Background.—Epidemiologic studies link short sleep duration to obesity and weight gain. Insufficient sleep appears to alter circulating levels of the hormones leptin and ghrelin, which may promote appetite, although the effects of sleep restriction on caloric intake and energy expenditure are unclear. We sought to determine the effect of 8 days/8 nights of sleep restriction on caloric intake, activity energy expenditure, and circulating levels of leptin and ghrelin.

Methods.—We conducted a randomized study of usual sleep vs a sleep restriction of two-thirds of normal sleep time for 8 days/8 nights in a hospital-based clinical research unit. The main outcomes were caloric intake, activity energy expenditure, and circulating levels of leptin and ghrelin.

Results.—Caloric intake in the sleep-restricted group increased by +559 kcal/d (SD, 706 kcal/d, $P = .006$) and decreased in the control group by −118 kcal/d (SD, 386 kcal/d, $P = .51$) for a net change of +677 kcal/d (95% CI, 148-1, 206 kcal/d; $P = .014$). Sleep restriction was not associated with changes in activity energy expenditure ($P = .62$). No change was seen in levels of leptin ($P = .27$) or ghrelin ($P = .21$).

Conclusions.—Sleep restriction was associated with an increase in caloric consumption with no change in activity energy expenditure or leptin and ghrelin concentrations. Increased caloric intake without any accompanying increase in energy expenditure may contribute to obesity in people who are exposed to long-term sleep restriction.

▶ Obesity is a challenge Americans continue to face. The growing (no pun intended) numbers of patients, particularly youth, with obesity and obesity-related diseases is astonishing. I frequently see patients who have insufficient sleep times for different reasons (eg, shift work) who report weight gain. Hence, this article is quite timely in this regard. There is increasing interest in changes in hormones, like leptin and ghrelin, and their responses to sleep deprivation. This topic is important, because a pathway identified could lead to targeted therapies at a hormonal or even molecular level to lose weight (or prevent weight gain).

Although this study was conducted in young healthy patients, it gives important insight in to understanding the impact of sleep restriction on calorie intake. Without any change in the energy expenditure, a 500-kcal/d increase could lead to a weight gain of one pound per week! It is interesting the lack of any change in ghrelin or leptin levels in this study. As obesity continues to become a public problem, expect to see additional studies in this area.

S. F. Jones, MD, FCCP, DABSM

Self-reported Sleep and β-Amyloid Deposition in Community-Dwelling Older Adults

Spira AP, Gamaldo AA, An Y, et al (The Johns Hopkins Bloomberg School of Public Health, Baltimore, MD; Natl Insts of Health, Baltimore, MD; et al)
JAMA Neurol 70:1537-1543, 2013

Importance.—Older adults commonly report disturbed sleep, and recent studies in humans and animals suggest links between sleep and Alzheimer disease biomarkers. Studies are needed that evaluate whether sleep variables are associated with neuroimaging evidence of β-amyloid (Aβ) deposition.

Objective.—To determine the association between self-reported sleep variables and Aβ deposition in community-dwelling older adults.

Design, Setting, and Participants.—Cross-sectional study of 70 adults (mean age, 76 [range, 53-91] years) from the neuroimaging substudy of the Baltimore Longitudinal Study of Aging, a normative aging study.

Exposure.—Self-reported sleep variables.

Main Outcomes and Measures.—β-Amyloid burden, measured by carbon 11-labeled Pittsburgh compound B positron emission tomography distribution volume ratios (DVRs).

Results.—After adjustment for potential confounders, reports of shorter sleep duration were associated with greater Aβ burden, measured by mean cortical DVR (B = 0.08 [95% CI, 0.03-0.14]; $P = .005$) and precuneus DVR (B = 0.11 [0.03-0.18]; $P = .007$). Reports of lower sleep quality were associated with greater Aβ burden measured by precuneus DVR (B = 0.08 [0.01-0.15]; $P = .03$).

Conclusions and Relevance.—Among community-dwelling older adults, reports of shorter sleep duration and poorer sleep quality are associated with greater Aβ burden. Additional studies with objective sleep measures are needed to determine whether sleep disturbance causes or accelerates Alzheimer disease.

▶ It is known that patients with Alzheimer disease suffer from poor sleep and frequent awakenings, but this study is unique in that authors report an increase in the amount of β-amyloid plaques in patients who reported short sleep duration. The population studied includes community-dwelling older patients. Even after exclusion of subjects with mild cognitive impairment and dementia, a signal still was observed between sleep duration β-amyloid plaque burden. Could short sleep duration predispose or increase one's risk of Alzheimer disease development? We don't know. The study's cross-sectional design does not allow one to assess for cause and effect. I expect to see more research in this area. Longitudinal follow-up of subjects is needed to determine if poor sleep duration precedes the development of plaque burden and symptoms of disease. Although it will be a while from now, if these findings are replicated and poor sleep is a precursor to Alzheimer disease, interventional studies examining effects of increasing sleep on disease progression would be expected.

S. F. Jones, MD, FCCP, DABSM

Pediatric Sleep-Disordered Breathing

Morbidity and mortality in children with obstructive sleep apnoea: a controlled national study

Jennum P, Ibsen R, Kjellberg J (Danish Ctr for Sleep Medicine, Glostrup, Denmark; Itracks, Aarhus, Denmark; Danish Inst for Local and Regional Government Res, Copenhagen, Denmark)
Thorax 68:949-954, 2013

Background.—Little is known about the diagnostic patterns of obstructive sleep apnoea (OSA) in children. A study was undertaken to evaluate morbidity and mortality in childhood OSA.

Methods.—2998 patients aged 0–19 years with a diagnosis of OSA were identified from the Danish National Patient Registry. For each patient we randomly selected four citizens matched for age, sex and socioeconomic status, thus providing 11 974 controls.

Results.—Patients with OSA had greater morbidity at least 3 years before their diagnosis. The most common contacts with the health system arose from infections (OR 1.19, 95% CI 1.01 to 1.40); endocrine, nutritional and metabolic diseases (OR 1.30, 95% CI 0.94 to 1.80); nervous conditions (OR 2.12, 95% CI 1.65 to 2.73); eye conditions (OR 1.43, 95% CI 1.07 to 1.90); ear, nose and throat (ENT) diseases (OR 1.61, 95% CI 1.33 to 1.94); respiratory system diseases (OR 1.78, 95% CI 1.60 to 1.98); gastrointestinal diseases (OR 1.34, 95% CI 1.09 to 1.66); skin conditions (OR 1.32, 95% CI 1.02 to 1.71); congenital malformations (OR 1.56, 95% CI 1.31 to 1.85); abnormal clinical or laboratory findings (OR 1.21, 95% CI 1.06 to 1.39); and other factors influencing health status (OR 1.29, 95% CI 1.16 to 1.43). After diagnosis, OSA was associated with incidences of endocrine, nutritional and metabolic diseases (OR 1.78, 95% CI 1.29 to 2.45), nervous conditions (OR 3.16, 95% CI 2.58 to 3.89), ENT diseases (OR 1.45, 95% CI 1.14 to 1.84), respiratory system diseases (OR 1.94, 95% CI 1.70 to 2.22), skin conditions (OR 1.42, 95% CI 1.06 to 1.89), musculoskeletal diseases (OR 1.29, 95% CI 1.01 to 1.64), congenital malformations (OR 1.83, 95% CI 1.51 to 2.22), abnormal clinical or laboratory findings (OR 1.16, 95% CI 1.06 to 1.27) and other factors influencing health status (OR 1.35, 95% CI 1.20 to 1.51). The 5-year death rate was 70 per 10 000 for patients and 11 per 10 000 for controls. The HR for cases compared with controls was 6.58 (95% CI 3.39 to 12.79; $p < 0.001$).

Conclusions.—Children with OSA have significant morbidities several years before and after their diagnosis.

▶ The authors used the Danish National Patient registry to report on an increase in morbidity for 3 years before the diagnosis of obstructive sleep apnea (OSA). This is not too surprising because an evaluation for another disease like attention deficit disorder or recurrent pharyngitis prompts consideration for OSA. However, there are certain disease-related groups that are associated with OSA in children in this study that are less understood: gastro-intestinal and musculoskeletal disease. Cause and effect cannot be delineated from this study.

After diagnosis of OSA, there are still high rates of comorbid diseases and, even more alarming, a higher rate of death in children with OSA compared with controls. Although we cannot estimate the death attributed to OSA in this study, it does lead one to consider a few points. Because childhood OSA is often underdiagnosed, are the numbers of comorbid diseases and deaths actually higher? Would the rates of comorbid diseases remain increased, and to what degree in the subset who received treatment (adenotonsillectomy)?

S. F. Jones, MD, FCCP, DABSM

A Randomized Trial of Adenotonsillectomy for Childhood Sleep Apnea
Marcus CL, for the Childhood Adenotonsillectomy Trial (CHAT) (Univ of Pennsylvania, Philadelphia; et al)
N Engl J Med 368:2366-2376, 2013

Background.—Adenotonsillectomy is commonly performed in children with the obstructive sleep apnea syndrome, yet its usefulness in reducing symptoms and improving cognition, behavior, quality of life, and poly-somnographic findings has not been rigorously evaluated. We hypothe-sized that, in children with the obstructive sleep apnea syndrome without prolonged oxyhemoglobin desaturation, early adenotonsillec-tomy, as compared with watchful waiting with supportive care, would result in improved outcomes.

Methods.—We randomly assigned 464 children, 5 to 9 years of age, with the obstructive sleep apnea syndrome to early adenotonsillectomy or a strategy of watchful waiting. Polysomnographic, cognitive, behavio-ral, and health outcomes were assessed at baseline and at 7 months.

Results.—The average baseline value for the primary outcome, the atten-tion and executive-function score on the Developmental Neuropsychologi-cal Assessment (with scores ranging from 50 to 150 and higher scores indicating better functioning), was close to the population mean of 100, and the change from baseline to follow-up did not differ significantly according to study group (mean [±SD] improvement, 7.1 ± 13.9 in the early-adenotonsillectomy group and 5.1 ± 13.4 in the watchful-waiting group; $P = 0.16$). In contrast, there were significantly greater improvements in behavioral, quality-of-life, and polysomnographic findings and signifi-cantly greater reduction in symptoms in the early-adenotonsillectomy group than in the watchful-waiting group. Normalization of polysomno-graphic findings was observed in a larger proportion of children in the early-adenotonsillectomy group than in the watchful-waiting group (79% vs. 46%).

Conclusions.—As compared with a strategy of watchful waiting, surgical treatment for the obstructive sleep apnea syndrome in school-age children did not significantly improve attention or executive function as measured by neuropsychological testing but did reduce symptoms and improve secondary outcomes of behavior, quality of life, and polysomnographic findings, thus providing evidence of beneficial effects of early adenotonsillectomy. (Funded by the National Institutes of Health; CHAT ClinicalTrials.gov number, NCT00560859.)

▶ When behavioral problems are noted, concerned parents, teachers, and health care professionals evaluate whether the child has childhood obstructive sleep apnea syndrome, particularly when tonsillar enlargement is noted on the examination and a history of snoring is elicited. When obstructive sleep apnea is diagnosed, clinicians are faced with considering treatment with adenotonsillectomy. This study is important in that it examines a large cohort of children 5 to 9 years of age (the age at which tonsillectomy is considered probably most efficacious) with apnea–hypopnea index (AHI) of 2 or more without oxyhemoglobin desaturation. This study examined the natural history of polysomnographic outcomes over a 7-month period with watchful waiting vs the effect of early adenotonsillectomy but also, and importantly, cognitive and behavioral outcomes measured by psychometrist, parents, and teachers. Although the authors found no difference in attention and executive function score, greater behavioral improvement and symptoms of obstructive sleep apnea noted by parents and teachers were observed in those receiving early adenotonsillectomy. Although technically this is a negative study because the primary outcome was the measurement of attention and executive functioning by psychometrist evaluation, I think it does have clinical relevance. How a child behaves at home and at school (real life settings) are what drive the evaluation for childhood obstructive sleep apnea in many cases. Benefits in these outcomes are important clinically. The fact is that children who received early adenotonsillectomy had moderate to large improvements in these components plus the improvements in polysomnography that indicate fewer arousals, improved AHI, and lighter stages of sleep.

The complication rate was low with early adenotonsillectomy. It is important to note that watchful waiting is still a reasonable option, particularly because spontaneous regression of polysomnographic outcomes occurred in nearly 40%. But follow-up is emphasized, and adenotonsillectomy should be reconsidered if improvements are not observed within a reasonable timeframe.

S. F. Jones, MD, FCCP, DABSM

8 Critical Care Medicine

Introduction

This has been another great year of reading in Critical Care. Included are some wonderful state-of-the-art articles ranging from ARDS to VAP to COPD. In addition, there is an excellent article on use of ECMO. I encourage you to read each and every excellent article. All apply to those of us who are actively practicing Pulmonary/Critical Care.

James A. Barker, MD, CPE, FACP, FCCP, FAASM

Acute Respiratory Disorder Syndrome

Acute Respiratory Distress Syndrome After Spontaneous Intracerebral Hemorrhage
Elmer J, Hou P, Wilcox SR, et al (Univ of Pittsburgh Med Ctr, PA; Brigham and Women's Hosp, Boston, MA; Harvard Med School, Boston, MA; et al)
Crit Care Med 41:1992-2001, 2013

Objectives.—Acute respiratory distress syndrome develops commonly in critically ill patients in response to an injurious stimulus. The prevalence and risk factors for development of acute respiratory distress syndrome after spontaneous intracerebral hemorrhage have not been reported. We sought to determine the prevalence of acute respiratory distress syndrome after intracerebral hemorrhage, characterize risk factors for its development, and assess its impact on patient outcomes.

Design.—Retrospective cohort study at two academic centers.

Patients.—We included consecutive patients presenting from June 1, 2000, to November 1, 2010, with intracerebral hemorrhage requiring mechanical ventilation. We excluded patients with age less than 18 years, intracerebral hemorrhage secondary to trauma, tumor, ischemic stroke, or structural lesion; if they required intubation only during surgery; if they were admitted for comfort measures; or for a history of immunodeficiency.

Interventions.—None.

Measurements and Main Results.—Data were collected both prospectively as part of an ongoing cohort study and by retrospective chart review.

Of 1,665 patients identified by database query, 697 met inclusion criteria. The prevalence of acute respiratory distress syndrome was 27%. In unadjusted analysis, high tidal volume ventilation was associated with an increased risk of acute respiratory distress syndrome (hazard ratio, 1.79 [95% CI, 1.13–2.83]), as were male sex, RBC and plasma transfusion, higher fluid balance, obesity, hypoxemia, acidosis, tobacco use, emergent hematoma evacuation, and vasopressor dependence. In multivariable modeling, high tidal volume ventilation was the strongest risk factor for acute respiratory distress syndrome development (hazard ratio, 1.74 [95% CI, 1.08–2.81]) and for inhospital mortality (hazard ratio, 2.52 [95% CI, 1.46–4.34]).

Conclusions.—Development of acute respiratory distress syndrome is common after intubation for intracerebral hemorrhage. Modifiable risk factors, including high tidal volume ventilation, are associated with its development and in-patient mortality (Table 2).

▶ Neurogenic pulmonary edema is a relatively common form of noncardiogenic pulmonary edema. How often it progresses to acute respiratory distress syndrome (ARDS) has been heretofore unknown. Similarly, it has long been known that a significant number of patients with subarachnoid hemorrhage or intracerebral hemorrhage will develop ARDS, yet the precise incidence and risk factors have not been well elucidated before this study.

Twenty-seven percent, or roughly one-quarter of these patients, developed ARDS. And clearly that combination was associated with worse mortality. I was also surprised at the prevalence of male vs female patients. Likewise, the inverse relationship to age surprised me. Not discussed here but probably important is whether triple H therapy was done (hypervolemia, hypertension, hypernatremia), as this has also been previously associated with an increased ARDS rate in neurologically injured patients.

As in many other pathologic states associated with ARDS, these patients likely do have capillary leak phenomenon. This probably helps explain the high correlation with high tidal volume ventilation (eg, volutrauma is worse

TABLE 2.—Multivariable Model of Risk Factors for Development of Acute Respiratory Distress Syndrome

Characteristic	Multivariable Hazard Ratio	P
Tidal volume >8 mL/kg	1.74 (1.08–2.81)	0.02
Male	1.70 (1.27–2.28)	0.02
Vasopressor dependence	1.70 (1.24–2.24)	0.001
Obesity	1.67 (1.25–2.24)	<0.001
Hypoxemia at presentation	1.59 (1.18–2.10)	<0.001
Packed RBC exposure (per unit)	1.20 (1.13–1.28)	<0.001
Fluid balance (per liter)	1.10 (1.02–1.18)	0.01
Fresh frozen plasma exposure (per unit)	1.04 (1.01–1.08)	0.03
Intracerebral hemorrhage volume		
<30 mL	Reference	
30 to <60 mL	0.81 (0.57–1.14)	0.23
60 to <90 mL	0.72 (0.47–1.11)	0.14
≥90 mL	0.41 (0.24–0.71)	0.001

with volume overload) and with overall volume overload. Table 2 nicely identifies these risk factors.

Several of these factors could theoretically be altered by different care strategies.

J. A. Barker, MD, FACP, FCCP

Acute Respiratory Failure

Fatal Neurological Respiratory Insufficiency Is Common Among Viral Encephalitides
Wang H, Siddharthan V, Kesler KK, et al (Utah State Univ, Logan)
J Infect Dis 208:573-583, 2013

Background.—Neurological respiratory insufficiency strongly correlates with mortality among rodents infected with West Nile virus (WNV), which suggests that this is a primary mechanism of death in rodents and possibly fatal West Nile neurological disease in human patients.

Methods.—To explore the possibility that neurological respiratory insufficiency is a broad mechanism of death in cases of viral encephalitis, plethysmography was evaluated in mice infected with 3 flaviviruses and 2 alphaviruses. Pathology was investigated by challenging the diaphragm, using electromyography with hypercapnia and optogenetic photoactivation.

Results.—Among infections due to all but 1 alphavirus, death was strongly associated with a suppressed minute volume. Virally infected mice with a very low minute volume did not neurologically respond to hypercapnia or optogenetic photoactivation of the C4 cervical cord. Neurons with the orexin 1 receptor protein in the ventral C3−5 cervical cord were statistically diminished in WNV-infected mice with a low minute volume as compared to WNV-infected or sham-infected mice without respiratory insufficiency. Also, WNV-infected cells were adjacent to neurons with respiratory functions in the medulla.

Conclusions.—Detection of a common neurological mechanism of death among viral encephalitides creates opportunities to create broad-spectrum therapies that target relevant neurological cells in patients with types of viral encephalitis that have not been treatable in the past.

▶ This mouse and rat model nicely shows that respiratory failure does occur at a high rate in various viral encephalitidies. The possible mechanisms are also shown.

J. A. Barker, MD, CPE, FACP, FCCP, FAASM

Clinical correlates, outcomes and healthcare costs associated with early mechanical ventilation after kidney transplantation
Yuan H, Tuttle-Newhall JE, Dy-Liacco M, et al (Saint Louis Univ School of Medicine, MO; et al)
Am J Surg 206:686-692, 2013

Background.—Information is lacking on the frequency, clinical implications, and costs of respiratory failure requiring mechanical ventilation after kidney transplantation.

Methods.—U.S. Renal Data System records for Medicare-insured kidney transplant recipients (1995 to 2007; n = 88,392) were examined to identify post-transplantation mechanical ventilation from billing claims within 30 days after transplantation.

Results.—Post-transplantation mechanical ventilation was required among 2.1% of the cohort. Independent correlates of early mechanical ventilation included recipient age, low body mass index, coronary artery disease, and cerebrovascular disease. Post-transplantation mechanical ventilation was twice as likely with delayed graft function (adjusted odds ratio, 2.13; $P < .001$) and 35% lower among recipients of living versus deceased donor allografts. Patients needing early mechanical ventilation experienced 5-fold higher 1-year mortality, as well as significantly higher Medicare costs during the transplant hospitalization and first post-transplantation year.

Conclusions.—Recognition of patients at risk for post-transplantation respiratory failure may help direct protocols for reducing the incidence and consequences of this complication.

▶ Kidney transplants (along with liver) have become commonplace and have excellent 5- and 10-year survival. However, as intensivists we realize that those who have acute respiratory failure in the time immediately after transplant do worse. This study confirms that opinion. Not only do these patients have a worse survival acutely, but their evidence of graft failure and long-term results are significantly worse than others. The predisposing factors are hardly surprising but of course are useful. As in many other transplants, living-related donor recipient transplants do by far the best.

J. A. Barker, MD, FACP, FCCP

Emerging Indications for Extracorporeal Membrane Oxygenation in Adults with Respiratory Failure
Abrams D, Brodie D (Columbia Univ College of Physicians and Surgeons/New York—Presbyterian Hosp)
Ann Am Thorac Soc 10:371-377, 2013

Recent advances in technology have spurred the increasing use of extracorporeal membrane oxygenation (ECMO) in patients with severe hypoxemic respiratory failure. However, this accounts for only a small percentage of patients with respiratory failure. We envision the application of ECMO in many other forms of respiratory failure in the coming years. Patients with less severe forms of acute respiratory distress syndrome, for instance, may benefit from enhanced lung-protective ventilation with the very low tidal volumes made possible by direct carbon dioxide removal from the blood. For those in whom hypercapnia predominates, extracorporeal support will allow for the elimination of invasive mechanical ventilation in some cases. The potential benefits of ECMO may be further enhanced by improved techniques, which facilitate active mobilization. Although ECMO for these and other expanded applications is under active investigation, it has yet to be proven beneficial in these settings in rigorous controlled trials. Ultimately, with upcoming and future technological advances, there is the promise of true destination therapy, which

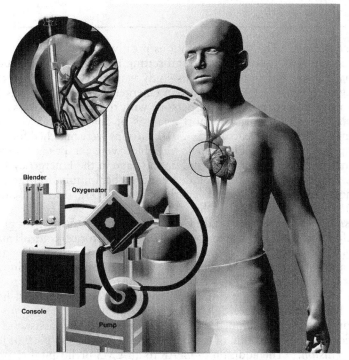

FIGURE 1.—Single-site approach to venovenous extracorporeal membrane oxygenation (ECMO) in the ambulatory patient. A dual-lumen cannula inserted in the internal jugular vein permits both the withdrawal of venous blood from the vena cavae and the reinfusion of oxygenated blood into the right atrium. Avoidance of femoral cannulation, in combination with more compact circuit components that can be easily mobilized, facilitates ambulation and physical rehabilitation in patients with respiratory failure requiring extracorporeal support. *Inset:* deoxygenated blood is withdrawn through ports positioned in both the superior and inferior vena cavae. The reinfusion port is oriented such that oxygenated blood is directed toward the tricuspid valve. Illustration used with permission from COACHsurgery.com and Columbia University. (Reprinted from Abrams D, Brodie D. Emerging indications for extracorporeal membrane oxygenation in adults with respiratory failure. *Ann Am Thorac Soc.* 2013;10:371-377, with permission from the American Thoracic Society.)

could lead to a major paradigm shift in the management of respiratory failure (Fig 1).

▶ Extracorporeal membrane oxygenation (ECMO) is hitting mainstream in medical intensive care units now. These authors push the envelope on ECMO use. In other words, ECMO can be used for several types of respiratory failure. Newer setups (see Fig 1) enable ambulation and extubation.

J. A. Barker, MD, FACP, FCCP

Assessment of the addition of prehospital continuous positive airway pressure (CPAP) to an urban emergency medical services (EMS) system in persons with severe respiratory distress
Aguilar SA, Lee J, Castillo E, et al (Univ of California San Diego (UCSD) Med Ctr; Scripps Mercy Hosp, San Diego, CA; et al)
J Emerg Med 45:210-219, 2013

Background.—The use of continuous positive airway pressure (CPAP)-assisted ventilation in the prehospital setting has not been well studied.

Objectives.—The purpose of this study was to measure the efficacy of adding prehospital CPAP to an urban emergency medical services (EMS) respiratory distress protocol for persons with respiratory distress.

Methods.—An historical cohort analysis of consecutive EMS patients presenting during the years 2005–2010. Groups were matched for severity of respiratory distress. Physiologic variables were the primary outcomes obtained from first responders and upon triage in the Emergency Department. Additional outcomes included endotracheal intubation rate, hospital mortality, overall hospital length of stay (LOS), intensive care unit (ICU) admission, and ICU LOS.

Results.—There were a total of 410 consecutive patients with predetermined criteria for severe respiratory distress, 235 historical controls matched with 175 post-implementation patients, entered in the study. The average age was 67 years; 54% were men. There were significant median differences in heart and respiratory rates favoring the historical cohort (all $p < 0.05$). There were no significant differences in intubation rate, overall hospital LOS, ICU admission rate, ICU LOS, or hospital mortality (all $p > 0.05$). Patients who were continued on non-invasive ventilatory assistance had a significantly improved rate of intubation and ICU LOS (all $p < 0.05$).

Conclusion.—The addition of CPAP to an EMS prehospital respiratory distress protocol resulted in improved heart and respiratory rates. Though not statistically significant, decrease in overall and ICU LOS were observed. Patients with continued ventilatory assistance seemed to have improved rates of intubation and ICU LOS.

▶ Is the intensive care unit (ICU) a set area of a hospital or is it a state of mind? With modern technology and innovation, it is clearly possible to take the ICU to the patient. This is a fascinating study in which the practitioners decided to try something new. After all, we know that patients with chronic obstructive pulmonary disease exacerbations and respiratory failure do better with noninvasive ventilation rather than endotracheal tube intubation. Trying continuous positive airway pressure in the field for similar patients is the logical extension of that. It probably works. I say probably because there weren't definitive findings here, but they suggest that it isn't dangerous if done right and that for some it probably does make a difference. A larger study powered to answer these questions is in order. I suspect they are already diagramming it out.

J. A. Barker, MD, FACP, FCCP

Airway Management

A Randomized, Double-Blind Comparison of Licorice Versus Sugar-Water Gargle for Prevention of Postoperative Sore Throat and Postextubation Coughing

Ruetzler K, Fleck M, Nabecker S, et al (Vienna Med Univ, Austria; et al)
Anesth Analg 117:614-621, 2013

Background.—One small study suggests that gargling with licorice before induction of anesthesia reduces the risk of postoperative sore throat. Double-lumen tubes are large and thus especially likely to provoke sore throats. We therefore tested the hypothesis that preoperative gargling with licorice solution prevents postoperative sore throat and postextubation coughing in patients intubated with double-lumen tubes.

Methods.—We enrolled 236 patients having elective thoracic surgery who required intubation with a double-lumen endotracheal tube. Patients were randomly assigned to gargle 5 minutes before induction of anesthesia for 1 minute with: (1) Extractum Liquiritiae Fluidum (licorice 0.5 g); or (2) Sirupus Simplex (sugar 5 g); each diluted in 30 mL water. Sore throat and postextubation coughing were evaluated 30 minutes, 90 minutes, and 4 hours after arrival in the postanesthesia care unit, and the first postoperative morning using an 11-point Likert scale by an investigator blinded to treatment.

Results.—The incidence of postoperative sore throat was significantly reduced in patients who gargled with licorice rather than sugar-water: 19% and 36% at 30 minutes, 10% and 35% at 1.5 hours, and 21% and 45% at 4 hours, respectively. The corresponding estimated treatment effects (relative risks) were 0.54 (95% CI, 0.30–0.99, licorice versus sugar-water; $P = 0.005$), 0.31 (0.14–0.68) ($P < 0.001$), and 0.48 (0.28–0.83) ($P < 0.001$).

Conclusion.—Licorice gargling halved the incidence of sore throat. Preinduction gargling with licorice appears to be a simple way to prevent a common and bothersome complication.

▶ Sometimes simple pleasures are the best. Sore throat after intubation is almost universal. And, one would think, it has to be definitely more likely in those who have a double lumen tube inserted, as these are considerably larger than standard ETTs. Liquid licorice appears to actually work in decreasing sore throat in these patients!

As long as we don't see a sudden surge of use (or abuse, oh my goodness), hopefully there won't be a resurgence of that other obscure but known side effect of glycyrrhizic acid: pseudohyperaldosteronism and metabolic alkalosis.

J. A. Barker, MD, FACP, FCCP

Accuracy of ultrasound-guided marking of the cricothyroid membrane before simulated failed intubation
Mallin M, Curtis K, Dawson M, et al (Univ of Utah, Salt Lake City; Univ of Kentucky, Lexington)
Am J Emerg Med 32:61-63, 2014

Background.—Interest in the use of dynamic ultrasound (US) for crico-thyrotomy has sparked a debate regarding its applicability in a crash air-way situation. Ultrasound-guided marking of the cricothyroid membrane (CTM) as a preintubation procedure may be better than the dynamic method. No prior study has evaluated the accuracy of using US to premark the CTM before attempted intubation.

Objectives.—To determine the feasibility of US-guided marking of the CTM before attempted simulated intubation so that this marking may be used as the location for the initial incision after failed intubation.

Methods.—Resident and attending physicians participated. Ultrasound was used to identify and mark the CTM with an invisible pen. Failed intubation was simulated, and the same operator then identified the CTM with US and marked the location with a black pen. The difference in the prein-tervention and postintervention markings was measured in millimeters. The length of the CTM was also measured as a reference.

Results.—Twenty-three models and operators were used for data collec-tion. The average CTM sagittal length was 13.9 mm (95% confidence interval [CI], 13.4-14.4). The average sagittal and axial differences before and after simulated intubation were found to be 0.91 mm (95% CI, 0.35-1.47) and 1.04 mm (95% CI, 0.38-1.7), respectively. The sagittal variabil-ity is 1/15 the total length of the CTM.

Conclusions.—Ultrasound marking of the CTM of healthy volunteers before simulated intubation accurately identifies the CTM after neck manipulation expected during a failed intubation. Further research is indi-cated to determine the clinical applicability of this model (Fig 2).

▶ Ultrasound scan is becoming a sixth vital sign in intensive care unit and emergency medicine. This unique study shows that ultrasound scan can be used in crash emergency intubations and cricothyrotomies to locate the airway at the level of the cricothyroid membrane. Even volunteers can quickly learn this. (See Fig 2 to view the ease of locating and marking the cricothyroid membrane.)

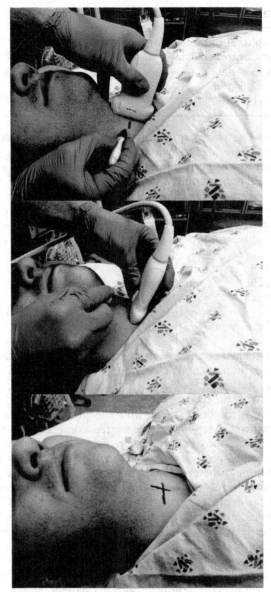

FIGURE 2.—Method of marking the CTM with US guidance. (Reprinted from Mallin M, Curtis K, Dawson M, et al. Accuracy of ultrasound-guided marking of the cricothyroid membrane before simulated failed intubation. *Am J Emerg Med*. 2014;32:61-63, Copyright 2014, with permission from Elsevier Inc.)

I have done emergency cricothyrotomies and would have found this technique very helpful. I believe this approach will soon enhance emergency airway therapy.

J. A. Barker, MD, FACP, FCCP

Cardiopulmonary Interactions

Central or Peripheral Catheters for Initial Venous Access of ICU Patients: A Randomized Controlled Trial

Ricard J-D, Salomon L, Boyer A, et al (Hôpital Louis Mourier, Colombes, France; Hôpital Pellegrin—Tripode, Bordeaux, France; et al)
Crit Care Med 41:2108-2115, 2013

Objectives.—The vast majority of ICU patients require some form of venous access. There are no evidenced-based guidelines concerning the use of either central or peripheral venous catheters, despite very different complications. It remains unknown which to insert in ICU patients. We investigated the rate of catheter-related insertion or maintenance complications in two strategies: one favoring the central venous catheters and the other peripheral venous catheters.

Design.—Multicenter, controlled, parallel-group, open-label randomized trial.

Setting.—Three French ICUs.

Patients.—Adult ICU patients with equal central or peripheral venous access requirement.

Intervention.—Patients were randomized to receive central venous catheters or peripheral venous catheters as initial venous access.

Measurements and Results.—The primary endpoint was the rate of major catheter-related complications within 28 days. Secondary endpoints were the rate of minor catheter-related complications and a composite score-assessing staff utilization and time spent to manage catheter insertions. Analysis was intention to treat. We randomly assigned 135 patients to receive a central venous catheter and 128 patients to receive a peripheral venous catheter. Major catheter-related complications were greater in the peripheral venous catheter than in the central venous catheter group (133 vs 87, respectively, $p = 0.02$) although none of those was life threatening. Minor catheter-related complications were 201 with central venous catheters and 248 with peripheral venous catheters ($p = 0.06$). 46% (60/128) patients were managed throughout their ICU stay with peripheral venous catheters only. There were significantly more peripheral venous catheter-related complications per patient in patients managed solely with peripheral venous catheter than in patients that received peripheral venous catheter and at least one central venous catheter: 1.92 (121/63) versus 1.13 (226/200), $p < 0.005$. There was no difference in central venous catheter-related complications per patient between patients initially randomized to peripheral venous catheters but subsequently crossed-over to central venous catheter and patients randomized to the central venous catheter group. Kaplan—Meier estimates of survival probability did not differ between the two groups.

Conclusion.—In ICU patients with equal central or peripheral venous access requirement, central venous catheters should preferably be inserted: a strategy associated with less major complications.

▶ This is a very important study. The rate of peripherally inserted central catheter (PICC) lines in inpatients has increased phenomenally over the last decade. Yet, these lines are not actually safer than central lines, as shown very nicely by these French investigators. PICC lines still get infected if left in for several days, and they also carry a relatively high upper extremity venous thrombosis rate as well. This very well done study confirms these findings. PICC lines may also decrease viability of one upper extremity for dialysis access as well.

In addition, subclavian lines are much more comfortable for the awake and moving patient. Think twice about a PICC in an intensive care unit patient!

J. A. Barker, MD, FACP, FCCP

Agreement Between ICU Clinicians and Electrophysiology Cardiologists on the Decision to Initiate a QTc-interval Prolonging Medication in Critically Ill Patients with Potential Risk Factors for Torsade de Pointes: A Comparative, Case-Based Evaluation

Fongemie JM, Al-Qadheeb NS, Mark Estes NA III, et al (Tufts Med Ctr, Boston, MA; Northeastern Univ, Boston, MA; et al)

Pharmacotherapy 33:589-597, 2013

Study Objectives.—To measure concordance between different intensive care unit (ICU) clinicians and a consensus group of electrophysiology (EP) cardiologists for use of a common rate-corrected QT interval (QTc)-prolonging medication in cases containing different potential risk factor(s) for torsade de pointes (TdP).

Design.—Prospective case-based evaluation.

Setting.—Academic medical center with 320 beds.

Subjects.—Medical house staff (MDs) and ICU nurses (RNs) from one center and select critical care pharmacists (PHs).

Intervention.—Completion of a survey containing 10 hypothetical ICU cases in which patients had agitated delirium for which a psychiatrist recommended intravenous haloperidol 5 mg every 6 hours. Each case contained different potential risk factor(s) for TdP in specific combinations. A group of five EP cardiologists agreed that haloperidol use was safe in five cases and not safe in five cases.

Measurements and Main Results.—For each case, participants were asked to document whether they would administer haloperidol, to provide a rationale for their decision, and to state their level of confidence in that decision. Most clinicians (92 of 115 [80%]) invited to participate completed the cases. Among the five cases where EP cardiologists agreed that haloperidol was not safe, 29% of respondents felt that haloperidol was safe. Conversely, in the five cases where EP cardiologists felt haloperidol was safe, 21% of respondents believed that it was not safe. Overall respondent-EP cardiologist agreement for haloperidol use across the 10 cases was moderate ($\kappa = 0.51$). MDs and PHs were in agreement with the EP cardiologists more than RNs (p = 0.03). Interprofessional variability existed for the TdP risk factors each best identified. Clinician confidence correlated with EP cardiologist concordance for MDs (p = 0.002) and PHs (p = 0.0002), but not for RNs (p = 0.69).

Conclusion.—When evaluating use of a QTc interval-prolonging medication, ICU clinicians often fail to identify the TdP risk factors that EP cardiologists feel should prevent its use. Clinician-EP cardiologist concordance varies by the specific risk factor(s) for TdP and the ICU professional conducting the assessment.

▶ Many medications prolong common rate-corrected QT interval (QTc) and may be of use in critical care. Haloperidol is commonly used for intensive care unit (ICU) delirium and does have known risk for prolonging QTc and inducing the Torsade de Pointes form of ventricular tachycardia. This survey model shows that both experts (electrophysiology cardiologists) and ICU practitioners (pharmacists and trainees) are inconsistent in application of definitions of prolonged QTc and, thus, risk. More formal training and practical definitions of this concept are in order.

J. A. Barker, MD, FACP, FCCP

Removing nonessential central venous catheters: evaluation of a quality improvement intervention
Ilan R, Doan J, Cload B, et al (Queen's Univ, Kingston, Ontario, Canada; Royal Univ Hosp, Saskatoon, Saskatchewan, Canada; et al)
Can J Anesth 59:1102-1110, 2012

Introduction.—Nonessential central venous catheters (CVCs) should be removed promptly to prevent adverse events. Little is known about effective strategies to achieve this goal. The present study evaluates the effectiveness of a quality improvement (QI) initiative to remove nonessential CVCs in the intensive care unit (ICU).

Methods.—A prospective observational study was performed in two ICUs following a QI intervention that included a daily checklist, education, and reminders. During 28 consecutive days, all CVCs were identified and the presence of ongoing indications for CVC placement was recorded. The proportions of nonessential CVCs and CVC days were compared with pre-intervention proportions and between the participating units. Rates of central line-associated bloodstream infections (CLABSI) were measured separately through Ontario's Critical Care Information System.

Results.—One hundred and ten patients and 159 CVCs were reviewed. Eighty-eight (11%) of 820 catheter days showed no apparent indication for CVC placement, and compared with the pre-intervention period, the

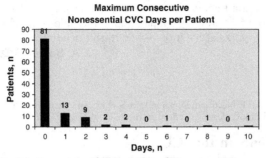

FIGURE 1.—Maximum consecutive nonessential CVC days per patient. CVC, central venous catheter. (With kind permission from Springer Science+Business Media. Ilan R, Doan J, Cload B, et al. Removing nonessential central venous catheters: evaluation of a quality improvement intervention. *Can J Anesth.* 2012;59:1102-1110.)

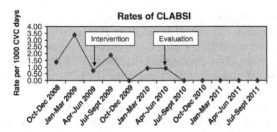

FIGURE 3.—CLABSI rates before, during and after the intervention. * CLABSI, central line associated bloodstream infection; CVC, central venous catheter. (With kind permission from Springer Science+Business Media. Ilan R, Doan J, Cload B, et al. Removing nonessential central venous catheters: evaluation of a quality improvement intervention. *Can J Anesth.* 2012;59:1102-1110.)

proportion of patients with any number of nonessential CVC days decreased from 51% to 26% (relative risk 0.51; 95% confidence interval 0.34 to 0.74; $P < 0.001$). There was no significant difference in the proportion of nonessential catheter days between participating units. Reported rates of CLABSI decreased substantially during the intervention.

Discussion.—A checklist tool supported by a multifaceted QI intervention effectively ensured prompt removal of nonessential CVCs in two ICUs (Figs 1 and 3).

▶ The importance of diligent care for central lines has been previously proven by Pronovost et al.[1] One of the most important features of the central line care bundle devised by Pronovost was the prompt removal of lines that are no longer needed. It stands to reason that lines can't become infected or thrombose veins if they are no longer in the patient. Yet this part of the bundle is frequently overlooked. No doubt that venous access is truly the lifeline for the intensive care unit patient. Thus, it can also become the death knell.

These Canadian investigators show very nicely how quality improvement can yield real results. Fig 1 shows the rapid decrease in nonessential catheter days once the focus is placed on the issue. The important data are presented in Fig 3.

Namely, the run chart shows the intervention followed by decrease in central line—associated infection rates culminating in multiple zero infection months. It is simple! It works! Take it out when it isn't needed.

J. A. Barker, MD, FACP, FCCP

Reference

1. Pronovost P, Needham D, Berenholtz S, et al. An intervention to decrease catheter-related bloodstream infections in the ICU. *N Engl J Med.* 2006;355:2725-2732.

COPD Patients in the ICU

A Patient With Acute COPD Exacerbation and Shock

Narula T, Raman D, Wiesen J, et al (Cleveland Clinic, OH)
Chest 144:e1-e3, 2013

Background.—Venous air embolism is rare but can complicate central venous catheterization. Emboli as small as 20 mL can cause severe complications, although most cases of air embolism are benign. A patient with acute chronic obstructive pulmonary disease (COPD) developed air emboli related to positive end-expiratory pressure (PEEP) treatment.

Case Report.—Elderly man with a history of COPD arrived at the emergency department reporting shortness of breath over the past 2 days. Physical examination noted jugular venous distension and distant breath sounds (no rales) bilaterally. Leukocytosis, acute renal failure, and a troponin T level of 0.44 ng/mL were found on laboratory evaluation. An electrocardiogram (ECG) revealed incomplete right bundle branch block and no significant ST segment or T-wave alterations. Radiographically, the patient had hyperinflated lung fields with bibasilar atelectasis and no focal opacity. Analysis of his arterial blood gases indicated combined hypoxemic and hypercapnic respiratory failure. Treatment was begun with bilevel positive airway pressure ventilation, but the patient developed hypotension and required endotracheal intubation. Despite aggressive intravenous (IV) fluid administration, his systolic blood pressure was 70 to 80 mm Hg. A femoral central venous catheter (CVC) was placed to allow a norepinephrine drip. He was diagnosed with acute respiratory failure resulting from an acute exacerbation of COPD and shock. In the intensive care unit (ICU), mechanical ventilator graphics analysis revealed intrinsic PEEP (PEEPi) was significant. Adjustments to ventilator modes and resolution of PEEPi diminished but did not eliminate the need for vasopressors. A bedside echocardiogram (ECHO) was done, and measures instituted to determine the cause of the right ventricular (RV) dilation and RV systolic failure. No thrombus was found on bedside lower extremity ultrasound. A careful examination of all the patient's IV accesses was done to determine the source of air entry into the venous system, identifying the femoral CVC as the culprit. The CVC was capped, and the patient's hemodynamics improved so he could be weaned from vasopressor therapy. Follow-up ECHO done 20 minutes later found no bubbles. Influenza A was diagnosed on the basis of a nasopharyngeal swab, and treatment with oseltamivir was begun. Extubation was successful the following day, and no further complications developed, permitting the patient to be discharged 3 days later.

Conclusions.—The ECHO was essential in identifying the dilated right ventricle and moderate to severe reduced RV systolic function in this patient with acute respiratory failure. It also identified a continuous stream of air bubbles, visible as hyperechoic freely mobile structures. Correcting the PEEPi and embolic load caused by the air bubbles allowed improved hemodynamics. It is important to recognize the significant effects of positive pressure ventilation on preload and afterload and the resulting hemodynamic consequences.

▶ This case report shows just how much we can learn from our patients. Shock is relatively common in chronic obstructive pulmonary disease exacerbations. Usually we are thinking of excess auto or intrinsic positive end-expiratory pressure. That was the case here, but the shock did not resolve with improving that.

Astutely, the authors looked for pulmonary emboli and deep vein thromboses. But instead they found air emboli. They then tracked back to find the source and realized that the central line was defective and the cause.

Air emboli are uncommon but life threatening. They must be included in the differential diagnosis in patients with invasive lines or open wounds and shock. Therapy can be high-flow oxygen or hyperbaric oxygen, positioning, and to close the source.

Bedside ultrasound scan is becoming standard of care in emergency medicine and critical care. This shows that it also should be routinely used in pulmonary medicine as well.

J. A. Barker, MD, FACP, FCCP

Influence of ICU Case-Volume on the Management and Hospital Outcomes of Acute Exacerbations of Chronic Obstructive Pulmonary Disease

Dres M, on behalf of the CUB-REA Group (Univ Paris Descartes, France; et al)
Crit Care Med 41:1884-1892, 2013

Objectives.—To study the relationship between case-volume and the use of noninvasive ventilation during acute exacerbations of chronic obstructive pulmonary disease in ICUs.

Design.—A 13-year multicenter retrospective cohort study of prospectively collected data.

Setting.—Medical ICUs.

Patients.—From 1998 to 2010, patients with acute exacerbations of chronic obstructive pulmonary disease were identified through a regional database.

Interventions.—The characteristics of hospitalization (including the type of mechanical ventilation) and demographic data of the patients were analyzed. ICUs were categorized into tertiles of the running mean annual volume of admissions. A logistic model performed a conditional multivariate analysis of prognostic factors after matching on a propensity score of being admitted to a high-volume unit and on the year of admission.

Measurements and Main Results.—Fourteen thousand four hundred forty acute exacerbations of chronic obstructive pulmonary disease were identified. The Simplified Acute Physiology Score II and ICU mortality increased during the study period (36 to 41 and 12% to 14%, respectively). The proportion of patients receiving any mechanical ventilation support also increased during the study period (from 64% to 86%), with a marked increase in the use of noninvasive ventilation (from 18% to 49%) and a decrease in the use of invasive ventilation (from 34% to 19%). Participating units were distributed into low-volume (<25 patients per year), medium-volume (26—47 patients per year), and high-volume (>47 patients per year) tertiles. There was a significant association between case-volume and 1) the proportion of patients receiving noninvasive ventilation (highest vs lowest case-volume tertiles: odds ratio, 1.43 [95% CI, 1.23—1.66]) and 2) lower mortality.

Conclusions.—Between 1998 and 2010, severity and mortality of acute exacerbations of chronic obstructive pulmonary disease admitted to Collège des Utilisateurs de Données en Réanimation ICUs increased. There was an increasing use of noninvasive ventilation and a decreasing use of invasive ventilation. Use of noninvasive ventilation was related to case-volume, suggesting that increasing experience favors the use of noninvasive ventilation and was associated with a strong trend toward decreased mortality.

▶ This is one of my favorite forms of studies. It is not as rigorous as a double-blind, randomized study but still beautiful in its simplicity and tremendously useful information. There has been a steady increase in the use of noninvasive ventilation for hypercarbic chronic obstructive pulmonary disease (COPD) exacerbations since a couple of seminal studies found decreased length of stay and increased survival for those patients. These French investigators take a look back to see what has happened in their own hospitals.

First, they confirm that COPD exacerbations are now treated more and more frequently with noninvasive ventilation and that this leads to increased survival.

Second, however, the smaller hospitals or those with fewer COPD patients, lagged behind. The concept of Centers of Excellence is real.

J. A. Barker, MD, FACP, FCCP

Miscellaneous

Acute Kidney Injury Secondary to Exposure to Insecticides Used for Bedbug (*Cimex lectularis*) Control

Bashir B, Sharma SG, Stein HD, et al (Abington Memorial Hosp, PA; and Columbia Univ, NY)

Am J Kidney Dis 62:974-977, 2013

Bedbug (*Cimex lectularis*) infestation is becoming a worldwide epidemic due to the emergence of insecticide-resistant strains. Pyrethroids are approved by the US Environmental Protection Agency for use against bedbugs and are considered minimally toxic to humans, with known respiratory, neurologic, and gastrointestinal effects. We present the first reported case of pyrethroid-induced toxic acute tubular necrosis (ATN). A 66-year-old healthy woman receiving no prior nephrotoxic medications presented with extreme weakness, decreased urine output, and acute kidney injury. She had administered multiple applications of a bedbug spray (permethrin) and a fogger (pyrethrin), exceeding the manufacturer's recommended amounts. She was found to have severe nonoliguric acute kidney injury associated with profound hypokalemia. Kidney biopsy revealed toxic ATN with extensive tubular degenerative changes and cytoplasmic vacuolization. With conservative management, serum creatinine level decreased from 13.0 mg/dL (estimated glomerular filtration rate, 3 mL/min/1.73 m^2) to 1.67 mg/dL (estimated glomerular filtration rate, 37 mL/min/1.73 m^2) within 6 weeks. Literature review uncovered no prior report of pyrethroid insecticide—induced ATN in humans, although there are reports of ATN with similar tubular vacuolization in rats exposed to this agent. Bedbug insecticides containing pyrethroids should be used with caution due to the potential development of toxic ATN after prolonged exposure.

▶ This report just goes to show that there is always something new to learn! I did know that bedbugs were becoming resistant to therapy. These insecticides are definitely toxic. We now need to add this to possible causes of acute tubular necrosis and acute renal failure.

J. A. Barker, MD, FACP, FCCP

Are Routine Intensive Care Admissions Needed after Endovascular Treatment of Unruptured Aneurysms?

Burrows AM, Rabinstein AA, Cloft HJ, et al (Mayo Clinic, Rochester MN)

Am J Neuroradiol 34:2199-2201, 2013

Routine intensive care unit monitoring is common after elective embolization of unruptured intracranial aneurysms. In this series of 200 consecutive endovascular procedures for unruptured intracranial aneurysms, 65% of patients were triaged to routine (non-intensive care unit) floor care based on intraoperative findings, aneurysm morphology, and absence of major co-morbidities. Only 1 patient (0.5%) required subsequent transfer to the intensive care unit for management of a perioperative complication. The authors conclude that patients without major co-morbidities, intraoperative complications, or complex aneurysm morphology can be safely observed in a regular ward rather than being admitted to the intensive care unit.

▶ Just because it is what we have always done, we should keep doing it, right? Not!

Neurosurgical care of aneurysms has radically changed over the last 10 years. Most patients are now undergoing interventional neuroradiology procedures such as coiling. Not surprisingly, these investigators have turned that concept (that all postoperative aneurysm patients need to be in the intensive care unit) on its head. Bravo!

These are heady days with rapidly progressive technology and limited resources. Change must happen.

J. A. Barker, MD, FACP, FCCP

Severe Sepsis and Septic Shock
Angus DC, van der Poll T (Univ of Pittsburgh School of Medicine, PA; Univ of Amsterdam, The Netherlands)
N Engl J Med 369:840-851, 2013

Background.—The definition of sepsis has evolved over generations. Today, the view is that sepsis is a systemic inflammatory response to infection that can follow multiple infectious causes and does not require the presence of septicemia. Severe sepsis and sepsis are terms often used interchangeably to describe infection complicated by acute organ dysfunction. The current state of knowledge about severe sepsis and septic shock was outlined.

Incidence and Causes.—US data indicate that 2% of patients admitted to the hospital have severe sepsis, and half of these are treated in the intensive care unit (ICU), accounting for 10% of ICU admissions. Similar data on ICU patients are found in other high-income countries. Both community-acquired and health care-n-associated infections precede severe sepsis, with pneumonia that most common cause, followed by intra-abdominal and urinary tract infections. Only a third of patients have positive blood cultures, and up to a third have negative cultures from all sites. The most common gram-positive isolates are *Staphylococcus aureus* and *Streptococcus pneumoniae*; with *Escherichia coli*, klebsiella species, and *Pseudomonas aeruginosa* the most common gram-negative isolates. Sixty-two percent of patients with severe sepsis had positive cultures for gram-negative bacteria, 47% for gram-positive bacteria, and 19% for fungi.

Clinical Features.—Clinical manifestations are a function of the initial site of infection, causative organism, pattern of acute organ involvement, patient's underlying health status, and wait before treatment begins. Signs of infection and organ dysfunction can be subtle, so the list of warning signs is long. Classic manifestations include acute dysfunction of the respiratory and cardiovascular systems; central nervous system dysfunction occurring as obtundation or delirium; and kidney injury indicated by decreased urine output and increased serum creatinine levels.

Pathophysiology.—Evidence indicates that infection triggers a complex, variable, and prolonged host response involving pro-inflammatory and anti-inflammatory mechanisms. The specific response depends on the causative pathogen, the host, and the location. Pathogens activate immune cells, including inflammasomes and alarmins. Severe sepsis is usually associated with altered coagulation as well. The humoral, cellular, and neural mechanisms in the immune system can attenuate the potentially harmful effects of pro-inflammatory response mechanisms. Patients who survive early sepsis but remain in the ICU have immunosuppressed systems. As a result, they often have sustained infectious foci or latent viral infections that can be reactivated. Their blood leukocytes have reduced responsiveness to pathogens and demonstrate impaired spleen cells and immunosuppression of the lungs. Impaired tissue oxygenation plays a key role in organ dysfunction, accompanied by contributions from hypotension, reduced red blood cell deformability, and microvascular thrombus. Mitochondrial damage caused by oxidative stress and other mechanisms alters cellular oxygen use. Alarmins in the extracellular environment can activate neutrophils and cause more tissue injury.

Treatment and Outcomes.—The guidelines for treatment recommend two bundles of care that are associated with improved outcomes for sepsis patients. The initial management bundle is accomplished in the first 6 hours after presentation, whereas the management bundle is done in the ICU. Patients are provided with cardiorespiratory resuscitation and mitigate immediate threats of uncontrolled infection during the initial phase. A probable diagnosis is formed, cultures are obtained, and empirical antimicrobial therapy and source control are done. Once the patient moves to a site for ongoing care, he or she is closely monitored and receives organ function support. The goal is to avoid complications and step care down as appropriate. The initial broad-spectrum therapy is de-escalated to minimize the emergence of resistant organisms, the risk of drug toxicity, and the cost. A short course of hydrocortisone (200 to 300 mg/day for up to 7 days or until vasopressor support is discontinued) can be helpful for patients with refractory septic shock. With advanced training, surveillance and monitoring, and prompt initiation of therapy for the underlying infection, along with support for failing organs, mortality is about 20% to 30% for many patients. However, patients who survive to discharge are at increased risk for death for several months or years thereafter.

Conclusions.—Clinicians can reduce the risk of death associated with sepsis through advances in intensive care, awareness of the problem, and the widespread availability of evidence-based treatment. However, patients who survive sepsis appear to be an increased risk for death in the next few months or years. New therapeutic agents and better approaches to the design and execution of clinical trials are needed.

▶ The authors are experts in this field and do an excellent job of outlining the current thought in the area. Figs 1 and 2 in the original article are invaluable in cartooning the current concepts of pathophysiology as to why sepsis and septic shock occur—in some, but not all, patients. Clearly, however, there is still great need for further knowledge in pathophysiology and therapy, as the mortality rate remains unacceptably high.

J. A. Barker, MD, FACP, FCCP

Choosing and Using Screening Criteria for Palliative Care Consultation in the ICU: A Report From the Improving Palliative Care in the ICU (IPAL-ICU) Advisory Board
Nelson JE, behalf of the Improving Palliative Care in the ICU (IPAL-ICU) Project Advisory Board (Icahn School of Medicine at Mount Sinai, NY; et al)
Crit Care Med 41:2318-2327, 2013

Objective.—To review the use of screening criteria (also known as "triggers") as a mechanism for engaging palliative care consultants to assist with care of critically ill patients and their families in the ICU.

Data Sources.—We searched the MEDLINE database from inception to December 2012 for all English-language articles using the terms "trigger," "screen," "referral," "tool," "triage," "case-finding," "assessment," "checklist," "proactive," or "consultation," together with "intensive care" or "critical care" and "palliative care," "supportive care," "end-of-life care," or "ethics." We also hand-searched reference lists and author files and relevant tools on the Center to Advance Palliative Care website.

Study Selection.—Two members (a physician and a nurse with expertise in clinical research, intensive care, and palliative care) of the interdisciplinary Improving Palliative Care in the ICU Project Advisory Board presented studies and tools to the full Board, which made final selections by consensus.

Data Extraction.—We critically reviewed the existing data and tools to identify screening criteria for palliative care consultation, to describe methods for selecting, implementing, and evaluating such criteria, and to consider alternative strategies for increasing access of ICU patients and families to high-quality palliative care.

Data Synthesis.—The Improving Palliative Care in the ICU Advisory Board used data and experience to address key questions relating to: existing screening criteria; optimal methods for selection, implementation, and evaluation of such criteria; and appropriateness of the screening approach for a particular ICU.

Conclusions.—Use of specific criteria to prompt proactive referral for palliative care consultation seems to help reduce utilization of ICU resources without changing mortality, while increasing involvement of palliative care specialists for critically ill patients and families in need. Existing data and resources can be used in developing such criteria, which should be tailored for a specific ICU, implemented through an organized process involving key stakeholders, and evaluated by appropriate measures. In some settings, other strategies for increasing access to palliative care may be more appropriate.

▶ Twenty percent or more of tertiary medical intensive care unit patients have chronic conditions or terminal conditions that will not be solved by critical care. Palliative care is appropriate for these and others. How do we decide which patients are in those categories? How do we choose which patients need palliative care consultations?

This consensus group has advanced our knowledge greatly in this area.

J. A. Barker, MD, FACP, FCCP

Do Windows or Natural Views Affect Outcomes or Costs Among Patients in ICUs?

Kohn R, Harhay MO, Cooney E, et al (Massachusetts General Hosp, Boston; Ctr for Clinical Epidemiology and Biostatistics, Philadelphia, PA; et al)
Crit Care Med 41:1645-1655, 2013

Objective.—To determine whether potential exposure to natural light via windows or to more pleasing views through windows affects outcomes or costs among critically ill patients.

Design.—Retrospective cohort study.

Setting.—An academic hospital in Philadelphia, PA.

Patients.—Six thousand one hundred thirty-eight patients admitted to a 24-bed medical ICU and 6,631 patients admitted to a 24-bed surgical ICU from July 1, 2006, to June 30, 2010.

Interventions.—Assignment to medical ICU rooms with vs. without windows and to surgical ICU rooms with natural vs. industrial views based on bed availability.

Measurements and Main Results.—In primary analyses adjusting for patient characteristics, medical ICU patients admitted to rooms with ($n = 4,093$) versus without ($n = 2,243$) windows did not differ in rates of ICU ($p = 0.25$) or in-hospital ($p = 0.94$) mortality, ICU readmissions ($p = 0.37$), or delirium ($p = 0.56$). Surgical ICU patients admitted to rooms with natural ($n = 3,072$) versus industrial ($n = 3,588$) views experienced slightly shorter ICU lengths of stay and slightly lower variable costs. Instrumental variable analyses based on initial bed assignment and exposure time did not show any differences in any outcomes in either the medical ICU or surgical ICU cohorts, and none of the differences noted in primary analyses remained statistically significant when adjusting for multiple comparisons. In a prespecified subgroup analysis among patients with ICU length of stay greater than 72 hours, MICU windows were associated with reduced ICU ($p = 0.02$) and hospital mortality ($p = 0.04$); these results did not meet criteria for significance after adjustment for multiple comparisons.

Conclusions.—ICU rooms with windows or natural views do not improve outcomes or reduce costs of in-hospital care for general populations of medical and surgical ICU patients. Future work is needed to determine whether targeting light from windows directly toward patients influences outcomes and to explore these effects in patients at high risk for adverse outcomes.

▶ Natural light exposure is necessary for human happiness as well as day/night timing and sleep. However, does that truly extrapolate to the need for windows in every intensive care unit room? There is a mandate for windows in newly constructed hospitals.

These investigators have shown that extrapolations and what seems to be the right thing to do may, in fact, just be urban myth. This nicely done study shows no difference in any parameter for patients with or without windows.

J. A. Barker, MD, FACP, FCCP

Prediction of Death in Less Than 60 Minutes Following Withdrawal of Cardiorespiratory Support in ICUs

Brieva J, Coleman N, Lacey J, et al (HNEAHS, Newcastle, NSW, Australia; et al)
Crit Care Med 41:2677-2687, 2013

Objectives.—Half of all ICU patients die within 60 minutes of withdrawal of cardiorespiratory support. Prediction of which patients die before and after 60 minutes would allow changes in service organization to improve patient palliation, family grieving, and allocation of ICU beds. This study tested various predictors of death within 60 minutes and explored which clinical variables ICU specialists used to make their prediction.

Design and Settings.—Prospective longitudinal cohort design (n = 765) of consecutive adult patients having withdrawal of cardiorespiratory support, in 28 ICUs in Australia. Primary outcome was death within 60 minutes following withdrawal of cardiorespiratory support. A random split-half method was used to make two independent samples for development and testing of the predictive indices. The secondary outcome was ICU Specialist prediction of death within 60 minutes.

Measurements and Main Results.—Death within 60 minutes of withdrawal of cardiorespiratory support occurred in 377 (49.3%). ICU specialist opinion was the best individual predictor, with an unadjusted odds ratio of 15.42 (95% CI, 9.33–25.49) and an adjusted odds ratio of 8.44 (4.30–16.58). A predictive index incorporating the ICU specialist opinion and clinical variables had an area under the curve of 0.89 (0.86–0.92) and 0.84 (0.80–0.88) in the development and test sets, respectively; and a second index using only clinical variables had an area under the curve of 0.86 (0.82–0.89) and 0.78 (0.73–0.83). The ICU specialist prediction of death within 60 minutes was independently associated with five clinical variables: pH, Glasgow Coma Scale, spontaneous respiratory rate, positive end-expiratory pressure, and systolic blood pressure.

Conclusion.—ICU specialist opinion is probably the current clinical standard for predicting death within 60 minutes of withdrawal of cardiorespiratory support. This approach is supported by this study, although predictive indices restricted to clinical variables are only marginally inferior. Either approach has a clinically useful level of prediction that would allow ICU service organization to be modified to improve care for patients and families and use ICU beds more efficiently.

▶ I agree with the authors that this seemingly morbid topic is of practical value. Families universally ask this. I believe that it is part of the natural coping method. Prediction allows many practical events to occur, such as attention by chaplains, transfer planning, and support of family and staff.

I have only been able to predict rapid death after withdrawal of life support in the extreme cases and even then have often been wrong. This is an impressive study, but further investigation is warranted.

J. A. Barker, MD, FACP, FCCP

Epidemiology of Obstetric-Related ICU Admissions in Maryland: 1999–2008
Wanderer JP, Leffert LR, Mhyre JM, et al (Vanderbilt Univ, Nashville, TN; Massachusetts General Hosp, Boston; The Univ of Michigan Health System, Ann Arbor; et al)
Crit Care Med 41:1844-1852, 2013

Objective.—To define the prevalence, indications, and temporal trends in obstetric-related ICU admissions.

Design.—Descriptive analysis of utilization patterns.

Setting.—All hospitals within the state of Maryland.

Patients.—All antepartum, delivery, and postpartum patients who were hospitalized between 1999 and 2008.

Interventions.—None.

Measurements and Main Results.—We identified 2,927 ICU admissions from 765,598 admissions for antepartum, delivery, or postpartum conditions using appropriate *International Classification of Diseases*, 9th Revision, Clinical Modification codes. The overall rate of ICU utilization was 419.1 per 100,000 deliveries, with rates of 162.5, 202.6, and 54.0 per 100,000 deliveries for the antepartum, delivery, and postpartum periods, respectively. The leading diagnoses associated with ICU admission were pregnancy-related hypertensive disease (present in 29.9% of admissions), hemorrhage (18.8%), cardiomyopathy or other cardiac disease (18.3%), genitourinary infection (11.5%), complications from ectopic pregnancies and abortions (10.3%), nongenitourinary infection (10.1%), sepsis (7.1%), cerebrovascular disease (5.8%), and pulmonary embolism (3.7%). We assessed for changes in the most common diagnoses in the ICU population over time and found rising rates of sepsis (10.1 per 100,000 deliveries to 16.6 per 100,000 deliveries, $p = 0.003$) and trauma (9.2 per 100,000 deliveries to 13.6 per 100,000 deliveries, $p = 0.026$) with decreasing rates of anesthetic complications (11.3 per 100,000 to 4.7 per 100,000, $p = 0.006$). The overall frequency of obstetric-related ICU admission and the rates for other indications remained relatively stable.

Conclusions.—Between 1999 and 2008, 419.1 per 100,000 deliveries in Maryland were complicated by ICU admission. Hospitals providing obstetric services should plan for appropriate critical care management and/or transfer of women with severe morbidities during pregnancy (Table 2).

▶ Obstetric intensive care unit patients strike fear in our hearts. The patients are generally young and healthy prenatally. The prevalence of admissions is low enough (except in rare centers at Women and Children hospitals) to

TABLE 2.—Occurrence of Maternal Conditions and Organ Dysfunction, Obstetric Intensive Care Admissions Versus Obstetric Non-ICU Admissions

Variable	Obstetric ICU Admissions (n = 2,927) (%)	Obstetric Non-ICU Admissions (n = 762,671) (%)
Maternal conditions		
Hypertensive disorders of pregnancy	875 (29.9)	68,159 (8.9)
Hemorrhage	551 (18.8)	39,397 (5.2)
Cardiomyopathy or other cardiac disease	536 (18.3)	3,723 (0.5)
Genitourinary infection	335 (11.4)	47,037 (6.2)
Complications from ectopic pregnancy or abortion	300 (10.3)	18,349 (2.4)
Nongenitourinary infection	296 (10.1)	7,566 (1.0)
Sepsis	207 (7.1)	853 (0.1)
Cerebrovascular disease	170 (5.8)	475 (0.06)
Pulmonary embolism	109 (3.7)	535 (0.07)
Aspiration	89 (3.0)	245 (0.03)
Trauma	87 (3.0)	598 (0.08)
Anesthetic complications	66 (0.4)	3,090 (2.3)
Hyperemesis	63 (2.2)	9,617 (1.3)
Status asthmaticus	56 (1.9)	343 (0.04)
Status epilepticus	14 (0.5)	18 (< 0.01)
Blood transfusion reaction	11 (0.4)	58 (0.01)
Organ dysfunction		
Respiratory failure	721 (24.6)	659 (0.1)
Coagulopathy	289 (9.9)	2,092 (0.3)
Liver failure	206 (7.0)	8,487 (1.1)
Shock	201 (6.9)	197 (0.03)
Acute renal failure	176 (6.0)	437 (0.06)
Pulmonary edema	56 (1.9)	204 (0.03)
Coma	14 (0.5)	12 (<0.01)

Differences between non-ICU and ICU admissions were statistically significant ($p \leq 0.01$ on chi-square analysis) for all comparisons between each group.

make true expertise in their care difficult. Table 2 outlines the incidence of disorders. I would not have guessed hypertension as the most common reason for admission.

It is reassuring to see that admission rates are not increasing. Yet, we somehow must lower maternal mortality to levels commiserate with other developed countries.

J. A. Barker, MD, FACP, FCCP

A Systematic Review of Evidence-Informed Practices for Patient Care Rounds in the ICU
Lane D, Ferri M, Lemaire J, et al (Univ of Calgary, Canada)
Crit Care Med 41:2015-2029, 2013

Objectives.—Patient care rounds are a key mechanism by which healthcare providers communicate and make patient care decisions in the ICU but no synthesis of best practices for rounds currently exists. Therefore, we systematically reviewed the evidence for facilitators and barriers to patient care rounds in the ICU.

Data Sources.—Search of Medline, Embase, CINAHL, PubMed, and the Cochrane library through September 21, 2012.

Study Selection.—Original, peer-reviewed research studies (no methodological restrictions) were selected, which described current practices, facilitators, or barriers to healthcare provider rounding in the ICU.

Data Extraction.—Two authors with methodological and content expertise independently abstracted data using a prespecified abstraction tool.

Data Synthesis.—The literature search identified 7,373 citations. Reviews of abstracts led to the retrieval of 136 full text articles for assessment; 43 articles in three languages (English, German, Spanish) were selected for review. Of these, 13 were ethnographic studies and 15 uncontrolled before-after studies. Six studies used control groups, including one cross-over randomized, one time-series, three cohort, and one controlled before-after study. A total of 13 facilitators and 9 barriers to patient care rounds were identified through a narrative and meta-synthesis of included studies. Identified facilitators suggest that the quality of rounds is improved when conducted by a multidisciplinary group of providers, with explicitly defined roles, using a standardized structure and goal-oriented approach that includes a best practices checklist. Barriers to quality patient care rounds include poor information retrieval and documentation, interruptions, long rounding times, and allied healthcare provider perceptions of not being valued by rounding physicians.

Conclusions.—Although the evidence base for best practices of patient care rounds in the ICU is limited, several practical and low-risk practices can be considered for implementation Table 4.

▶ It stands to reason that we should attempt to improve our own practice by scientific analysis. These authors have thoroughly reviewed the world literature

TABLE 4.—Evidence-Informed Practices for Patient Care Rounds in the ICU

Best Practice	Strength of Recommendation[a] (*JAMA* GRADE[b])
Implement multidisciplinary rounds (including at least a medical doctor, registered nurse, and pharmacist)	Strong—definitely do it ($\uparrow\uparrow$A)
Standardize location, time, and team composition	Strong—definitely do it ($\uparrow\uparrow$B)
Define explicit roles for each HCP participating on rounds	Strong—definitely do it ($\uparrow\uparrow$B)
Develop and implement structured tool (best practices checklist)	Strong—definitely do it ($\uparrow\uparrow$B)
Reduce nonessential time wasting activities	Strong—definitely do it ($\uparrow\uparrow$B)
Minimize unnecessary interruptions	Strong—definitely do it ($\uparrow\uparrow$C)
Focus discussions on development of daily goals and document all discussed goals in health record	Strong—definitely do it ($\uparrow\uparrow$C)
Conduct discussions at bedside to promote patient-centeredness	Weak—probably do it ($\uparrow$?A)
Conduct discussions in conference room to promote efficiency and communication	Weak—probably do it ($\uparrow$?C)
Establish open collaborative discussion environment	Weak—probably do it ($\uparrow$?C)
Ensure clear visibility between all HCP	Weak—probably do it ($\uparrow$?D)
Empower HCP to promote team-based approach to discussions	Weak—probably do it ($\uparrow$?D)
Produce visual presentation of patient information	No specific recommendation (??D)

Table sorted by strength of recommendation.

GRADE = Grades of Recommendation Assessment, Development, and Evaluation, HCP = healthcare provider.

[a]Based on the GRADE system, evaluating the efficacy of the intervention, balance between desirable and undesirable effects, costs (resource allocation), and quality of evidence (detailed summary of grading available on request).

[b]$\uparrow\uparrow$ = strong recommendation, $\uparrow$? = weak recommendation, ?? = no recommendation. Quality of evidence: A = very strong, B = strong, C = moderate, D = weak.

and come up with some excellent and practical recommendations. These are best summarized in Table 4. They really look like what those in the military or the airline industry would call Crew Resource Management: round at predictable times, make sure all members know their roles and responsibilities, allow all to speak during rounds, make data available and transparent.

There are those who fear the standardization of medical practice. They express a variety of (unfounded) fears of loss of autonomy, being forced to use "cookbook medicine," and loss of the "art." I say "poppycock!"

The more we standardize what is possible, the better we communicate, and the more scientific our approach, the better results our patients will experience.

J. A. Barker, MD, FACP, FCCP

Clostridium difficile Infection: A Multicenter Study of Epidemiology and Outcomes in Mechanically Ventilated Patients

Micek ST, Schramm G, Morrow L, et al (Barnes-Jewish Hosp, St Louis, MO; Mayo Clinic, Rochester, MN; Creighton Univ School of Medicine, Omaha, NE; et al)
Crit Care Med 41:1968-1975, 2013

Objectives.—*Clostridium difficile* is a leading cause of hospital-associated infection in the United States. The purpose of this study is to assess the prevalence of *C. difficile* infection among mechanically ventilated patients within the ICUs of three academic hospitals and secondarily describe the influence of *C. difficile* infection on the outcomes of these patients.

Design.—A retrospective cohort study.

Setting.—ICUs at three teaching hospitals: Barnes-Jewish Hospital, Mayo Clinic, and Creighton University Medical Center over a 2-year period.

Patients.—All hospitalized patients requiring mechanical ventilation for greater than 48 hours within an ICU were eligible for inclusion.

Interventions.—None.

Measurements and Main Results.—A total of 5,852 consecutive patients admitted to the ICU were included. Three hundred eighty-six (6.6%) patients with development of *C. difficile* infection while in the hospital (5.39 cases/1,000 patient days). Septic shock complicating *C. difficile* infection occurred in 34.7% of patients. Compared with patients without *C. difficile* infection (n = 5,466), patients with *C. difficile* infection had a similar hospital mortality rate (25.1% vs 26.3%, p = 0.638). Patients with *C. difficile* infection were significantly more likely to be discharged to a skilled nursing or rehabilitation facility (42.4% vs 31.9%, p < 0.001), and the median hospital (23 d vs 15 d, p < 0.001) and ICU length of stay (12 d vs 8 d, p < 0.001) were found to be significantly longer in patients with *C. difficile* infection.

Conclusions.—*Clostridium difficile* infection is a relatively common nosocomial infection in mechanically ventilated patients and is associated with prolonged length of hospital and ICU stay, and increased need for skilled nursing care or rehabilitation following hospital discharge (Tables 1 and 2).

▶ This is a useful and important article. The investigators confirm that *Clostridium difficile* superinfection is on the increase. The epidemiology (Table 1) surprised me somewhat. I did not realize the preponderance of women over men with this complication. Likewise, I was surprised at the high number of patients

TABLE 1.—Patient Demographics and Comorbidities

	CDI (n = 386)	No CDI (n = 5,466)	P
Age, yr	62.6 ± 16.8	60.1 ± 16.8	0.003
Gender: female, *n* (%):	236 (61.1)	3193 (58.4)	0.276
Ethnicity, *n* (%)			
Caucasian	296 (76.5)	3981 (72.8)	0.117
African American	80 (20.7)	1248 (22.8)	0.325
Medical patient, *n* (%):	189 (48.9)	2783 (50.9)	0.442
Diabetes, *n* (%):	82 (21.2)	1189 (21.8)	0.815
Class III or IV congestive heart failure, *n* (%)	73 (18.9)	1093 (20.0)	0.606
Chronic obstructive pulmonary disease, *n* (%)	62 (16.1)	1083 (19.8)	0.073
Active malignancy, *n* (%)	73 (18.9)	989 (18.1)	0.687
End-stage renal disease, *n* (%)	18 (4.7)	561 (10.3)	<0.001
End-stage liver disease, *n* (%)	32 (8.3)	190 (3.5)	<0.001
Acute Physiology and Chronic Health Evaluation II Score	19.6 ± 6.9	21.1 ± 7.6	<0.001

CDI = Clostridium difficile infection.
Values are expressed as mean ± sd.

TABLE 2.—Pharmacologic Risk Factors for *Clostridium difficile* Infection Patients ($n = 386$)

Prior antibiotics[a] (%)	358 (92.7)
Vancomycin	263 (68.1)
Cephalosporin	236 (61.1)
Other	195 (50.5)
Penicillin class	114 (29.5)
Fluoroquinolone	110 (28.5)
Carbapenem	97 (25.1)
Aminoglycoside	30 (7.8)
Linezolid	29 (7.5)
Prior acid-suppression therapy[a] (%)	
Proton-pump inhibitor	264 (68.4)
Histamine H2-receptor antagonist	70 (18.1)
Antacids	15 (3.9)

[a]Antibiotics and acid-suppression therapy administered for at least 24 hours prior to the diagnosis of *Clostridium difficile* Infection.

with the infection who had received intravenous vancomycin. I really expected carbapenems to be higher up on the antibiotic-associated list. As described in recent years, proton pump inhibitors lead those in the nonantibiotic category, which are associated with *C difficile* colitis.

Sadly, hospital length of stay, morbidity, and mortality remain elevated with this nosocomial infection in intensive care unit patients. I predict that we will solve the problem of *C difficile* overgrowth infection within the next decade. Just a wild guess, please don't come for my grandchildren or house if I am wrong!

J. A. Barker, MD, FACP, FCCP

Pulmonary Hypertension in the ICU

Capnography as a Diagnostic Tool for Pulmonary Embolism: A Meta-Analysis

Manara A, D'Hoore W, Thys F (Université Catholique de Louvain, Brussels, Belgium)
Ann Emerg Med 62:584-591, 2013

Study Objective.—Multiple studies have evaluated capnography for the diagnosis of pulmonary embolism; accordingly, we conduct a meta-analysis of these trials.

Methods.—We performed a systematic search from 1990 to 2011, using MEDLINE, EMBASE, and the Cochrane Library, including studies evaluating capnography as a diagnostic tool alone or in conjunction with other tests. After study quality evaluation, we calculated the pooled sensitivity, specificity, likelihood ratios, and diagnostic odds ratios.

Results.—We included 14 trials with 2,291 total subjects, with a 20% overall prevalence of pulmonary embolism. The pooled diagnostic accuracy for capnography was sensitivity 0.80 (95% confidence interval [CI] 0.76 to 0.83), specificity 0.49 (95% CI 0.47 to 0.51), negative likelihood ratio 0.32 (*95%* CI 0.23 to 0.45), positive likelihood ratio 2.43 (*95%* CI 1.70 to 3.46), and diagnostic odds ratio 10.4 (*95%* CI 6.33 to 17.1). The area under the summary receiver operating characteristic curve was 0.84. To reach pulmonary embolism posttest probabilities less than 1%, 2%, or 5%, pulmonary embolism prevalence or pretest probability had to be less than 3%, 5%, or 10% respectively. Because of interstudy differences in dead space measurements methodologies, the best cutoff in alveolar dead space or end tidal CO_2 conferring the best negative likelihood ratio could not be evaluated.

Conclusion.—Pooled data suggest a potential diagnostic role for capnography when the pulmonary embolism pretest probability is 10% or less, perhaps after a positive D-dimer test result.

▶ Carbon dioxide level should increase precipitously after pulmonary embolism because of dead space physiology. There have been prior emergency department studies confirming this, especially when paired with D-dimer. This meta-analysis confirms that capnography can function as an excellent noninvasive indicator of pulmonary embolism.

J. A. Barker, MD, FACP, FCCP

Trauma Issues

A 40-Year-Old Woman With Cough and Dyspnea 2 Months After a Motorcycle Accident

Hoffman PJ, Cooke DT, Zeki AA, et al (Univ of California, Davis Med Ctr, Sacramento)
Chest 144:1720-1723, 2013

Background.—Most patients who suffer blunt tracheobronchial injury (TBI) in a motor vehicle accident or crushing event die at the scene of the trauma. However, coexisting traumatic injuries can mask TBI and delay the diagnosis. A patient with delayed diagnosis of traumatic right main bronchus disruption was reported.

> *Case Report.*—Woman, 40, reported experiencing 6 weeks of dyspnea and nonproductive cough. She was in a high-speed motorcycle accident 2 months earlier and spent 15 days in the hospital for multiple traumatic injuries, including facial cervical vertebral, rib, pelvic, and tibial fractures; pneumomediastinum; and right pneumothorax. She also experienced a prolonged air leak after chest tube thoracostomy; the chest tube was removed on the ninth day in the hospital. She also had type 2 diabetes mellitus and chronic pain syndrome, along with a history of alcohol abuse and tobacco dependence. Physical examination revealed a rightward deviation of the trachea, absent breath sound over the right hemithorax with increased dullness to percussion, and lessened tactile fremitus with no egophony. Her chest radiograph showed total opacification

of the right hemithorax and ipsilateral tracheal and mediastinal shift. Her current computed tomography (CT) scan showed right lung atelectasis, elevated right hemidiaphragm, and ipsilateral mediastinal shift. The right bronchi were not visible beyond the main carina. Her previous CT scan demonstrated pneumomediastinum, right pneumothorax, and subcutaneous emphysema, with compromise of the right mainstem bronchus. Bronchoscopy revealed an airway that ended blindly and normal mucosa. A band of white fibrotic tissue blocked the right mainstem bronchus. Thoracic surgery consultation was obtained for the suspected delayed diagnosis of traumatic right main bronchus disruption. Surgery confirmed complete right mainstem transection at the carina level, and repair was undertaken. Postrepair intraoperative bronchoscopy revealed a widely patent right mainstem bronchus. Her chest radiograph after surgery showed excellent re-expansion of her right lung, and subsequent recovery was uneventful.

Discussion.—The most common site of injury in TBI is the right mainstem bronchus, with 80% of these injuries occurring within 2 cm of the carina. Symptoms of acute TBI include tachypnea, dyspnea, and hemoptysis, although subcutaneous emphysema, pneumothorax, and/or pneumomediastinum are also common. Rib fractures involving any of the first three ribs occur in up to 90% of these patients. Up to 20% of patients have no abnormalities on chest radiographs, but a "fallen lung" sign is rarely seen. TBI may also be diagnosed based on a persistent, massive air leak after chest tube thoracostomy for pneumothorax. Bronchoscopy is the gold standard for determining the diagnosis of TBI, with common findings being obstruction of the airway with blood and inability to view the distal lobar bronchi because of proximal bronchial collapse. Finding a luminal tear confirms the diagnosis.

Conclusions.—Coexisting traumatic injuries can complicate the timely diagnosis of TBI. A median of 6 months can elapse between the time of injury and the diagnosis in patients with these confounding injuries, which usually consist of small noncircumferential tears or complete transections leaving the free bronchial ends near enough to permit normal ventilation early in the post-trauma course. The most common presentation in delayed diagnosis is exertional dyspnea or postobstructive pneumonia.

▶ This unique case has many important learning points. As the authors point out, most patients with blunt trauma severe enough to cause mainstem tear or rupture do not survive the immediate wreck. (They have simultaneous aortic tear and die in the field.) However, in those who do survive and have a pneumothorax, especially with a prolonged air leak, an inspection bronchoscopy is indicated.

Fig 1 in the original article shows what looks like either complete collapse of the right lung or a complete hydrothorax on the right. It would be quite logical to consider a posttraumatic pleural effusion or empyema in this patient, as they are 6 weeks posthospitalization for major trauma and had pulmonary involvement on the initial admission. However, in Fig 2 of the original article we see that the chest computed tomography scan now (b) shows a very small, collapsed right lung with herniation upward of diaphragm and liver. So the thought then might be of a diaphragm paralysis caused by phrenic nerve injury. Again, however, the initial injury pattern must be considered. Bronchoscopy, thus, revealed the occlusion.

This is one lucky patient. She survived blunt trauma that most would not. And then she survived a missed transection of the right mainstem bronchus (which would often lead to mediastinitis or empyema).

So the take-home lesson is straightforward: Inspect the airways in patients with blunt chest trauma!

J. A. Barker, MD, FACP, FCCP

Ventilator Weaning

ICU Early Mobilization: From Recommendation to Implementation at Three Medical Centers

Engel HJ, Needham DM, Morris PE, et al (Univ of California San Francisco Med Ctr; Johns Hopkins Univ, Baltimore, MD; Wake Forest Univ School of Medicine, Winston Salem, NC)
Crit Care Med 41:S69-S80, 2013

Objective.—To compare and contrast the process used to implement an early mobility program in ICUs at three different medical centers and to assess their impact on clinical outcomes in critically ill patients.

Design.—Three ICU early mobilization quality improvement projects are summarized utilizing the Institute for Healthcare Improvement framework of Plan-Do-Study-Act.

Intervention.—Each of the three ICU early mobilization programs required an interprofessional team-based approach to plan, educate, and implement the ICU early mobility program. Champions from each profession—nursing, physical therapy, physician, and respiratory care—were identified to facilitate changes in ICU culture and clinical practice and to identify and address barriers to early mobility program implementation at each institution.

Setting.—The medical ICU at Wake Forest University, the medical ICU at Johns Hopkins Hospital, and the mixed medical-surgical ICU at the University of California San Francisco Medical Center.

Results.—Establishing an ICU early mobilization quality improvement program resulted in a reduced ICU and hospital length of stay at all three institutions and decreased rates of delirium and the need for sedation for the patients enrolled in the Johns Hopkins ICU early mobility program.

Conclusion.—Instituting a planned, structured ICU early mobility quality improvement project can result in improved outcomes and reduced costs for ICU patients across healthcare systems (Table 3).

▶ I have long believed in early mobility for hospitalized patients, especially those in the intensive care unit (ICU). However, the barriers are considerable

TABLE 3.—Comparison of Three ICU Early Mobility Quality Improvement Projects

Quality Improvement for Early Mobility	Wake Forest	Johns Hopkins	University of California San Francisco
Objective	Reduce immobility and weakness with early PT for MICU patients	Optimize patient sedation Provide early PM&R in the ICU for MICU patients	Provide earlier and more frequent PT in the ICU for MICU and surgical ICU patients
Planning time frame		1 yr	1.5 yr
Comparison group	$n = 165$ control group	$n = 27$ retrospective comparison	$n = 179$ retrospective comparison
Intervention group and time frame	$n = 165$ patients on MV	$n = 30$ on MV	$n = 294$ all ICU patients
	2004–2006 7 days/week mobility	2007 6 days/week mobility	2010 5 days/week mobility
Number of added personnel and titles	1 registered nurse, 1 certified nursing assistant, 1 physical therapist, 1 project manager	1 physical therapist, 1 occupational therapist, 1 technician, 1 coordinator, 1 part-time assistant coordinator	1 physical therapist, 1 part-time aide
Equipment added	None	2 wheelchairs	ICU platform walker
Outcome measures	Days until out of bed Frequency of therapy ICU/hospital LOS Adverse events	Percentage of ICU patients receiving PT ICU/hospital LOS Pain/delirium scores Adverse events	Number of days to initiating PT ICU/hospital LOS Distance walked in ICU Discharge disposition Incident reports
Financial analysis performed?	Yes	Yes	No
Expanded to other ICU's?	Yes	Yes	Yes
Results	Safe and feasible earlier mobility Increased number of patients receive ICU PM&R Patients receive increased number of treatments Decreased ICU and hospital LOS Net cost savings	Same results as shown in Wake Forest plus: Decreased dosages of sedating medications Decreased patient delirium rates No change in patient reported pain scores	Same results as shown in Wake Forest plus: Applied to medical and surgical all ICU patients Increased distance patients walked in ICU Increased percentage of patients able to discharge to home rather than rehabilitation facility

PT = physical therapy, MICU = medical ICU, PM&R = physical medicine and rehabilitation, MV = mechanical ventilation, LOS = length of stay.

in ICU patients, and, of course, many patients are too unstable. But even patients that I thought were too instrumented or ill can be allowed to move. For example, in our cardiothoracic surgery ICU, it is commonplace for extracorporeal membrane oxygenation patients to be extubated and ambulated once they stabilize. Similarly, our hospital in South Carolina (Palmetto Richland) made early ambulation a priority, and we found, just as these authors did, that it actually saved money despite the initial manpower outlay for therapists.

Therapists may be physical therapists, respiratory therapists, nurses, or even CMAs.

Fig 2 in the original article shows the "how to" of these 3 sites. I found it heartening that all 3 found improved outcomes and cost savings despite being in very different locations and having somewhat different patient cohorts.

J. A. Barker, MD, FACP, FCCP

Ventilator-Associated Pneumonia

ICU-Acquired Pneumonia With or Without Etiologic Diagnosis: A Comparison of Outcomes

Giunta V, Ferrer M, Esperatti M, et al (Universitat de Barcelona, Spain; et al)
Crit Care Med 41:2133-2143, 2013

Objectives.—The impact of ICU-acquired pneumonia without etiologic diagnosis on patients' outcomes is largely unknown. We compared the clinical characteristics, inflammatory response, and outcomes between patients with and without microbiologically confirmed ICU-acquired pneumonia.

Design.—Prospective observational study.

Setting.—ICUs of a university teaching hospital.

Patients.—We prospectively collected 270 consecutive patients with ICU-acquired pneumonia. Patients were clustered according to positive or negative microbiologic results.

Interventions.—None.

Measurements and Main Results.—We compared the characteristics and outcomes between both groups. Negative microbiology was found in 82 patients (30%). Both groups had similar baseline severity scores. Patients with negative microbiology presented more frequently chronic renal failure (15 [18%] vs 11 [6%]; $p = 0.003$), chronic heart disorders (35 [43%] vs 55 [29%]; $p = 0.044$), less frequently previous intubation (44 [54%] vs 135 [72%]; $p = 0.006$), more severe hypoxemia (Pao_2/Fio_2: 165 ± 73 mm Hg vs 199 ± 79 mm Hg; $p = 0.001$), and shorter ICU stay before the onset of pneumonia (5 ± 5 days vs 7 ± 9 days; $p = 0.001$) compared with patients with positive microbiology. The systemic inflammatory response was similar between both groups. Negative microbiology resulted in less changes of empiric treatment (33 [40%] vs 112 [60%]; $p = 0.005$) and shorter total duration of antimicrobials (13 ± 6 days vs 17 ± 12 days; $p = 0.006$) than positive microbiology. Following adjustment for potential confounders, patients with positive microbiology had higher hospital mortality (adjusted odds ratio 2.96, 95% confidence interval 1.24–7.04, $p = 0.014$) and lower 90-day survival (adjusted hazard ratio 0.50, 95% confidence interval 0.27–0.94, $p = 0.031$), with a nonsignificant lower 28-day survival.

Conclusions.—Although the possible influence of previous intubation in mortality of both groups is not completely discarded, negative microbiologic findings in clinically suspected ICU-acquired pneumonia are associated with less frequent previous intubation, shorter duration of antimicrobial treatment, and better survival. Future studies should corroborate the presence of pneumonia in patients with suspected ICU-acquired pneumonia and negative microbiology.

▶ This is an important article. I think many of us felt that this was true, namely, that ventilator-associated pneumonia (VAP) with positive cultures behaves differently than culture-negative VAP. Now there is proof. However, the proviso is that aggressive attempts at microbiologic diagnosis are needed.

Why do the 2 groups fall out differently? Perhaps the culture-negative ones are actually *pneumonitis* (inflamed but not clearly infected lungs). Or perhaps VAP patients with positive cultures have more aggressive organisms or a higher bacteriologic burden.

We can also more comfortably shorten intravenous antibiotic courses now in those who are culture-negative.

J. A. Barker, MD, FACP, FCCP

Impact of Regular Collaboration Between Infectious Diseases and Critical Care Practitioners on Antimicrobial Utilization and Patient Outcome

Rimawi RH, Mazer MA, Siraj DS, et al (Brody School of Medicine—East Carolina Univ, Greenville, NC; et al)
Crit Care Med 41:2099-2107, 2013

Objective.—Antimicrobial stewardship programs have been shown to help reduce the use of unnecessary antimicrobial agents in the hospital setting. To date, there has been very little data focusing on high-use areas, such as the medical ICU. A prospective intervention was done to assess guideline compliance, antimicrobial expenditure, and healthcare cost when an infectious disease fellow interacts regularly with the medical ICU team.

Design.—A 3-month retrospective chart review was followed by a 3-month prospective intervention the following year. Two hundred forty-six total charts were reviewed to assess generally accepted guideline compliance, demographics, and microbiologic results.

Setting.—Twenty-four-bed medical ICU at an 861-bed tertiary care, university teaching hospital in North Carolina.

Subjects.—Patients receiving antibiotics in the medical ICU.

Intervention.—During the intervention period, the infectious disease fellow reviewed the charts, including physician notes and microbiology data, and discussed antimicrobial use with the medical ICU team.

Measurements and Main Results.—Antimicrobial use, treatment duration, Acute Physiology and Chronic Health Evaluation II scores, length of stay, mechanical ventilation days, and mortality rates were compared during the two periods.

Results.—No baseline statistically significant differences in the two groups were noted (i.e., age, gender, race, or Acute Physiology and Chronic Healthcare Evaluation II scores). Indications for antibiotics included healthcare-associated (53%) and community-acquired pneumonias (17%). Significant reductions were seen in extended-spectrum penicillins ($p = 0.0080$), car-bapenems ($p = 0.0013$), vancomycin ($p = 0.0040$), and metronidazole ($p = 0.0004$) following the intervention. Antimicrobial modification led to an increase in narrow-spectrum penicillins ($p = 0.0322$). The intervention group had a significantly lower rate of treatments that did not correspond to guidelines ($p < 0.0001$). There was a reduction in mechanical ventilation days ($p = 0.0053$), length of stay ($p = 0.0188$), and hospital mortality ($p = 0.0367$). The annual calculated healthcare savings was \$89,944 in early antibiotic cessation alone.

Conclusion.—Active communication with an infectious disease practitioner can significantly reduce medical ICU antibiotic overuse by earlier modification or cessation of antibiotics without increasing mortality. This in turn can reduce healthcare costs, foster prodigious education, and strengthen relations between the subspecialties.

▶ Collaboration works! In this beautifully simple study, the investigators collect pre- and postintervention data. The data are impressive: patients have improved survival, lower cost, and fewer ventilator days. Many centers talk about antibiotic stewardship. Those that do it, as shown here at East Carolina, succeed!

J. A. Barker, MD, FACP, FCCP

Article Index

Chapter 1: Asthma, Allergy, and Cystic Fibrosis

Bronchial thermoplasty: Long-term safety and effectiveness in patients with severe persistent asthma 5

Safety of bronchial thermoplasty in patients with severe refractory asthma 8

Severe adult-onset asthma: A distinct phenotype 11

Heliox-driven β_2-agonists nebulization for children and adults with acute asthma: a systematic review with meta-analysis 14

Update in Asthma 2012 15

Asthma During Pregnancy and Clinical Outcomes in Offspring: A National Cohort Study 17

Omalizumab: A review of its Use in Patients with Severe Persistent Allergic Asthma 18

A Proof-of-Concept, Randomized, Controlled Trial of Omalizumab in Patients With Severe, Difficult-to-Control, Nonatopic Asthma 20

Metabolic syndrome and incidence of asthma in adults: the HUNT study 22

Remission and Persistence of Asthma Followed From 7 to 19 Years of Age 24

Sex differences in asthma symptom profiles and control in the American Lung Association Asthma Clinical Research Centers 26

Prescription fill patterns in underserved children with asthma receiving subspecialty care 29

Phase II studies of nebulised Arikace in CF patients with *Pseudomonas aeruginosa* infection 30

Chapter 2: Chronic Obstructive Pulmonary Disease

Cardiovascular Risk, Myocardial Injury, and Exacerbations of Chronic Obstructive Pulmonary Disease 37

Cognitive Dysfunction in Patients Hospitalized With Acute Exacerbation of COPD 39

Bidirectional Associations Between Clinically Relevant Depression or Anxiety and COPD: A Systematic Review and Meta-analysis 41

Chronic Pain and Pain Medication Use in Chronic Obstructive Pulmonary Disease: A Cross-Sectional Study 42

COPD Surveillance—United States, 1999-2011 44

A meta-analysis on the prophylactic use of macrolide antibiotics for the prevention of disease exacerbations in patients with Chronic Obstructive Pulmonary Disease 46

High-Dose N-Acetylcysteine in Stable COPD: The 1-Year, Double-Blind, Randomized, Placebo-Controlled HIACE Study 47

Statin Use and Risk of COPD Exacerbation Requiring Hospitalization 49

Tiotropium Respimat Inhaler and the Risk of Death in COPD 50

Characteristics, stability and outcomes of the 2011 GOLD COPD groups in the ECLIPSE cohort 52

A New Approach to Classification of Disease Severity and Progression of COPD   54

Predictors of Mortality in Hospitalized Adults with Acute Exacerbation of Chronic Obstructive Pulmonary Disease: A Systematic Review and Meta-analysis   56

Acquired Cystic Fibrosis Transmembrane Conductance Regulator Dysfunction in the Lower Airways in COPD   57

Effects of Allergic Phenotype on Respiratory Symptoms and Exacerbations in Patients with Chronic Obstructive Pulmonary Disease   59

Pulmonary hypertension in COPD: results from the ASPIRE registry   60

Systematic Review of Supervised Exercise Programs After Pulmonary Rehabilitation in Individuals With COPD   62

Chapter 3: Lung Cancer

Cancer Statistics, 2013   68

Epidemic of Lung Cancer in Patients With HIV Infection   72

Asbestos, Asbestosis, Smoking, and Lung Cancer. New Findings from the North American Insulator Cohort   73

50-Year Trends in Smoking-Related Mortality in the United States   75

The Association Between Smoking Quantity and Lung Cancer in Men and Women   77

21st-Century Hazards of Smoking and Benefits of Cessation in the United States   78

Electronic cigarettes for smoking cessation: a randomised controlled trial   81

Screening for Lung Cancer: U.S. Preventive Services Task Force Recommendation Statement   83

Benefits and Harms of Computed Tomography Lung Cancer Screening Programs for High-Risk Populations   86

Selection Criteria for Lung-Cancer Screening   91

American Cancer Society Lung Cancer Screening Guidelines   95

Interstitial Lung Abnormalities in a CT Lung Cancer Screening Population: Prevalence and Progression Rate   96

Targeting of Low-Dose CT Screening According to the Risk of Lung-Cancer Death   98

Executive Summary: Diagnosis and Management of Lung Cancer, 3rd ed: American College of Chest Physicians Evidence-Based Clinical Practice Guidelines   100

Evaluation of Individuals With Pulmonary Nodules: When Is It Lung Cancer? Diagnosis and Management of Lung Cancer, 3rd ed: American College of Chest Physicians Evidence-Based Clinical Practice Guidelines   103

Recommendations for the Management of Subsolid Pulmonary Nodules Detected at CT: A Statement from the Fleischner Society   106

Radiation and Chest CT Scan Examinations: What Do We Know?   109

What Do You Mean, a Spot? A Qualitative Analysis of Patients' Reactions to Discussions With Their Physicians About Pulmonary Nodules   113

The Stage Classification of Lung Cancer: Diagnosis and Management of Lung Cancer, 3rd ed: American College of Chest Physicians Evidence-Based Clinical Practice Guidelines   114

Probability of Cancer in Pulmonary Nodules Detected on First Screening CT   116

Endobronchial Ultrasound-Guided Transbronchial Needle Aspiration for Differentiating N0 Versus N1 Lung Cancer   119

Physiologic Evaluation of the Patient With Lung Cancer Being Considered for Resectional Surgery: Diagnosis and Management of Lung Cancer, 3rd ed: American College of Chest Physicians Evidence-Based Clinical Practice Guidelines   121

Mechanism of Action of Conventional and Targeted Anticancer Therapies: Reinstating Immunosurveillance   124

American College of Chest Physicians and Society of Thoracic Surgeons Consensus Statement for Evaluation and Management for High-Risk Patients With Stage I Non-small Cell Lung Cancer   125

Targeted Therapy for Non–Small Cell Lung Cancer   127

The Impact of Genomic Changes on Treatment of Lung Cancer   129

Chapter 4: Pleural, Interstitial Lung, and Pulmonary Vascular Disease

The Toll-like Receptor 3 L412F Polymorphism and Disease Progression in Idiopathic Pulmonary Fibrosis   132

Patients with Idiopathic Pulmonary Fibrosis with Antibodies to Heat Shock Protein 70 Have Poor Prognoses   133

Echocardiographic and Hemodynamic Predictors of Mortality in Idiopathic Pulmonary Fibrosis   134

Morbidity and mortality in patients with usual interstitial pneumonia (UIP) pattern undergoing surgery for lung biopsy   136

Effect of ambulatory oxygen on exertional dyspnea in IPF patients without resting hypoxemia   137

Diagnosis and Treatment of Connective Tissue Disease-Associated Interstitial Lung Disease   139

Mycophenolate Mofetil Improves Lung Function in Connective Tissue Disease-associated Interstitial Lung Disease   141

Pleural Plaques and the Risk of Pleural Mesothelioma   142

Surgical decortication as the first-line treatment for pleural empyema   144

Preoperative Predictors of Successful Surgical Treatment in the Management of Parapneumonic Empyema   146

A Propensity-Matched Comparison of Pleurodesis or Tunneled Pleural Catheter in Patients Undergoing Diagnostic Thoracoscopy for Malignancy   147

Clinical Outcomes of Indwelling Pleural Catheter-Related Pleural Infections: An International Multicenter Study   149

Evaluation of the Predictive Value of a Clinical Worsening Definition Using 2-Year Outcomes in Patients With Pulmonary Arterial Hypertension: A REVEAL Registry Analysis   150

Treatment of patients with pulmonary arterial hypertension at the time of death or deterioration to functional class IV: Insights from the REVEAL Registry   151

A Novel Channelopathy in Pulmonary Arterial Hypertension   154

Correction of Nonsense *BMPR2* and *SMAD9* Mutations by Ataluren in Pulmonary Arterial Hypertension   155

Pulmonary Artery Denervation to Treat Pulmonary Arterial Hypertension: The Single-Center, Prospective, First-in-Man PADN-1 Study (First-in-Man Pulmonary Artery Denervation for Treatment of Pulmonary Artery Hypertension)   156

Riociguat for the Treatment of Pulmonary Arterial Hypertension   157

Riociguat for the Treatment of Chronic Thromboembolic Pulmonary Hypertension   159

Macitentan and Morbidity and Mortality in Pulmonary Arterial Hypertension   160

Chapter 5: Community-Acquired Pneumonia

Functional Disability, Cognitive Impairment, and Depression After Hospitalization for Pneumonia   164

Modifiable Risk Factors for Pneumonia Requiring Hospitalization of Community-Dwelling Older Adults: The Health, Aging, and Body Composition Study   166

Readmission Following Hospitalization for Pneumonia: The Impact of Pneumonia Type and Its Implication for Hospitals   167

Use of serum C reactive protein and procalcitonin concentrations in addition to symptoms and signs to predict pneumonia in patients presenting to primary care with acute cough: diagnostic study   168

Inhaled corticosteroids in COPD and the risk of serious pneumonia   170

The role of vitamin D supplementation in the risk of developing pneumonia: three independent case—control studies   172

Risk Factors for Drug-Resistant Pathogens in Community-acquired and Healthcare-associated Pneumonia   173

Risk factors for methicillin-resistant *Staphylococcus aureus* in patients with community-onset and hospital-onset pneumonia   175

Incidence and Risk Factors of *Legionella pneumophila* Pneumonia During Anti-Tumor Necrosis Factor Therapy: A Prospective French Study   176

U.S. Hospitalizations for Pneumonia after a Decade of Pneumococcal Vaccination   178

Geographic and Temporal Trends in Antimicrobial Nonsusceptibility in Streptococcus pneumoniae in the Post-vaccine era in the United States   179

Admission Decisions and Outcomes of Community-Acquired Pneumonia in the Homeless Population: A Review of 172 Patients in an Urban Setting   181

Use of an Electronic Health Record Clinical Decision Support Tool to Improve Antibiotic Prescribing for Acute Respiratory Infections: The ABX-TRIP Study   182

Chapter 6: Lung Transplantation

Lung Transplantation in Patients with Pretransplantation Donor-Specific Antibodies Detected by Luminex Assay   187

Acute antibody-mediated rejection after lung transplantation   188

Pre-transplant antibodies to Kα1 tubulin and collagen-V in lung transplantation: Clinical correlations   189

Gene Set Enrichment Analysis Identifies Key Innate Immune Pathways in Primary
Graft Dysfunction After Lung Transplantation   190

Disparities in lung transplantation before and after introduction of the lung
allocation score   191

Survival Benefit of Lung Transplant for Cystic Fibrosis since Lung Allocation Score
Implementation   193

The use of lung donors older than 55 years: A review of the United Network of
Organ Sharing database   194

Lung Transplantation After Lung Volume Reduction Surgery   195

Functional Status Is Highly Predictive of Outcomes After Redo Lung
Transplantation: An Analysis of 390 Cases in the Modern Era   197

Clostridium difficile infection increases mortality risk in lung transplant recipients   198

Decreased incidence of cytomegalovirus infection with sirolimus in a post hoc
randomized, multicenter study in lung transplantation   199

Effect of Cytomegalovirus Immunoglobulin on the Incidence of
Lymphoproliferative Disease After Lung Transplantation: Single-Center
Experience With 1157 Patients   201

Aspiration and Allograft Injury Secondary to Gastroesophageal Reflux Occur in
the Immediate Post-Lung Transplantation Period (Prospective Clinical Trial)   202

Acute Fibrinoid Organizing Pneumonia after Lung Transplantation   203

Pulmonary rehabilitation in lung transplant candidates   205

Chapter 7: Sleep Disorders

Randomized Controlled trial of Noninvasive Positive Pressure Ventilation (NPPV)
Versus Servoventilation in Patients with CPAP-Induced Central Sleep Apnea
(Complex Sleep Apnea)   208

An Official American Thoracic Society Clinical Practice Guideline: Sleep Apnea,
Sleepiness, and Driving Risk in Noncommercial Drivers: An Update of a 1994
Statement   209

Does autotitrating positive airway pressure therapy improve postoperative
outcome in patients at risk for obstructive sleep apnea syndrome? A randomized
controlled clinical trial   210

Impact of Group Education on Continuous Positive Airway Pressure Adherence   212

Maximizing Positive Airway Pressure Adherence in Adults: A Common-Sense
Approach   213

The Face of Sleepiness: Improvement in Appearance after Treatment of Sleep Apnea   214

5-Years APAP adherence in OSA patients – Do first impressions matter?   215

Impact of Treatment with Continuous Positive Airway Pressure (CPAP) on Weight
in Obstructive Sleep Apnea   217

Effect of CPAP on Blood Pressure in Patients With Obstructive Sleep Apnea and
Resistant Hypertension: The HIPARCO Randomized Clinical Trial   219

Defining Phenotypic Causes of Obstructive Sleep Apnea: Identification of Novel
Therapeutic Targets   220

Novel and Emerging Nonpositive Airway Pressure Therapies for Sleep Apnea 223

Health Outcomes of Continuous Positive Airway Pressure versus Oral Appliance Treatment for Obstructive Sleep Apnea: A Randomized Controlled Trial 225

Oral Appliance Versus Continuous Positive Airway Pressure in Obstructive Sleep Apnea Syndrome: A 2-Year Follow-up 226

Effectiveness of Lifestyle Interventions on Obstructive Sleep Apnea (OSA): Systematic Review and Meta-Analysis 228

Effects of Experimental Sleep Restriction on Caloric Intake and Activity Energy Expenditure 230

Self-reported Sleep and β-Amyloid Deposition in Community-Dwelling Older Adults 231

Morbidity and mortality in children with obstructive sleep apnoea: a controlled national study 232

A Randomized Trial of Adenotonsillectomy for Childhood Sleep Apnea 233

Chapter 8: Critical Care Medicine

Acute Respiratory Distress Syndrome After Spontaneous Intracerebral Hemorrhage 235

Fatal Neurological Respiratory Insufficiency Is Common Among Viral Encephalitides 237

Clinical correlates, outcomes and healthcare costs associated with early mechanical ventilation after kidney transplantation 238

Emerging Indications for Extracorporeal Membrane Oxygenation in Adults with Respiratory Failure 238

Assessment of the addition of prehospital continuous positive airway pressure (CPAP) to an urban emergency medical services (EMS) system in persons with severe respiratory distress 240

A Randomized, Double-Blind Comparison of Licorice Versus Sugar-Water Gargle for Prevention of Postoperative Sore Throat and Postextubation Coughing 241

Accuracy of ultrasound-guided marking of the cricothyroid membrane before simulated failed intubation 242

Central or Peripheral Catheters for Initial Venous Access of ICU Patients: A Randomized Controlled Trial 244

Agreement Between ICU Clinicians and Electrophysiology Cardiologists on the Decision to Initiate a QTc-interval Prolonging Medication in Critically Ill Patients with Potential Risk Factors for Torsade de Pointes: A Comparative, Case-Based Evaluation 245

Removing nonessential central venous catheters: evaluation of a quality improvement intervention 246

A Patient With Acute COPD Exacerbation and Shock 248

Influence of ICU Case-Volume on the Management and Hospital Outcomes of Acute Exacerbations of Chronic Obstructive Pulmonary Disease 249

Acute Kidney Injury Secondary to Exposure to Insecticides Used for Bedbug (*Cimex lectularis*) Control 251

Are Routine Intensive Care Admissions Needed after Endovascular Treatment of
Unruptured Aneurysms? 251

Severe Sepsis and Septic Shock 252

Choosing and Using Screening Criteria for Palliative Care Consultation in the ICU:
A Report From the Improving Palliative Care in the ICU (IPAL-ICU) Advisory
Board 254

Do Windows or Natural Views Affect Outcomes or Costs Among Patients in ICUs? 255

Prediction of Death in Less Than 60 Minutes Following Withdrawal of
Cardiorespiratory Support in ICUs 256

Epidemiology of Obstetric-Related ICU Admissions in Maryland: 1999–2008 257

A Systematic Review of Evidence-Informed Practices for Patient Care Rounds in
the ICU 259

Clostridium difficile Infection: A Multicenter Study of Epidemiology and
Outcomes in Mechanically Ventilated Patients 260

Capnography as a Diagnostic Tool for Pulmonary Embolism: A Meta-Analysis 262

A 40-Year-Old Woman With Cough and Dyspnea 2 Months After a Motorcycle
Accident 263

ICU Early Mobilization: From Recommendation to Implementation at Three
Medical Centers 265

ICU-Acquired Pneumonia With or Without Etiologic Diagnosis: A Comparison of
Outcomes 267

Impact of Regular Collaboration Between Infectious Diseases and Critical Care
Practitioners on Antimicrobial Utilization and Patient Outcome 268

Author Index

A

Abrams D, 238
Adachi T, 230
Aguilar SA, 240
Agusti A, 52
Ahya VN, 199
Al-Qadheeb NS, 245
Amelink M, 11
An Y, 231
Andersson M, 24
Angus DC, 252
Araghi MH, 228
Aramini B, 146
Armstrong ME, 132
Ascioti AJ, 147
Atlantis E, 41
Austin ED, 154

B

Badesch DB, 150
Bankier AA, 106
Barrera E Jr, 95
Bashir B, 251
Baz MA, 199
Beaty CA, 197
Beauchamp MK, 62
Belli A, 59
Berg CD, 98
Berger KI, 121
Bhama JK, 195
Bhargava A, 133
Bittle GJ, 194
Bjerg A, 24
Boldt A, 29
Bollinger ME, 29
Boyer A, 244
Bredenoord AJ, 202
Brieva J, 256
Brodie D, 238
Brown KK, 141
Brugière O, 187
Brumpton BM, 22
Brunelli A, 121
Budhiraja R, 217
Bullen C, 81
Burrows AM, 251

C

Cairns AA, 213
Calvin AD, 230
Camargo CA Jr, 22
Cantu E, 190
Cardarella S, 129
Carr LL, 127
Carter BD, 75
Carter RE, 230
Castillo E, 240
Castro-Rodriguez JA, 14
Chalmers JD, 56
Chang YS, 144
Charlton RA, 39
Chaudhry A, 46
Chawla A, 96
Chen S-L, 156
Chen Y-F, 228
Chervin RD, 214
Chiron R, 20
Chowdhury NA, 205
Christie JD, 193
Clancy JP, 30
Clarke DP, 217
Cload B, 246
Cloft HJ, 251
Cochrane B, 41
Coleman N, 256
Condliffe R, 60
Conner KE, 109
Cooke DT, 263
Cooney E, 255
Croft JB, 44
Curtis K, 242

D

Darendeliler MA, 225
Davydow DS, 164
Dawson M, 242
de Groot JC, 11
de Nijs SB, 11
deAndrade JA, 191
della Casa G, 146
Dellweg D, 208
Detterbeck FC, 100, 114
D'Hoore W, 262
Diaz-Guzman E, 54
Diekemper R, 100
Doan J, 246
Dodd JW, 39
Doff MHJ, 226
Donaldson GC, 37
Donath E, 46
Donington J, 103, 125
Drake KM, 155
Dransfield MT, 57

Dres M, 249
Du Bois RM, 141
Dunmore BJ, 155
Dy-Liacco M, 238

E

Eckert DJ, 220
Elliot CA, 60
Ellis S, 203
Elmer J, 235
Elze M, 136
Engel HJ, 265
Esperatti M, 267
Evans R, 62

F

Fahey P, 41
Farber HW, 151
Feller-Kopman D, 149
Ferrer M, 267
Ferri M, 259
Feskanich D, 75
Fischer A, 141
Flanagan B, 57
Fleck M, 241
Fongemie JM, 245
Fontham ETH, 95
Ford ES, 44
Forfia PR, 134
Freeman RK, 147
Frost AE, 150
Fukai Y, 137
Fysh ETH, 149

G

Galluzzi L, 124
Gamaldo AA, 231
Garcia G, 20
Gaut JP, 188
Gautam B, 189
Gay PC, 210, 223
Ghassemieh B, 199
Ghofrani H-A, 157, 159
Gilbert S, 195
Giunta V, 267
Gould MK, 103, 113
Griffin MR, 178
Griffin SM, 202

Grunstein RR, 225
Gundlapalli AV, 181

H

Harhay MO, 255
Harrington KF, 191
Hartert T, 15
Hartry A, 42
Hedman L, 24
Heilbrun ME, 109
Hernandez-Aya LF, 46
Hertz MI, 198
Hocking WG, 91
Hoehn E, 208
Hoekema A, 226
Hoffman PJ, 263
Hou P, 235
Hough CL, 164
Howe C, 81
Hubbard RB, 77
Hull M, 72
Hurdman J, 60

I

Ibsen R, 232
Ilan R, 246
Iyen-Omofoman B, 77

J

Jagielski A, 228
Jaksch P, 201
Jamieson DB, 59
Janaudis-Ferreira T, 62
Jemal A, 68
Jennum P, 232
Jett JR, 127
Jha P, 78
Jin GY, 96
Johnson BE, 129
Jones B, 181
Jones JP, 181
Jordan AS, 220
Juthani-Mehta M, 166

K

Kahloon RA, 133
Katki HA, 91

Kelly RF, 198
Kerl J, 208
Kesler KK, 237
Kilic A, 197
Kim AW, 121
Kim TH, 144
Kjellberg J, 232
Kocher A, 201
Kohn R, 255
Kon ZN, 194
Kovalchik SA, 98
Kowlessar BS, 37
Kreider M, 134

L

Lacey J, 256
Landsman V, 78
Lane D, 259
Lanternier F, 176
Lapi F, 170
Laugesen M, 81
Laurent F, 142
Lee J, 240
Lee JT, 198
Leffert LR, 257
Lemaire J, 259
Lettieri CJ, 212, 213
Levin SM, 73
Levine DA, 164
Lewis SZ, 100
Li M, 205
Link-Gelles R, 179
Litvin CB, 182
Lo Y-W, 49
Lynch D, 96
Lynch WR, 103
Lynfield R, 179

M

Ma L, 154
MacMahon H, 106
Magnan A, 20
Mahidhara RS, 147
Mal H, 193
Mallin M, 242
Man SFP, 72
Manara A, 262
Mannino DM, 44, 54
Mapel DW, 42
Marcus CL, 233
Mark Estes NA III, 245

Markowitz SB, 73
Martínez-García M-A, 219
Mathur S, 205
Matsui EC, 59
Mayo JR, 116
Mazer MA, 268
McCallister JW, 26
McKeage K, 18
McLean C, 203
McNelly LN, 155
McWilliams A, 116
Meltzer LA, 151
Merlo CA, 197
Mhyre JM, 257
Micek ST, 260
Miller A, 73
Miller DP, 150, 151
Miyajima H, 137
Moore MR, 178
Morgenthaler TI, 210
Morgenthaler TM, 223
Morris PE, 265
Morrow L, 260
Moyer VA, 83
Mudd KE, 29

N

Nabecker S, 241
Naidich DP, 106
Naishadham D, 68
Nakajima T, 119
Narula T, 248
Needham DM, 265
Nelson JE, 254
Nishiyama O, 137

O

O'Dwyer DN, 132
O'Gorman SM, 210
Olsen J, 17
Oosterheert JJ, 172
Ornstein SM, 182
Osei-Agyemang T, 136

P

Pairon J-C, 142
Paraskeva M, 203
Park JG, 223
Patel ARC, 37

Patenaude V, 170
Pavord ID, 8
Phillips CL, 225
Plönes T, 136
Pospisil J, 54
Postmus PE, 114
Powell HA, 77
Pulido T, 160

Q

Quan SF, 217

R

Rabinstein AA, 251
Raiteri L, 47
Raman D, 248
Ramasundarahettige C, 78
Reichley R, 167
Remmelts HHF, 172
Ricard J-D, 244
Rimawi RH, 268
Rinaldo M, 142
Rivera-Lebron BN, 134
Roberts MH, 42
Robertson AGN, 202
Rodrigo GJ, 14
Roman-Campos D, 154
Romundstad PR, 22
Ruetzler K, 241
Ruzicka DL, 214

S

Salomon L, 244
Sanchez PG, 194
Santos AC, 215
Sarma A, 109
Sarma NJ, 189
Schaffner E, 17
Schembri S, 56
Schramm G, 260
Severo M, 215

Sharma SG, 251
Shigemura N, 195
Shin JA, 144
Shindo Y, 173
Shorr AF, 167
Siddharthan V, 237
Siegel R, 68
Singanayagam A, 56
Siraj DS, 268
Smyth MJ, 124
Spira AP, 231
Spoorenberg SMC, 172
Stefani A, 146
Stein HD, 251
Strek ME, 139
Strohl KP, 209
Suberbielle C, 187
Suissa S, 170

T

Tammemagi M, 98
Tammemagi MC, 116
Tammemägi MC, 91
Tanoue LT, 114
Tegethoff M, 17
Thabut G, 187, 193
Thomas A, 179
Thun MJ, 75
Thys F, 262
Tiriveedhi V, 189
Tremblay A, 149
Trujillo G, 132
Tsai C-L, 49
Tse HN, 47
Tuttle-Newhall JE, 238

V

Vahabzadeh A, 214
van den Broek MD, 39
van der Poll T, 252
van Vugt SF, 168
van Zeller M, 215
Vij R, 139
von Mutius E, 15

W

Waddell T, 119
Walter RJ, 212
Wanderer JP, 257
Wang H, 237
Wang M-T, 49
Wechsler ME, 5
Wender R, 95
Wessell AM, 182
White DP, 220
Wickwire EM, 213
Wiedemann D, 201
Wiener RS, 113
Wiesen J, 248
Wijkstra PJ, 226
Wilcox SR, 235
Wilhelm AM, 57
Wille KM, 191
Winston LG, 175
Winstone TA, 72
Wise RA, 50
Witt CA, 188
Woloshin S, 113
Wong KY, 47
Wooten DA, 175

X

Xu J, 156
Xue J, 133

Y

Yasufuku K, 119
Yuan H, 238
Yusen RD, 188

Z

Zeki AA, 263
Zhang F-F, 156
Zhu Y, 178
Zilberberg MD, 167
Zitvogel L, 124

Edwards Brothers Malloy
Ann Arbor MI. USA
July 1, 2014